Better Births

Better Births

The Midwife 'with Woman'

Edited by

Anna M. Brown
School of Health Sciences
University of Surrey
Guildford, Surrey, UK

WILEY Blackwell

Registered Office(s)
John Wiley & Sons, Inc., 111 River Street, Hoboken, NJ 07030, USA
John Wiley & Sons Ltd, The Atrium, Southern Gate, Chichester, West Sussex, PO19 8SQ, UK

Editorial Office
9600 Garsington Road, Oxford, OX4 2DQ, UK

For details of our global editorial offices, customer services, and more information about Wiley products visit us at www.wiley.com.

Wiley also publishes its books in a variety of electronic formats and by print-on-demand. Some content that appears in standard print versions of this book may not be available in other formats.

Library of Congress Cataloging-in-Publication Data
Names: Brown, Anna (Anna Maria), editor.
Title: Better births : the midwife 'with woman' / edited by Anna M. Brown.
Description: Hoboken, NJ : Wiley-Blackwell, 2021. | Includes
    bibliographical references and index.
Identifiers: LCCN 2020051701 (print) | LCCN 2020051702 (ebook) |
    ISBN 9781119628743 (hardback) | ISBN 9781119628804 (adobe pdf) |
    ISBN 9781119628842 (epub)
Subjects: MESH: Nurse Midwives | Midwifery | Nurse-Patient Relations
Classification: LCC RG525 (print) | LCC RG525 (ebook) | NLM WY 157 | DDC
    618.2–dc23
LC record available at https://lccn.loc.gov/2020051701
LC ebook record available at https://lccn.loc.gov/2020051702

Cover Design: Wiley
Cover Illustration: © Harriet Lee-Merrion

Set in 9.5/12.5pt STIXTwoText by SPi Global, Pondicherry, India
Printed and bound by CPI Group (UK) Ltd, Croydon, CR0 4YY

C9781119628743_250321

This book is dedicated to my family, my colleagues and friends who have supported me during its creation.

I especially wish to thank all the women and midwives who have sent me their stories. Their contribution to this work is pivotal and I hope the content will inspire future generations of midwives, as well as those currently in the profession. A midwifery colleague wrote these lovely words below. When I read them, they resonated with me and the true essence and spirit of this book:
Holding Space
By kind permission of Emily Clark

What does it mean to hold space
For the pregnant/ birthing person
And the new parent?

To be a hundred percent present
Emotionally, physically and mentally.

To walk their journey with them
Without judgement or opinion.

To understand by opening
Your heart to them.

To give them space to feel
Their feelings and just be.

To be 'with woman'.

Finally, I wish to remember my parents Myriam and Paul who sadly are no longer with us, but who have always wholeheartedly supported my endeavours.

Anna M. Brown

Contents

Preface

I have been a midwife for 35 years. Throughout this time, I have witnessed the impact and implications of childbirth. However, more recent events have encouraged me to examine childbirth experiences which have involved close family members. Heartfelt comments have ranged from desperate pleas such as 'nobody tells you the reality of becoming a mother . . . I feel overwhelmed' to 'I feel abandoned'. Such observations have urged me to explore the concept of what it means to women and midwives to be 'with woman'. In addition, new standards for the profession were published in November 2019, one of which requires midwives to be able to provide and promote continuity of care and carer. This is not a new phenomenon but seen through the concept of being 'with woman' would provide a safer and more effective delivery of maternity care.

'With woman' is an old term in the English language from which the word 'midwife' is derived. The meaning and concept of being 'with woman' may be interpreted as providing care and support in a physical, psychological, emotional and spiritual sense. Hunter (2002, p. 650), explored this concept to focus on the 'presence and support by a caregiver as desired by the labouring woman'. Early on, nurse-midwife core competencies in America emphasised the importance of human presence with the childbearing woman as a therapeutic and professional philosophy (ACNM 1979). More recently, Bradfield et al.'s (2018a) integrative review of the literature explored the 'with woman' phenomena to present an understanding and perspective of this concept. The authors suggest that being 'with woman' is an evolutionary construct, which is dynamic and continues to develop, and is fundamental to midwifery practices and professional philosophy.

An integrative review of the literature pertaining to midwives being 'with woman' (Bradfield et al. 2018a) suggests that this concept is a developing, integrative construct that is dynamic and ever evolving. Its philosophy underpins midwifery practice to identify and guide it in context, making it contemporary and creating spaces for innovation and further research, enhancing an ever-growing body of knowledge. 'With woman' requires building mutually trusting relationships between the woman, her partner and the midwife and the complexities and challenges that this entails. It needs to take into consideration the expectations and decisions of women in partnership with the midwife. This relationship 'with woman' ought to be empowering for both woman and midwife, but sadly women's stories are a disappointing testament to a lack of control in what should be a safe and happy life-changing event.

The purpose of this textbook is to provide an arena of enquiry and debate for those interested in the concept of being 'with woman' in the childbearing context. Recent publications from the Royal College of Midwives (RCM) on Better Births (NHS England 2016a), followed by the implementation of research (NHS England 2017), explored what women want from the childbearing experience. This National Maternity Review (NHS England 2016b) set out a five-year plan to ensure that NHS maternity services in England are safer and more personal and that women's expectations of the childbearing experience is as close as is reasonably possible. The Better Births vision is to ensure that women are able to build a trusting relationship with their named midwife based on mutual trust and respect in line with the woman's decisions and fulfilling a true philosophy of being 'with woman'. This can only be achieved through a personal relationship of continuity of carer over the childbearing. Such a relationship has been found to have positive effects on women's birthing experience and safer outcomes for mothers and neonates (Hunter 2009; Dahlberg and Aune 2013; Sandall 2014; Rayment-Jones et al. 2015).

A national Maternity Transformation Programme (NHS England 2016b) has been created to achieve the Better Births (NHS England 2016a) vision through its implementation and establish transformed maternity services. This is to be achieved by providing consistency of care throughout the antenatal, intrapartum and postnatal periods by a known midwife or obstetrician. The named midwife would take responsibility for coordinated care throughout the childbearing continuum and develop a mutually trusting relationship with the woman and her family. In attempting to fulfil the 'with woman' concept, the provision of care will impact on models of midwifery care and how midwives work.

A wide range of literature documents the different models of midwifery care that have underpinned midwifery practice over the past few decades. Much debate has resulted from these publications (Hatem et al. 2008; McLachlan et al. 2012; Walsh and Devane 2012; Tracy et al. 2013; Sandall et al. 2015; Brady et al. 2019; Gidaszewski et al. 2019). The recommendations in the Five Year Forward View for Implementing Better Births: Continuity of Carer (NHS England 2017) suggest two models that could be most effective in promoting this concept: team continuity and case loading. Much of the literature available presents benefits but also highlights the impact that these models of care can have on midwives attempting to delivery maternity services with the capacity to be 'with woman' (Leinweber and Rowe 2010; Yoshida and Sandall 2013; Davis and Homer 2016; Bradfield et al. 2018b). Ultimately, the aim is to ensure safe and personalised care to meet all women's needs, whatever their circumstances, through the most effective midwifery model of care. I see the 'with woman' concept as the fundamental building block for these recommendations and in a sense it has always been the true philosophy underpinning holistic midwifery practice.

The thread of being 'with woman' is explored in each chapter in this textbook through an examination of the literature focused on an aspect or situation in the journey of childbearing women or their neonate. The different chapters explore attributes of the concept to be 'with woman' to bring together a more in-depth understanding, thus generating discussion of what this concept means to women and midwives in differing situations and environments. The aim of each chapter is to illustrate the different attributes of the overall 'with woman' concept. The objective is to generate debate and discussion in a classroom or clinical setting to further examine current practice and create a space in which contemporary practice could be developed to inform future midwifery care.

Chapters explore the focused literature for a specific aspect of midwifery care; for example, pregnant women in prison and the maternity care that is available to them. Rodgers' phases of Evolutionary Concept Analysis (1989, Rodgers and Knafl 2000) will be the framework on which each chapter is based to identify attributes of the concept (Foster 2017) and it provides a different perspective from which the evidence can be explored. Integral to each chapter, individual situations will be illustrated with examples from practice. The reality and feasibility of being 'with woman' in a variety of situations is illustrated by midwives from their daily clinical experiences. Women are also invited to share their stories, which will help to analyse the concept of interest pertinent to these women's needs and the focus of each specific chapter. An asterisk next to the midwife/woman's name indicates a changed given name to maintain anonymity.

This textbook seeks to present the evidence of 'with woman' in different circumstances and viewed from women's and midwives' perspectives, to engender understanding and learning and ensure better births for all women. In addition, I believe that the content will inform and re-ignite the passion for midwifery, in students and midwives, which sadly has seen a decline in the last two decades. Students engaging with the content will develop reflective skills to successfully inform their knowledge and clinical competence. I hope that the content is relevant to practitioners and those interested in women's position in society, those interested in women's human rights around birth and motherhood and those who strive to promote the legalisation and protection of the midwifery profession.

References

American College of Nurse-Midwives (1979). *The Core Competencies of Basic Midwifery Practice*. Washington DC: ACNM.

Bradfield, Z., Duggan, R., Hauck, Y., and Kelly, M. (2018a). Midwives being "with woman": an integrative review. *Women and Birth* 31: 143–152.

Bradfield, Z., Kelly, M., Hauck, Y., and Duggan, R. (2018b). Midwives "with woman" in the private obstetric model: where divergent philosophies meet. *Women and Birth* http://doi.org/10.1016/j.wombi.2018.07.013.

Brady, S., Lee, N., Gibbons, K., and Bogossian, F. (2019). Women-centred care: an integrative review of the empirical literature. *International Journal of Nursing Studies* 94: 107–119.

Dahlberg, U. and Aune, I. (2013). The woman's birth experience- the effects of interpersonal relationships and continuity of care. *Midwifery* 29: 407–415.

Davis, D.L. and Homer, C.S.E. (2016). Birthplace as the midwife's work place: how does place of birth impact on midwives? *Women and Birth* 29: 407–415.

Foster, J. (2017). Using research to advance nursing practice: a guide to concept analysis. *Clinical Nurse Specialist* 31 (2): 70–73. http://www.cns-journal.com.

Gidaszewski, B., Khajehei, M., Gibbs, E., and Chai Chua, S. (2019). Comparison of the effect of caseload midwifery program and standard midwifery-led care on pimiparous birth outcomes: a retrospective cohort matching study. *Midwifery* 69: 10–16.

Hatem, M., Sandall, J., DeVane, D. et al. (2008). Midwife-led versus other models of care for childbearing women. *Cochran Database Systematic Review* (4) (Art. No.: CD004667).

Hunter, L.P. (2002). Being with woman: a guiding concept for the care of labouring women. *Journal of Obstetric, Gynaecological and Neonatal Nursing* 31: 650–657.

Hunter, L.P. (2009). A descriptive study of "being with woman" during labour and birth. *Journal of Midwifery & Women's Health* 54 (2): 111–118.

Leinweber, J. and Rowe, H.J. (2010). The cost of "being with woman": secondary traumatic stress in midwifery. *Midwifery* 26: 76–87.

McLachlan, H.L., Foster, D.A., Davey, M.A. et al. (2012). Effects of continuity of care by a primary midwife (caseload midwifery) on caesarean section rates in women of low obstetric risk: the COSMOS randomised controlled trial. *BJOG An International Journal of Obstetrics and Gynaecology*. https://doi.org/10.1111/j.1471-0528.2012.03446.x.

NHS England (2016a). Better Births: Improving outcomes of maternity services in England. A five year forward view for maternity care. https://www.england.nhs.uk/wp-content/uploads/2016/02/national-maternity-review-report.pdf (accessed 23 January 2019).

NHS England (2016b). Maternity Transformation Programme. https://www.england. nhs.uk/mat-transformation (accessed 23 January 2019).

NHS England (2017). Implementing Better Births: Continuity of carer. https://www. england.nhs.uk/wp-content/uploads/2017/12/implementing-better-births.pdf (accessed 23 January 2019).

Rayment-Jones, H., Murrells, T., and Sandall, J. (2015). An investigation of the relationship between the caseload model of midwifery for socially disadvantaged women and childbirth outcomes using routine data–a retrospective, observational study. *Midwifery* 31 (4): 409–417.

Rodgers, B.L. (1989). Concepts, analysis and the development of nursing knowledge: the evolutionary cycle. *Journal of Advanced Nursing* 14: 330–335.

Rodgers, B.L. and Knafl, K.A. (2000). *Concept Development in Nursing: Foundations, Techniques and Applications*. Philadelphia, PA: WB Saunders Co.

Sandall, J. (2014). The contribution of continuity of midwifery care to high quality maternity care. London: The Royal College of Midwives [online]. www.rcm.org. uk/sites/default/files/Continuity%20of%20Care%20A5%20Web.pdf (accessed 23 January 2019).

Sandall, J., Soltani, H., Gate, S. et al. (2015). Midwife-led continuity models versus other models of care for childbearing. *The Cochrane Database of Systematic Reviews* (8): https://doi.org/10.1002/14651858.CD004667.pub5.

Tracy, S.K., Hartz, D.L., Tracy, M.B. et al. (2013). Caselaod midwifery care versus standard maternity care for women of any risk: M@NGO, a randomised controlled trial. *The Lancet* 23 (382): 1723–1732.

Walsh, D. and Devane, D. (2012). A metasynthesis of midwife-led care. *Qualitative Health Research* 22 (7): 897.

Yoshida, Y. and Sandall, J. (2013). Occupational burnout and work factors in community and hospital midwives: a survey analysis. *Midwifery* 29: 921–926.

Foreword

I am delighted to welcome you to this essential text: *Better Births: The Midwife 'with Woman'*. I know the passion and dedication shown by the Lead Author and Editor, Dr Anna M. Brown as I have been fortunate to work with her for many (nearly 20) years! Many of the other authors are also colleagues and practice partners which gives me a real sense of pride in the enthusiasm shown by the clinicians who I work alongside.

The introductory chapter sets the scene clearly for the focus of the book, detailing the stories from Midwives on being 'with women.' The importance of sharing our experiences is paramount in supporting the learning and reflection of our colleagues, students and the generation of professionals. Indeed, the voice of women also comes through clearly; thank you to all those who have shared their personal experiences of pregnancy and birth, your courage and honesty will support learning for the profession.

I would personally like to thank the contributors of this book as I know it will form a valuable resource for all who access it. I look forward to seeing our Surrey students 'thumbing' through it, knowing that it is being opened more widely across the next generation of this vibrant group of professionals.

Professor Melaine Coward
Head of School, School of Health Sciences, University of Surrey
Interim Executive Dean, Faculty of Health and Medical Sciences

1

An Evolutionary Concept Analysis

Anna M. Brown, Kath Lawton, Lauren Brown; Victoria Wulker,
Lucy Jane, Paruit Cass (midwives); and Emily and Victoria (women)

This exploration of the 'with woman' concept stems from a need to understand the perceptions of women and midwives of its meaning. It is hoped that a broader understanding of the concept will encourage midwives to work towards engagement with women to fulfil the true meaning of the concept. Hunter (2002) suggests that the 'with woman' concept involves emotional, physical, spiritual and psychological events or phenomenon and its meaning fluctuates according to process, behaviour or environment towards the purpose that its serves (Rodgers 1989; Higgins et al. 2017).

Higgins et al. (2017, p. 30) identified that many concepts in healthcare can have different meaning to individual professions and likewise to the patients themselves, '*shaped by the relationship between the patient and the provider and the environment in which healthcare delivery takes place*'. In bringing together a mutual understanding, by midwife and woman, it will improve the process and outcomes or consequences of the concept. In addition, a brief historic review will place the 'with woman' concept in its context.

A Historic Review of Being 'with Woman'

Contemporary British midwifery education often includes a consideration of the historical context of midwifery, and as such many midwives will be aware that the term 'midwife' derives from Anglo-Saxon, meaning 'with woman'. This terminology itself identifies the role of the midwife, and the importance it puts on the person whom the midwife attends. However, it is acknowledged that the voice of this woman has historically been unheard (Evenden 2000), as has the voice of the midwife (Harley 1993). This lack of voice generally stems from a lack of strong historic evidence, resulting in the historic misrepresentation of midwives (McIntosh 2012; Marland 1993; Harley 1990). Oral histories such as Leap and Hunter (1993) and collected letters such as Llewelyn Davies (1915) do give us an insight into the more recent past, but to go further back presents challenges. What evidence we do have, in terms of parish registers (Allison 2016) or material from early midwives' licenses (Evenden 2000; Harley 1990), does not directly inform us about the relationship between midwife and woman.

Taking all this into account, then much of how early midwives were viewed by the woman they cared for must be inferred from such records. Evenden (2000) acknowledges that childbirth practices of seventeenth-century midwives often comes from second-hand sources, or *'prescriptive information from non-partici-pating males'* (p. 79), and these are often more a direction as to what the midwife should do; for example, how to prepare the bed, the lighting within the room, and how to examine the woman and physically care for her in labour. There isn't any evidence of the relationship between mother and midwife beyond this care given. This does not appear to be unusual, with a textbook written in 1671 by Jane Sharpe, a midwife, also focusing on the physical care given. What does give an indication of satisfaction of the care provided is the *'repeat business'* that Evenden (2000) found in her exploration of midwives in seventeenth-century London, with women often recommending their midwife to family and friends.

Where we do have direct evidence of midwives' attitudes to women, it can appear alien to the concept of women-centred care and being 'with woman'. Leap and Hunter (1993) describe how their *'romantic expectations about our midwifery heritage'* were dashed by the authoritarian stance of some of the midwives they interviewed for their oral history, with these midwives taking a somewhat patron-ising approach to the woman in their care, one being quoted as saying *'They had to be taught to be good mothers. Some of them were very foolish and irresponsible'* (Leap and Hunter 1993, p. 193). It is perhaps not suprising that this was the point of view of this midwife, when it is considered that midwifery textbooks at the time when she was likely to have been in training were prescriptive in the expectations of pregnant woman – down to what was appropriate clothing (Myles 1953).

A more humanistic approach to the mother–midwife relationship in a 'with woman' phenomenon is central to midwifery practice today. This is a physical manifestation of the relationship created by midwives with women. On the other hand, the 'with woman' concept is a mental construct, conceived and created in midwifery practice, to capture the essence, values, behaviours and functions of this special relationship. The 'with woman' concept is explored more closely in the fol-lowing chapters and is specifically examined through a theoretical framework in the next section.

Rodgers' Concept Analysis Framework

Rodgers (1989) suggests that defining a concept can be difficult if the attributes that shape the concept are not clear. The author suggests that the different aspects of a concept are created through an evolutionary view, associated with its attributes, through the process of concept change and development. Such development can only occur if the 'with woman' concept is significant to both midwife and mother, is used to fulfil physical, emotional, spiritual and psychological needs and is applied through midwifery skills and shared knowledge in this partnership. In addition, such a concept is influenced by a set of internal and external factors before it can be achieved (Burgess 2014; Sheen et al. 2016; Foster 2017). The woman–midwife relationship is a key factor in fulfilling the aims of the 'with woman' concept and must include attributes of confidence, competence and compassion demonstrated by the midwife (Menage et al. 2017; Knapp 2017a; BenZion 2018), the environment in which care is given (i.e. woman and midwife focused place of birth, such as the woman's home or a birth centre/midwifery-led unit) (Davis and Homer 2016), and the resources and cost that will affect the birth outcome (Leinweber and Rowe 2010). This 'with woman' concept is increasingly significant depending on such factors and how effectively it is achieved considering the extent and frequency of its use. The antecedents or events/phenomenon of this concept therefore precede and shape an aspect of the concept which has meaning to either the midwife and/or the woman herself.

In her presentation of how concepts can be analysed, Rodgers (1989) indicates a seven-stage process or framework that will assist this investigation (Table 1.1). An examination of the literature will explore the historical use and linguistic interpretation of the term 'with woman' and identify the antecedents to being 'with woman' which can be viewed from physical, emotional, spiritual and psychological perspectives and carried out through knowledge and care skills by the professional. The next stage in Rodgers' (1989) framework is to identify the attributes which articulate the concept through common use of the 'with woman' term and identify references to the application in events and situations as a

Table 1.1 Rodgers' Evolutionary Conceptual Analysis framework (1989).

1) Identify and name the concept 'with woman'
2) Identify surrogate terms and relevant use of the concept
3) Identify databases and search term for 'with woman'
4) Identify the attributes of the concept
5) Identify the references, antecedents and consequences of the concept (Table 1.3)
6) Identify concepts related to the 'with woman' concept
7) Midwives' and women's stories to illustrate the concept

phenomenon. The antecedents generally precede a perspective or instance of the concept. Consequences of a 'with woman' concept follow as a result or an occurrence of the concept. A final stage in Rodgers' (1989) Conceptual Analysis framework is to clarify and illustrate the attributes of the concept through presentation of cases, as examples from everyday clinical practice and stories as told by midwives and women.

Search Strategy and Inclusion/Exclusion Criteria

A literature review was carried out using a search strategy identified by the editor and a midwife reviewer and applied to the following databases and the search terms as identified in Table 1.2. A range of literature in English, from academic journals and which were published in full text between 2009 and 2019, was identified and retrieved for review. Key search terms were 'with woman', midwifery, midwife, midwives, and mid* and related terms such as 'with woman', 'being with woman', 'continuity of carer', 'known mid*' and therapeutic relationship synonyms and abbreviations applied within the context of childbirth, such as 'women centred care' and combined with the Boolean operators of 'AND' and 'OR'.

The following databases were accessed in the searches for literature published up to 2019 resulting in CINAHL, Medline, British Nursing Index, PsychINFO, Internurse and Nursing & Allied Health as working databases. The resulting

Table 1.2 Databases searched and number of articles selected for final review.

Database	Number of hits after application of search terms	Number of articles selected for review	Articles accepted after review
CINAHL	96	15	5
Medline	71	16	6
BNI	137	15	2
PsychINFO	48	8	5
Internurse	22	3	1
Nursing & Allied Health	10	2	2
	Screened for relevance and filters applied	Duplications removed	Total = 21

literature was read for abstract content and then selected papers were scrutinised in full text to be included in the final number of papers identified. The results included an interpretation of the 'with woman' term which can sometimes be interchanged or used as a surrogate term. As identified in search terms, 'with woman' was associated with terms such as 'continuity of care and carer', 'therapeutic relationship', 'woman centred care', 'doula or spiritual companion' and 'midwife led care' or 'known midwife'.

Data Extraction and Analysis

Two reviewers carried out the literature search and almost identical publications were listed in the final search. Titles containing the 'with woman', one-to-one care/carer, continuity of care/carer, doula and birth companion were combined with search terms of midwives, midwifery practice/care. Abstracts were also screened for these words or terms. The resulting studies were then scanned for attributes of behaviour, process or environment pertaining to the concept of being 'with woman'. A second screening sought words or terms that expressed or described the consequence or result of the 'with woman' concept. Search results which contained none of the above criteria were excluded.

Both reviewers assessed the final papers selected and entered details of year of publication, reason for selection – i.e. 'with woman' term or associated terms in the title, abstract, or text content – on a simple data extraction sheet. The resulting literature was further analysed using the antecedents of emotional, psychological, spiritual and physical health, midwifery skills and knowledge and organisational working patterns, resulting in attributes pertaining to the behaviour, process and environment of the 'with woman' concepts and the resulting subsequent consequences as per Table 1.3 below.

Characteristics of the 'with Woman' Concept

Limited literature exists on the 'with woman' concept and mostly presents a professional point of view and the implications for midwives in attempting to fulfil the concept. Much of the research implies that the midwife 'with woman' has physical, mental and resource implications (Leap 2009; Hunter 2009; Leinweber and Rowe 2010; Aune et al. 2014; Hunter 2015; Astrup 2016; Power et al. 2016; Reed et al. 2016; Knapp 2017a; Hunter et al. 2017; Amir and Reid 2018; Bradfield et al. 2019b, c; Brady et al. 2019).

A dearth of literature on this topic, from women's perspectives, exists; particularly in publications outside the UK (Dahlberg and Aune 2013; Bradfield et al. 2018a).

Table 1.3 Antecedents, attributes and consequences of the 'with woman' concept resulting from Rodgers' Evolutionary Concept Analysis framework.

'With woman' antecedents	Attributes (behaviour)	Consequences
Emotional wellbeing Hunter (2009) Huber and Sandall (2009) Aune et al. (2014) Hunter (2015)	Positive presence and calm Listening Acknowledging feelings Empathy Reassurance Affirmation Sensitivity	Relational continuity MW compassion MW understanding Mutual recognition Therapeutic space Respect for woman Empowerment
Psychological health Bradfield et al. (2019c) Perriman et al. (2018) Nystedt et al. (2014)	Trusting relationship Woman-centred care Known midwife Continuity of midwifery care Co-participation Nurturance Helpfulness	Impact on MW and woman Greater satisfaction Personalised care Psychological and physical support Decreased anxiety/fear Courage to give birth
Spiritual health Hunter et al. (2017) Dahlberg and Aune (2013)	Giving of self Engagement/connectedness Mindfulness Intuitive Awareness/ recognition	Empowered woman Provides confidence Positive birth experience Holistic care provision Acknowledging expectations

'With woman' antecedents	Attributes (process)	Consequences
Midwifery knowledge Bradfield et al. (2018a,b) Brady et al. (2019) Leap (2009)	Dynamic developing construct Control and empowerment Woman-centred care Midwifery guidance	Partnership Empowers women Supports/hinders behaviours Safe, supportive and gentle
Midwifery skills Power et al. (2016) Bradfield et al. (2019b) Astrup (2016)	Responsibility to the woman Advocacy Communication Professional expertise, identity Midwifery responsibility and flexibility	Teaches competence and confidence Better birth experience Greater maternal satisfaction

Table 1.3 (Continued)

'With woman' antecedents	Attributes (environmental)	Consequences
Physical wellbeing McDonald (2011) Reed et al. (2016)	Continuous support Birth aids/equipment Sustaining strength Comfort Touch or closeness/support Companion/doula One-to-one care/carer Ritual companion	Reduced pain, less analgesia Shorter labour, fewer operative outcomes Maternal satisfaction Personal attention Continuous labour support Being there Better birth experience
Resources: organisational factors and costs Leinweber and Rowe (2010) Yoshida and Sandall (2013) Knapp (2017a,b) Amir and Reid (2018)	Staff shortages/lack of time Reduced maternity services Cost to midwives Burnout	Serious incidences Morbidity/mortality Midwifery burnout Midwifery dissatisfaction

The evidence suggests that although some women document the various benefits for childbearing women when the midwife is 'with them' in various situations and aspects, many express differing views of the 'continuity of care' and carer concept (Huber and Sandal 2009; Nystedt et al. 2014; Perriman et al. 2018). Their childbirth outcomes are also affected in terms of morbidity, such as birth trauma – both physical and psychological – and neonatal outcomes (Yoshida and Sandall 2013; McDonald 2011).

As identified from the literature above, the 'with woman' concept is a complex phenomenon and includes a range of antecedents. These consider emotional, psychological and spiritual wellbeing, physical health, midwifery knowledge and skills and resource implication to fulfil the concept. Each of these antecedents will be considered in turn and the attributes pertaining to behaviour, process and environment are examined for the subsequent consequences.

Wellbeing and Health Through Positive Behaviour

The terms 'emotional wellbeing' and 'psychological and spiritual health' were identified from the literature as antecedents to the 'with woman' concept (Hunter 2009; Huber and Sandall 2009; Aune et al. 2014; Hunter 2015 for emotional wellbeing and Bradfield et al. 2019c; Perriman et al. 2018; Nystedt et al. 2014 for psychological and spiritual health). The study by Hunter (2009) suggests that a Positive Presence Index (PPI) administered to women during labour and birth, either in a hospital or a birth centre environment, resulted in a higher PPI scores for those women in the birth centre due to improved interaction and personal quality of midwifery care. A meaningful relationship based on trust through continuity of midwifery care (Perriman et al. 2018) and a shared philosophy between a woman and midwife has an impact of satisfaction on both (Bradfield et al. 2019c) and is a consequence of this approach. Support during childbirth results in reduced anxiety and fear, and courage of the woman to give birth (Nystedt et al. 2014).

A calm and positive midwifery presence as described by Huber and Sandall (2009), and provision of continuous support through relational competence Aune et al. (2014), are other attributes of the 'with woman' concept. The midwife demonstrates behaviour of listening, acknowledging the woman's feelings, displays empathy and sensitivity and provides reassurance and affirmation of the woman's ability to birth her baby. Hunter (2015) suggests that a therapeutic space is created through mutual recognition and respect as attributes, which consequently empower both the woman and the midwife (Dahlberg and Aune 2013; Andrews 2017). Hunter et al. (2017) found that the attribute of mindfulness can provide a way for midwives to contain levels of stress. This can be achieved through a reconnection with self and the woman to improve job satisfaction and provide holistic 'with woman' care.

Processing Midwifery Knowledge and Skills

A 'with woman' concept demands antecedents of sound midwifery knowledge and competent skills. The integrative review by Bradfield et al. (2018a,b) of this concept has identified the attribute of a dynamic developing process of this construct. The authors suggest a transference of power to the woman through effective informed decision making and facilitation of 'space' by the midwife that enables this process (Dolin 2017). However, much of the literature that explores related concepts, such as 'women centred care', can have a wide variation in how this is interpreted. Leap (2009) suggests that whilst contesting meanings of the term, the focus should be on shifting the locus of control to the woman, in meeting her individual needs through safe, supportive and gentle care.

The phenomenological study by Bradfield et al. (2019b) indicates that midwives consider the 'with woman' phenomenon as an essential element to the practice and identity of their profession. Midwifery knowledge and experience informs their skills underpinned by a 'with woman' philosophy that defines and identifies them as experts in their field. Being 'with woman' in contemporary midwifery as best practice needs to be recognised, maintained and disseminated to future generations of midwives (Power et al. 2016). In addition, maintaining a therapeutic partnership with women and their families requires advanced, effective communication skills to provide advocacy for women with knowledge and confidence (Bradfield et al. 2019a, Bradfield et al. 2019b). The mother and midwife relationship through continuity of care provides midwives with greater flexibility and responsibility, leading to improved maternal satisfaction (Astrup 2016).

Physical Wellbeing Through Environmental Factors

The interpretation of continuous support during labour has changed over time. Women have been cared for and supported physically and psychologically, across the ages, by other women during childbirth. Changes in models of care during labour have impacted the way women are supported during this life-changing event. Consequently, a rise in hospital births in the post-war era has medicalised childbirth and interrupted the relationship of midwives with women in the home environment. However, a move towards provision of continuity of support in labour, by midwives as 'ritual companions', over the last few decades, has had an impact on birth outcomes (Reed et al. 2016). Physical, psychological and spiritual support has resulted in a reduced risk of caesarean section, instrumental delivery and need for analgesia (McDonald 2011).

Innovations such as birthing pools, improved equipment and alternative therapies for pain relief used in labour have changed midwifery practices to ameliorate the birthing environment. However, organisational factors such as rising costs, shortage of staff and resources have had an impact on the provision and quality of maternity services. Over time, these have collectively had a significant bearing on women's satisfaction with their childbirth experiences and have 'cost' midwives and healthcare professionals in terms of their health and wellbeing (Leinweber and Rowe 2010; Amir and Reid 2018).

The new standards for the midwifery profession (NMC 2019, p. 16) state that a midwife must '*Provide safe and effective midwifery care: promoting and providing continuity of care and carer*'. It is unclear how midwives will be able to fulfil the expectation of continuity of carer when the midwifery workforce is depleted to a risk level that needs addressing urgently. Consequently, midwives are suffering from occupational burnout, experiencing stress and anxiety and need organisational and peer/colleague support (Yoshida and Sandall 2013). The Department of Health has recognised these shortfalls and currently changes are in progress. There is a move to improve and balance life/work conditions (Knapp 2017a) and change to bursaries for students entering the profession as a way forward for those who struggle, at personal cost, to provide safe and effective midwifery care.

Conclusion

This chapter has examined the literature that cites the 'with woman' concept and presented the findings through Rodgers' Concept Analysis framework. Further searches were carried out at the start of each subsequent chapter to add terms and associated concepts or surrogate terms specific to the chapter title; for example, the With Woman in Prison Chapter 9 (Shlafer et al. 2014) included word searches such as 'with woman' AND/OR pregnant, imprisoned, incarcerated, pregnant in prison, childbearing women in prison and maternity services in prison.

Stories from midwives and women complete the final stage of Rodgers' Concept Analysis framework to illustrate the findings from the analysis. Identified attributes of a positive calming presence, reassurance and nurturance through a therapeutic relationship resulted in empowerment and control for the woman and her partner and a positive birth experience.

Midwives' Story

Victoria's Story

Lisa's birth story:* As a midwife I try to maintain a relaxing and calm atmosphere for the woman and her partner as it promotes a positive birth experience.

Lisa and David came into the midwife-led birth centre for a labour assessment. Lisa was 40 weeks and four days pregnant with her second baby. All of her observations were within normal limits and she was contracting three times in 10 minutes, which felt moderate on palpation. Her waters were intact and the fetal heartrate was normal when I listened in. I took her into a room and encouraged her to eat, drink and mobilise. At this point, her contractions were regular, and I did not feel that there was any indication to offer a vaginal examination.

Whilst they waited for labour to progress, David put some music on a speaker and I turned the lights down low. Lisa breathed calmly through her contractions for a couple of hours whilst I quietly observed her and listened to the fetal heart (FH) every 15 minutes. I also offered aromatherapy, which was accepted. Lisa inhaled frankincense and black pepper oils from a cloth whilst her contractions increased in strength and frequency.

As she began to feel pressure, her waters broke, and she requested to use the birthing pool. She visibly relaxed as she entered the warm water and began to bear down in an all fours position. Aside from quietly listening in every five minutes and checking Lisa's pulse, the room was quiet. David moved a chair closer to the pool and held his wife as she began to have expulsive contractions.

The atmosphere in the room remained calm and primal as the vertex became visible. Lisa listened as I calmly guided her to stop pushing as baby's head crowned. She reached down to touch her baby's head before the body was born with the next contraction. I passed her pink and crying baby girl up to her chest. Lisa held her baby for 10 minutes until the cord stopped pulsating and as baby was keenly searching for her breast. David cut the baby's cord and had some skin to skin with his new daughter whilst I helped his wife out of the pool. The placenta was delivered passively on the toilet into a bowl and, as Lisa had an intact perineum, she began breastfeeding within 30 minutes of birth. As a midwife I helped to facilitate this birth for this couple; however, the woman and her partner were fully in control of the environment and their own experience.

Lucy's Story

***Fiona*'s birth story:** To me, midwifery-led care is about being with woman – not just in the physical sense, but holistically engaging with her, understanding her story and actively listening. I feel extremely privileged, within the National Health Service (NHS), to work in a home birth team, case-loading and providing community to our clients. Through this level of continuity, I feel I have been able to give the best care of my career, because for the first time I am getting to know the women we care for. As a team we care for mothers throughout their pregnancy, and spend time understanding them as an individual. What motivates her? What are her fears? What are her preferences and why? What does she find supportive and obstructive? Listen carefully to a mother and she will tell you her story; engage with her and you will understand it.*

One evening I was first on call, about five months into my career with the team, and about 18 months post qualification. I received a phone call from Fiona, a term mother, at about 9 p.m. to say her waters had broken. This mother was someone I had booked under the team's care when she transferred to us in the third trimester from another location. She had a previous home birth elsewhere and was incredibly calm as a person. Her first birth had been straightforward and had been the quicker side of 'normal'. I confirmed her waters were clear, and baby was moving well. Fiona reported feeling very comfortable, with just a few 'niggles' so far. Guided by this information and her relaxed manner on the phone, I suggested she rest and call back when things changed or if she had any concerns.

(Continued)

A few hours passed, and I received another phone call. Still calm and relaxed, Fiona told me that she was now having two contractions every 10 minutes. She felt they were mild to moderate in strength but could feel they were beginning to spread from previously being low and crampy to now up and across her abdomen. They were lasting about 40 seconds. By textbook definition, I knew that this indicated that Fiona was not in 'active' labour, as her contractions were not yet regular or occurring 3:10 lasting 60 seconds. But on hearing her pause and breathe through a contraction on the phone, I felt that I should make my way to her.

When I arrived, Fiona was quietly pacing in her room using a TENS machine and listening to a relaxation track. I checked my kit and quietly set up my resuscitation equipment – the family had a full discussion with us at a 36 weeks antenatal appointment and knew what kit would be present. So this was not alarming. I completed a full assessment – observations, abdominal palpation, began regular auscultations and then sat back and observed her. Liquor remained clear, and baby was still moving well; all was well. We do not routinely perform vaginal examinations, unless requested or unless there are any deviations from normal, for at least the first four hours – within which time many mothers have birthed or are close to birthing.

Fiona continued to pace, and I observed as she paused to breathe through each contraction. I noticed she was now contracting about three times in every 10 minutes, but reflected on how on an average triage shift, a mother as stoic as her would likely have midwives saying 'she's not in labour' 'she can't be in labour' – and yet here she was, and signs implied otherwise. In hospital, perhaps a vaginal examination may have surprised a midwife. But in reality, that information would not change this picture at all. What was important was that Fiona was contracting regularly – she required midwifery support, it didn't matter if she was 4 or 8 cm. With no interruptions to her hormonal and physiological progress in labour, I knew her dilation was likely to be advancing rapidly, especially as a multiparous mother. Her partner, Rob inflated the birthing pool and began to fill it.

Occasionally, I reminded Fiona to stay hydrated and she began sipping water after contractions. I asked when she last passed urine, and she thought it had been a few hours. She mobilised to the bathroom. I documented and phoned my second midwife to attend – I knew her drive was a bit further than mine and felt the mother was so calm and stoic we could be having a baby here soon. Shortly after coming off the phone, I heard a quiet 'grunt' from behind the bathroom door.

I asked to enter the bathroom and found Fiona beginning to spontaneously push at the height of her contraction. With Rob speedily filling the pool, which was just about 20 cm deep, I suggested we move off the toilet and make her more comfortable. I was now auscultating baby central and low, where we had previously been listening in at the left occipito anterior (LOA) position. A steady 130–135 bpm baseline remained post contraction. This implied that the baby was progressing down through the mechanisms of labour and was ready to be born. As Fiona moved back into the bedroom, she spontaneously knelt on her bedroom floor, leaning on the bed, and I placed pillows under her knees.

As the next contraction came, there was a forewater rupture and vertex was visible. I grabbed my 'delivery kit' – a small zip-lock bag with cord clamps, sterile scissors, swabs and, if needed, syntometrine. (We carry full delivery kits, but this is an easy grab bag when baby comes quickly.) I began five-minute fetal heart (FH) auscultation and told Rob to stop filling the pool – the baby was coming! I asked instead for a bowl of the pool warm water and used this for my warm compress to protect Fiona's perineum, with consent, as baby advanced. I reassured her that everything was progressing well and to keep listening to her body. At this moment, her son woke up and came into the room – Rob quickly reassured him, and I greeted a hello as we had met throughout her pregnancy. The child sat excitedly with his father and supported the mother – even clapping hands in excitement! As Fiona's baby's head crowned I reminded her to blow and control her breathing, as we had discussed at the 36 weeks antenatal appointment, to allow baby's head to birth slowly – she calmly blew long breaths as baby delivered – head then body within three minutes of vertex being visible. I passed Fiona's baby through her legs and she held her close to her chest maintaining skin to skin whilst I rubbed baby and covered them both in a warm towel. The second midwife arrived shortly afterwards, and Fiona went on to have a physiological birth of the placenta also.

On reflection, I was relieved I had attended at the time I did, despite the fact that, at the time, Fiona was reporting mild to moderate tightening. Fiona's labour was not typical as she was so stoic throughout; I'm not sure she would have ever sounded like a textbook 'actively labouring' mother over the phone. In hindsight, knowing the mother as I did, meant I had an understanding of her nature, and knew she would likely be incredibly calm in labour. This had a huge influence on my decision making, based on my relationship with Fiona and knowing her as an individual, which I intuitively considered when attending to her and providing care as her midwife.

Women's Stories

Emily's Story

On the morning of my due date, I had a few mild cramps which came and went with me hardly even noticing them. I put it down to 'due date excitement'! I had a sweep booked in with Emily (my midwife was also called Emily!) at around mid-day and I was excited at the prospect of it possibly starting things off. I took my toddler to nursery and my husband and I went out for breakfast to enjoy some child-free time before the next baby came along. Emily and a student midwife came over after lunch at around 1:30 p.m., and after a cup of tea and a lovely chat she did the sweep for me. She said I was already 3 cm dilated and my cervix was fully effaced!! What!? My body had been up to all sorts of things without me even knowing! Emily said that we would very likely have our baby today and said to call the team when things ramped up and advised that we inflate the birthing pool. Having the sweep at home was much more relaxing than at hospital (if you can call a sweep relaxing!?).

Once Emily and the student midwife left, I couldn't quite believe that we might meet our baby today. I felt absolutely fine except for now having a few more strong cramps. My previous labour and delivery was about five hours long so I expected something similar this time around ... (how wrong I was!)

My husband and daughter blew up the birthing pool in the front room (which she found such great fun!) and lit some candles. By now I was having fairly regular, strong contractions but as it wasn't that long since Emily had left, I didn't think I needed to phone the midwives just yet.

I phoned my mum and asked her to come and collect our daughter so that we could concentrate on the labour. I did hip circles on my birthing ball, as advised by Emily, to help dilate my cervix. After my mum left, I was struggling to talk through contractions. They were coming every two and a half to three minutes. It had only been about an hour and a half since I had my sweep, so I thought surely I'd still have ages left. I phoned Emily to let her know that things had ramped up, but I told her I felt as though I was coping well at the moment. She advised that my husband should start filling up the pool with water and I could get in to use it for pain relief if I wanted. She also informed Heather who was on call for births that day.

Heather phoned me a few minutes after I had got off the phone to Emily to check how I was doing, and even though it was only a few minutes later, I suddenly couldn't cope with the pain anymore. I couldn't talk and was crying through contractions. She stayed on the phone to me to listen and gauge how I was labouring and said that she was going to drive over immediately. I still thought that I probably had ages to go until I delivered the baby.

Heather arrived and by this stage I was on all fours in my lounge and I was 'mooing' loudly to get through the pain! I suddenly felt as though I couldn't go through with the delivery and remembered that feeling from my last labour as being incredibly close to having the baby. I still couldn't believe that it was all happening so quickly.

Heather helped me take my underwear off and asked my husband to get our birth kit ready and put the shower curtain out on the floor as the baby was likely to be out a bit quicker than we all thought! The contractions were becoming unbearable and I felt a huge urge to push. I asked for gas and air and my husband stayed with me and kept talking to me the whole time, encouraging me to keep going. My body seemed to do most of the work as each contraction felt so strong and made me involuntarily push. The position I was in really helped and was the most 'comfortable' one to be – leant forwards over the arm of an armchair. By now Kirsty had also arrived who I had seen at all of my antenatal appointments. It was so nice to have two familiar faces at my delivery.

Heather had a mirror which she put on the floor between my legs so that she could see how close the baby was to coming out. Every step of the way she was incredible and told me exactly what to do. When to push and when not to push. She was so reassuring and if I felt panicked or scared, she seemed to read my mind and told me exactly what was going on, which was hugely calming.

Once the baby's head was out she told me to reach down and put my hand on his head. It was the most incredible and emotional feeling I have ever experienced. I burst into tears and felt so much relief that he was nearly out. To be able to feel his head there was just amazing! With the next push he was out, and Heather helped pass him to me as I sat back and brought him to my chest whilst I sobbed (with relief and happiness!).

Just after our baby was born and as I brought him to my chest, Kirsty used my husband's phone to take a few photos of the three of us. I hadn't realised they were being taken at the time and they are the most precious photos! I'm so grateful to her for taking them for us!!

I opted for physiological management of the placenta, so I didn't have the injection. About five minutes after delivering my baby I felt a lot of pressure down below and Heather helped me deliver the placenta, which was quick and pain-free. Heather and Kirsty helped clean me up, covered my sofa in towels and protective sheets and helped me lie back on the sofa and enjoy skin to skin with my baby. I put him to the breast straight away. I then realised the birthing pool was still

(Continued)

filling up! My husband hadn't had time to switch the tap off, but luckily it was only half full.

The cherry on top was when the midwives brought me a cup of tea and a brownie to enjoy whilst I chilled on the sofa with my husband and our gorgeous new baby in the comfort of our own home. They really do go the extra mile.

Heather, Kirsty and all the members of the team we met along the way were absolutely amazing: kind, compassionate and incredibly professional. I am forever grateful that they made our home birth experience so special. I can't recommend the Homebirth Team enough.

Victoria's Story

Every night in my 39th week of pregnancy I kept going to bed thinking: is this it, will we get to meet our baby tonight? It's such a weird feeling having absolutely no control of your body and not knowing when such a big life change will happen.

I'll be honest: it felt really lonely waiting, especially as my husband was working all week. I kept telling myself you just have let it go and trust my body will do what it needs to do when it's ready to do it. As I knew from practising hypnobirthing, my body would not begin the process of birth until it was fully relaxed and ready.

On the Thursday of that week, I was woken just after midnight by my waters breaking. It wasn't the big surge of water you imagine but enough to know that things were starting. I took myself to the bathroom, told my husband James and headed back into bed to try and get some rest. The surges began slowly so I started timing them using a brilliant app called 'Freya'. Every time a surge (contraction) would start, I would press the button on the app and it would count through my surges. I messaged my midwife an hour later to let her know and also my student midwife, Maddy, who had been following my journey through pregnancy since my first appointment with the community midwife.

After a few hours, I decided to curl up on the sofa under a blanket with only a candle for light (Jo Malone London – Mimosa & Cardamom – a scent I'd been drawn to through my pregnancy) and listened to my birthing playlist through my headphones. Still counting and breathing through my surges.

Ollie (our three year-old) woke up around 6.00 a.m. and by this time my surges were getting stronger but were still comfortable. He and my husband James started getting all the things needed for the birthing pool – old towels, waterproof sheets, the pool, hose, etc. He even got a chair from his room to put inside the pool, so I had somewhere to sit; this was particularly funny.

About this time one of my best friends messaged me this perfect quote: 'My job is simply to relax and allow my body to birth my baby.' Reading that along with my prepared positive affirmations, I was feeling strong and powerful at this point. I found walking around the house and taking myself from room to room to experience the surges really lovely. At one point I opened the front door to breathe in the sunlight and spring air. I remember looking out of my bedroom window a lot at our garden and spraying some of my Basil & Neroli Jo Malone London fragrance. It reminds me of bright spring mornings, and this was exactly what it was like this particular morning as the sun was rising.

I asked James to call the midwives around 8 a.m. as the surges were more powerful and he would be having to take Ollie to playschool at 9 a.m. and I didn't want to be on my own. They arrived around 8.30 and the pool started to be filled. Again, Ollie enjoyed helping with this job, as well as getting out his doctor's kit to show the midwives and playing them some tunes on his guitar. He kept them highly entertained. And I was so happy he was around for this part of the labour.

The midwives arrived so quietly, just coming into my bedroom to listen to baby's heartrate and taking my blood pressure. Apart from that they completely left me alone. I remember thinking I should offer them a cup of tea, but they just helped themselves which was perfect. I also remember thinking they must be so bored; but they were great, so patient and so calm and quiet, just letting my body do its thing. I really appreciated not having that transition to the hospital this time round (as I had done with Ollie).

Whilst James was taking Ollie to playgroup, I heard the midwives getting pots and pans of water on the cooker so they could help fill the pool up quicker, as they said now that Ollie had gone my surges would probably get stronger. They were right, my body felt more relaxed now he wasn't there, and things really kicked in. By the time James got home I was needing him for the surges and found standing backwards leaning on his hands for him to take my weight was the most comfortable way to get through them. I finally got into the pool around 9.30 and it was heavenly. The warmth of the water definitely helped with the strength of the surges I was experiencing, and I enjoyed floating there.

Sometime not much later, I lay floating on my side and holding my student midwife, Maddy's, hand. I burst into tears for some reason and just had a massive cry. They say this is common when a woman is in the 'transition' phase. That feeling of 'I can't do this' takes over. However, I knew to expect this so told myself this must be transition. That means I'm about to enter the pushing phase of the birth so needed all the strength I could get. Soon my body had the pushing sensations (think of an involuntary surge when you're sick), your body completely takes over

(Continued)

and sort of feels like it has convulsions. This is where my animal instincts took over and my mooing sounds erupted (my poor neighbours). I knew the baby was getting lower and lower as the midwives were checking the pulse with a Doppler and that was getting lower and lower. I didn't need to ask them; I just knew.

The strongest pushes soon came, and I could feel the head appearing. But it almost came out and popped back up again. I definitely had a feeling that I wouldn't be doing this again at that point. Then in the next push the head was out. I actually felt down and just felt a full head of hair which was an unforgettable moment.

In the next push the whole body was out, Maddy caught the baby underwater and brought it up and out and into my arms to Coldplay's song 'A Sky Full of Stars'. I felt numb holding this little body, I just couldn't move my arms or body to even see if it was a boy or a girl.

James announced it was a baby girl.

Well, I just cried and cried, and the midwives shed a little tear too. I just couldn't believe it. I honestly didn't think I had a preference, but I was overjoyed to have a girl. She wouldn't open her eyes to start with as the sun was shining in at her through the window, but when she finally did she looked straight at us.

I hadn't even noticed another midwife had arrived to support us and unbeknown to us she had filmed it. This sounds gross and weird, but you just see Isla coming out the water; it is incredible to watch back and relive this moment again and again. The next few hours were so calm and relaxed. I stayed in the water for a little while just holding her until the placenta was delivered, and I handed her to James at that point.

The midwives helped me get out of the pool and onto the sofa where I pretty much stayed all afternoon drifting in and out of sleep and cuddling my baby daughter.

Lessons Learnt

The above stories demonstrate some wonderful aspects of the 'with woman' concept and highlight some valuable lessons that can be learnt from midwives' and women's birth experiences. Victoria's (the midwife) account perfectly illustrates how the woman's physical wellbeing is preserved though the attributes of a calm, relaxed and quiet atmosphere. A therapeutic relationship between the woman and midwife is portrayed through the woman's perceptions of empowerment. She is fully in control of her environment and the birth experience through minimal intervention by the midwife (no vaginal examination and a physiological third stage) resulting in an intact perineum and early initiation of breastfeeding.

Lucy's account highlights the value of continuity of carer using her intuitive knowledge. This is beautifully illustrated when despite being told that the rate and strengths of contraction were not indicative of active labour, Lucy actively listened to Fiona and engaged fully with her to understand how events were unfolding. Lucy's quote is illuminative of the wonderful attributes that she displays in truly being 'with woman'. Lucy says, *'listen carefully to a mother and she will tell you her story; engage with her and you will understand it'*.

Finally, the women's stories demonstrate the value of continuity of carer in their own home environment. The attributes of 'known' midwives, whose presence offers reassurance, decreased anxiety and fear, were perceived by the women as *'kindness, compassion and incredibly professional'*. This presence encouraged a self-belief in the women, affirming that their own bodies can birth naturally. This is wonderfully reaffirmed by Victoria's friend when she messaged, *'My job is simply to relax and allow my body to birth my baby'*. Victoria acknowledged the midwives' intuition in getting ready for the birth and states, *'they were right'*. They remained patient and calm, giving of self through a balance of engagement with Victoria but affording her therapeutic space when needed, *'and completely left me alone'*. These attributes and consequences of being 'with woman' are clearly identified through Rodgers' Concept Analysis of the literature, but the stories above, speak for themselves.

References

Allison, J. (2016). Midwives of sixteenth-century rural East Anglia. *Rural History* 27 (1): 1–19.

Amir, Z. and Reid, A.J. (2018). The cost of being "with women": the impact of traumatic perinatal events on burnout rates amongst midwives. *MIDIRS Midwifery Digest* 28 (3): 307–308.

Andrews, N. (2017). Holding space: with women in a labyrinth. *Midwifery* 121: 9–11.

Astrup, J. (2016). In safe hands. *Midwives* 20 (2): 46–51.

Aune, I., Amundsen, H., and Akaget Aas, L. (2014). Is a midwife's continuous presence during childbirth a matter of course? Midwives' experiences and thoughts about factors that may influence their continuous support of women during labour. *Midwifery* 30: 89–95.

BenZion, M. (2018). Learning to trust birth though continuity of care. *Midwifery* 125: 18–22.

Bradfield, Z., Duggan, R., Hauck, Y. et al. (2018a). Midwives being "with woman": an integrative review. *Women and Birth* 31: 143–152.

Bradfield, Z., Kelly, M., Hauck, Y., and Duggan, R. (2018b). Midwives "with woman" in the private obstetric model: where divergent philosophies meet. *Women and Birth* https://doi.org/10.1016/j.wombi.2018.07.013.

Bradfield, Z., Hauck, Y., Kelly, M., and Duggan, R. (2019a). Midwives' experiences of being "with woman" in a model where midwives are unknown. *Midwifery* 69: 150–157.

Bradfield, Z., Hauck, Y., Duggan, R. et al. (2019b). Midwives' perception of being "with woman": a phenomenological study. *BMC Pregnancy and Childbirth* 19: 363. https://doi.org/10.1186/s12884-019-2548-4.

Bradfield, Z., Hauck, Y., Kelly, M. et al. (2019c). "It's what midwifery is about": Western Australian midwives' experiences of being "with woman" during labour and birth in the known midwife model. *BMC Pregnancy and Childbirth* 19: 29. https://doi.org/10.1186/s12884-018-2144-z.

Brady, S., Lee, N., Gibbons, K., and Bogossian, F. (2019). Women-centred care: an integrative review of the empirical literature. *International Journal of Nursing Studies* 94: 107–119.

Burgess, A. (2014). An evolutionary concept analysis. *International Journal of Childbirth Education* 29 (2): 64–72.

Dahlberg, U. and Aune, I. (2013). The woman's birth experience- the effects of interpersonal relationship of continuity of care. *Midwifery* 29 (4): 407–415.

Davis, D.L. and Homer, C.S. (2016). Birthplace as the midwife's work place: how does place of birth impact on midwives? *Women & Birth* 29: 407–415.

Dolin, J. (2017). Thinking about the influences of informed choice. *Midwifery* 124: 50–51.

Evenden, E. (2000). *The Midwives of Seventeenth-Century London*. Cambridge: Cambridge University Press.

Foster, J. (2017). Using research to advance nursing practice: A guide to concept analysis. *Clinical Nurse Specialist* 31 (2): 70–73.

Harley, D. (1990). Historians as demonologists: the myth of the midwife- witch. *Social History of Medicine* 3 (1): 1–26.

Harley, D. (1993). Provincial midwives in England: Lancashire and Cheshire, 1660 – 1760. In: *The Art of Midwifery: Early Modern Midwives in Europe* (ed. H. Marland), 27–48. London/New York: Routledge.

Higgins, T., Larson, E., and Schnall, R. (2017). Unravelling the meaning of patient engagement: a concept analysis. *Patient Education and Counselling* 100: 30–36.

Huber, U.S. and Sandall, J. (2009). A qualitative exploration of the creation of calm in a continuity of carer model of maternity care in London. *Midwifery* 25: 613–621.

Hunter, L.P. (2002). Being with woman: a guiding concept for the care of labouring women. *Journal of Obstetric, Gynecologic, & Neonatal Nursing* 31: 650–657.

Hunter, P. (2009). A descriptive study of "Being with Woman" during labour and birth. *Journal of Midwifery & Women's Health* 54 (2): 111–118.

Hunter, L. (2015). Being with woman: claiming midwifery space. *Practising Midwife* 18 (3): 20–22.

Hunter, L., Snow, S., and Warriner, S. (2017). Being there and reconnecting: Midwives' perceptions of the impact of mindfulness training on their practice. *Journal of Clinical Nursing* 27: 1227–1238.

Knapp, R. (2017a). Wellbeing and resilience 1. The resilient midwife. *Practising Midwife* 20 (3): 26–28.

Knapp, R. (2017b). The resilient midwife 2: The self-compassionate midwife. *Practising Midwife* 20 (5): ePub.

Leap, N. (2009). Woman-centred or women-centred care: does it matter? *Midwifery* 17 (1): 12–16.

Leap, N. and Hunter, B. (1993). *The Midwife's Tale: An Oral History from Handy Woman to Professional Midwife*. London: Scarlet Press.

Leinweber, J. and Rowe, H.J. (2010). The cost of "being with woman": secondary traumatic stress in midwifery. *Midwifery* 26: 76–87.

Llewelyn Davies, M. (ed.) (1915, reprinted 1978). *Maternity: Letters from Working Women Collected by the Women's co-Operative Guild*. London: Virago.

Marland, H. (ed.) (1993). *The Art of Midwifery: Early Modern Midwives in Europe*. London/New York: Routledge.

McDonald, S. (2011). Women who receive continuous support during labour have reduced risk of caesarean, instrumental delivery or need for analgesia compared to usual care: systematic review. *Midwifery* 16 (2): 40–41.

McIntosh, T. (2012). *A Social History of Maternity and Childbirth: Key Themes in Maternity Care*. London/New York: Routledge.

Menage, D., Bailey, E., Lees, S., and Coad, J. (2017). A concept analysis of compassionate midwifery. *Journal of Advanced Nursing* 73 (3): 558–573.

Myles, M. (1953). *A Textbook for Midwives*. Edinburgh: E & S Livingstone Ltd.

Nursing & Midwifery Council (2019). Standards of proficiency for midwives. www.nmc.org.uk/globalassets/sitedocuments/standards/standards-of-proficiency-for-midwives.pdf (accessed 10 January 2020).

Nystedt, A., Kristiansen, L., Ehrenstrale, K. et al. (2014). Exploring some Swedish women's experiences of support during childbirth. *International Journal of Childbirth* 4 (3): 183. https://doi.org/10.1891/2156-5287.4.3.183.

Perriman, N., Davis, D.L., and Ferguson, S. (2018). What women value in the midwifery continuity of care model: a systematic review with meta-synthesis. *Midwifery* 62: 220–229.

Power, A., Davidson, S., and Patrick, K. (2016). Being "with woman" in contemporary midwifery practice: one Trust's response to the Francis report. *British Journal of Midwifery* 24 (10): 711–713.

Reed, R., Rowe, J., and Barnes, M. (2016). Midwifery practice during birth: ritual companionship. *Women and Birth* 29: 269–278.

Rodgers, B.L. (1989). Concepts, analysis and the development of nursing knowledge: the evolutionary cycle. *Journal of Advanced Nursing* 14: 330–335.

Sheen, K., Spiby, H., and Slade, P. (2016). The experience and impact of traumatic perinatal event experiences in midwives: a qualitative investigation. *International Journal of Nursing Studies* 53: 61–72.

Shlafer, R., Hellerstedt, W.L., Secor-Turner, M. et al. (2014). Doulas' perspective about providing support to incarcerated women: a feasibility study. *Public Health Nursing* 32 (4): 316–326.

Yoshida, Y. and Sandall, J. (2013). Occupational burnout and work factors in community and hospital midwives: a survey analysis. *Midwifery* 29: 921–926.

2

Ethical Perspectives of Being 'with Woman'

Anna M. Brown; Donna Hunt (midwife); and Emily (woman)

Introduction

This chapter considers ethical issues which impact women and maternity healthcare professionals as a result of care delivery during the childbearing continuum. Women have to make informed decisions and face a myriad of choices during their journey. Equally, care providers have an obligation to provide the best available evidence and information to enable women to make choices about the model of care that is available to them, places of birth and modes of delivery. Midwives seek to deliver care that is effective, ethical and takes into consideration their professional autonomy and responsibility (NMC 2018). New professional standards for midwifery proficiencies indicate that key domains include *'an accountable and autonomous midwife who provides safe and effective care as colleague, scholar and leader'* though models of continuity of care and carer (NMC 2018 p. 16). These expectations have ethical implications which can influence the outcomes of a woman's birthing experience and a midwife's scope of professional practice.

It is reasonable to suggest that women's experience of childbirth is influenced by the care providers and the environment in which the birth takes place. The power dynamics between the midwife's autonomy to provide care, which is embedded in knowledge, and a woman's input to the process is crucial to birth outcomes. The place of birth impacts on the woman giving birth and on the midwife's social and spatial relationship. This includes the dynamics of control in which the birth event takes place. A woman is empowered to feel in control in a 'home' environment where she is familiar and comfortable; whilst a midwife has knowledge of the complex settings in a hospital environment. The midwife is

Better Births: The Midwife 'with Woman', First Edition. Edited by Anna M. Brown.
© 2021 John Wiley & Sons Ltd. Published 2021 by John Wiley & Sons Ltd.

therefore perceived by the woman to be in control. As such, it has been argued that hospital births do not generally accommodate the midwifery construct of a belief in the competence of a woman's body to be able to birth a baby and be an active participant in the childbearing process (Davis and Walker 2010).

Midwifery Working Practices

A document published in 2011 (Birthplace in England Collaborative Group) supports evidence that considers the impact of midwife-led intrapartum care from the user perspective (Renfew et al. 2008; Smith et al. 2008; Cheyne et al. 2013). This report suggests that this model of care offers a better birth experience. Other evidence shows how this model of care also increases women's satisfaction and reduces medical interventions during childbirth (Thompson et al. 2016, p. 67; Ross-Davie and Cheyne 2014; Sandall et al. 2015). Walsh and Devane (2012, p. 897) suggest that the term midwife-led care has evolved to mean '*autonomous care by a midwife of women designated at entering the maternity services to be healthy and at low risk of complications for pregnancy and birth*'. A meta synthesis of related literature identified that a midwifery-led approach to care increased midwifery autonomy (Walsh and Devane 2012). This results in empathetic and nurturing care; a language of compassion and sensitivity which is facilitated through the midwife–woman relationship.

Previous literature, reporting the perspectives of service users, (CQC 2013; Janssen and Wiegers 2006) recognised the need for improvement in maternity care services and highlighted problems of lack of continuity of care, courtesy and professional competence. The findings from the 2013 Care Quality Commission (CQC) survey reported on missed essential elements of care as identified by women accessing maternity care services. These included lack of support and inconsistent information to women, which disempowered them when attempting to make decisions about their care. This was compounded by lack of continuity of care and carer. Unfortunately, these concerns are still relevant, as highlighted by the more recent Better Birth's report (NHS England 2016) which implies that maternity services improvements are still to be made, thus impeding optimal care in childbirth.

The publication by NHS England (2017) to implement Better Births and promote continuity of carer set out a guide to support maternity care providers to start up pilot schemes which encourage two main models of maternity care. The first, the Team Midwifery model, indicates that each woman has an individual midwife who is responsible for coordinating care whilst working in a team of four to eight midwives, with team members backing-up their colleagues. The second suggested model was that of Total Case Loading in which each midwife is allocated a number of women to care for and then arranges her working life around the needs of the caseload (Dunkley-Bent 2018). However, both schemes could impact on the work–life balance of midwives and have implications for health and wellbeing, resources and cost to staff and organisations. These findings are supported by Jepsen et al.'s (2016) study which suggests that midwives need to be prepared to provide a caseload service by balancing disadvantages of their work commitment and obligation, in return for appreciation and social recognition. The outcomes are a meaningful and satisfactory result for the midwife in fulfilling a woman's expectations through a positive birth experience. However, such a commitment and obligation must surely impact on the health and wellbeing of staff.

Taylor et al.'s survey (2018) and earlier literature (Yoshida and Sandall 2013) suggested that although midwives welcomed the focus on continuity of carer, they did raise issues of concern, such as confidence and safety in working across maternity settings and practical barriers such as caring responsibilities, transport and proximity to work and health issues. However, the study participants did provide helpful suggestions in support of the care models to include adequate staffing, organisation of roles and good leadership and management, induction, support and training for staff, and finally a change in the midwifery profession culture to provide continuity of care of a high standard which is safe (Sandall 2017). The survey concludes that these models of providing maternity care may not suit all midwives and would only be successful if midwives were supported at a local level (RCM 2017) to change the ways in which they practise whilst maintaining their own wellbeing. The above issues will be explored in greater depth in the next chapter. However, changing practice and ways in which midwives work to fulfil the concept of being 'with woman' through the models described above can have ethical implications for midwives and an impact on the maternity services for women they care for.

Ethics and Standards

It is often challenging for midwives to make decisions which are appropriate and right for the childbearing women and the families they care for (Katz Rothman 2013). Childbirth is a social phenomenon and is created through the midwife and mother relationship and responsibilities through this social process (MacLellan 2014). Moral actions, underpinning the childbirth phenomenon, are guided by ethical principles in clinical situations to support safe and effective care based on principles of ethics (McCormick 2013).

One approach to ethics, in relation to midwifery practice, is the four principles approach, as identified by Beauchamp and Childress (2013). The principles of respect for autonomy, beneficence (do good), non-maleficence (minimise harm) and justice (treat people fairly) map well onto the profession's code (NMC 2018). The Code (NMC 2018) specifically emphasises the preservation of safety through prioritising people, effective practice and promoting professionalism and trust. The ethical importance of safety (Chadwick 2015) for women is supported by the four ethical principles: *respect for autonomy* supports and respects autonomous decisions by both woman and midwife; an obligation not to cause harm through the principle of *non-maleficence;* avoiding harm and calculating risks to ensure positive and beneficial outcomes through *beneficence;* and *justice* which ensures a fair distribution of risks, benefits and costs (Foster and Lasser 2011).

An interesting approach to ethical midwifery practice is presented by MacLellan (2014), suggesting that the role of care and responsibility may be embedded in actions and judgements through an interpersonal relationship between mother and midwife within a relational model as an *'ethic of care'*, also known as care ethics (Gallagher 2017). This approach is concerned with contextual details within a valued social relationship that is individual to the mother (Newnham and Kirkham 2019). In this model, care is balanced with responsibility of the midwife to ensure compassion and adhere to the principle of non-maleficence and accountability. This relational support ensures that midwives seek to fulfil women's expectations of their birthing outcomes and is reinforced through the choices offered by midwives when women are in control and empowered through their experiences (Dodwell and Newburn 2010).

Choices, Autonomy and Decision Making

Childbearing women are entitled to make choices based on information and evidence provided by healthcare professionals in seeking the safest and best outcome during childbirth. On the other hand, midwives must consider relevant ethical principles that impact their autonomy in supporting childbearing women to make these choices. However, midwives as healthcare providers are held legally and professional accountable for the care they provide, not only within legal and professional regulations and frameworks, but also as primarily accountable to the woman and her birthing experience, their employing organisation and the community in which they practise (Jefford and Jomeen 2015). They are in a difficult position and must consider the consequences of their decisions, which places midwives in what is perceived to be a vulnerable position (MacLellan 2014). They may consider practising defensively, forgoing autonomous practice in the need to ensure that the accountability of midwifery practice is within the remit of 'safe' practice. Hastings-Tolsma and Nolte (2014) identified this concept as 'failure to rescue', which has ethical implications for a midwifery philosophy that promotes normality in childbirth but results in 'safe' interventions during childbirth.

Women have the right not to be harmed when in the care of midwives, and care professionals will be liable in the law of negligence if harm results during childbirth (Griffiths 2011). On the other hand, midwives make decisions based on evidence and logical rationale, from a hypothetic-deductive perspective, together with intuition resulting from experiences based on an intuitive-humanistic approach (Smith 2016; Jefford et al. 2010; Jefford and Fahy 2015). However, ethical decision making ought to include the emotions and feelings, needs and wishes of the woman (Weltens et al. 2019), as a result of engagement in the mother–midwife relationship, to reflect cognitive beliefs of integrity and justice (Thompson 2005). Ultimately, Daemers et al. (2017) suggest that shared decision making is shaped by experience, intuition and individual circumstance and is influenced by knowledge, attitude towards the natural physiology of childbearing, centring the woman in the event and collaboration with other professionals.

The woman's sense of control and the ability to make choices is informed through their awareness of physiological processes in conjunction with organisational and resource limitations. However, more recently, authors have suggested that hospital culture and policies affect the way that information is presented (Newnham et al. 2017). In these situations, information is not truly unbiased and consequently women are unable to give true informed consent to care that affects their and their baby's outcome. Influencing factors, expectations of the midwife's role and perceived safety have an impact on choices women make – especially in first-time mothers, as documented by Borelli et al. (2017). The authors suggest that choices such as choosing a place of birth are not influenced by women's perception of midwifery competence in different settings but by their preferences, prior knowledge and a need for a safe and fulfilling experience.

Towards a Relational Model with Confidence and Responsibility

The social context in which choices about care are made are not made in isolation but through an understanding of a professional's true autonomy. A relational model of autonomy is defined by Christman (2015) as the *'relatedness [that] plays in both persons' self-conceptions . . . and the dynamics of deliberation and reasoning'* and is relevant in relation to informed choices in decision making through the dynamics of shared knowledge and negotiation of shifting power between the woman and the midwife (Nieuwenhuijze et al. 2014). Both midwife and woman must become responsible for the consequences of choices made when engaging with and embracing their autonomy.

Relational autonomy creates a space in which women are supported to develop their skills, self-confidence and self-esteem to recognise the social context for their decisions (Meadow 2014). However, the principle of respect is key in enabling shared decision making in support of relational autonomy (Lewis 2019). Midwives need to recognise their capability to self-trust (McCourt and Stevens 2009), to have self-esteem, self-respect and act effectively, underpinned by their values and evidence-based professional knowledge. Women, on the other hand, must be aware of constraining factors, such as organisational resources, when making choices and decisions (Thompson 2013). However, the woman in labour needs to be free from pain and fear, unhindered by medical interventions and afforded her dignity through a relationship with midwives based on trust and sympathetic understanding of her individual needs in a caring and nurturing environment (Morad et al. 2013). Midwives must therefore seek alternative approaches to the care they provide through the value of relational autonomy in which the midwife's and the woman's autonomy is negotiated respectfully to reach an informed decision (Noseworthy et al. 2013). The resulting empowerment process is mutual within the context of midwives 'being with others' rather than fulfilling midwifery skills and tasks (Hermansson and Martensson 2011). Parents, once informed and made aware of available resources and possibilities, will be able to agree on choices and willingly participate in the decision-making process towards a safe and fulfilling birth experience (Halfdansdottir et al. 2015). In addition, Hall et al. (2018) indicate that women's dynamic experience of birth is influenced by the confidence felt in the belief that one's body is able to give birth, whilst drawing on emotional and physical support to cope with the experience and a sense of control over pain and pain relief to ensure comfort and increased relaxation.

The relational model also considers relational continuity which enables professionals to provide holistic care through their presence whilst providing emotional support in the woman–midwife relationship. Quality and content of care is perceived by women to be important in enabling a positive birthing experience (Dahlberg and Aune 2013), aided by the nurturing presence of the midwife as her advocate and companion. The concept of the 'ritual companion' has been explored from an Australian perspective and concludes that two contrasting types of midwifery practice were being facilitated: that of the 'rites of passage' during childbirth, in which the woman–midwife relationship is enabling and empowering and, the 'rites of protection' in which labour is perceived to be a time of danger and requires monitoring and assessment to provide a sense of control over the childbirth process (Reed et al. 2016).

Earlier literature advocates for a 'caring presence' in the true sense of 'with woman' that involves a personal connection between woman and midwife placing the woman at the centre of the relationship and creating an environment of security and trust (Pembroke and Pembroke 2008). With this commitment by midwives to positively enhance the birth experience, the authors suggest that the spirituality of midwifery is played out through the concepts of responsiveness and availability. It is viewed sensitivity and respects the uniqueness of each woman. As identified in the study by Brown (2012), midwives are 'with woman' when they are perceptive enough to read the situation and are responsive to her needs and values. This requires the midwife to be available as a ready listener and include herself in the protective sphere that women retreat to when in labour. In addition, it needs the midwife to understand and be actively involved in providing the information and skills to enable the woman to make the right decisions.

Women and midwives are generally in agreement about the need to achieve a positive outcome for every birthing experience. This agreement is based on shared values of solidarity which promote and champion physiological birth through social and mutual support and minimum intervention (Brown and Gallagher 2015). The concept of solidarity as applied to bioethics results in cohesion and integration connected through similar aspirations (Prainsack and Buyx 2011) of mother and midwife in an interdependent relationship to achieve a safe and effective birth outcome. An integration of solidarity with an ethos of midwifery practice can only be achieved through reciprocity of information, transparency and honesty between childbearing women and the health professional to maintain the 'with woman' concept (Dann 2007). In making rational choices, the midwife and woman must justify their decisions by considering the value that is placed on the birthing experience. This shared solidarity is demonstrated through mutually shared responsibility between mother and midwife who take on personal accountability for choices and decisions made.

Advocacy

Making decisions is challenging and complex, especially within midwifery practice, and has an impact on the type and standard of care that is provided (Smith 2016). Reasoned and safe choices based on evidence and intuition can be achieved through this partnership with women (Daemers et al. 2017). A sympathetic and empathetic approach to decisions is perceived by women to result in a more positive birth experience (Boyle et al. 2016). However, pain during childbirth is one aspect that can hinder the decision-making process (Whitburn et al. 2019) and requires midwives to exercise the concept of relational autonomy to protect the woman when she cannot make reasoned decisions (Brown and Salmon 2018). In this respect, autonomy (discussed earlier in this chapter) *'is a key concept in understanding advocacy'* (Cole et al. 2014, p. 576).

Advocacy has had an important role in professional/service user relationships. One of the 'key messages' in 'Midwifery 2020: Delivering expectations' is in the section 'Developing the midwife's role in public health and reducing inequalities' which states:

> *Midwives should use their advocacy role for influencing and improving the health and wellbeing of women, children, and families. This will include making the economic case for committing resources so that the midwife can deliver public health messages in the antenatal and postnatal periods and ensuring that there is a midwifery contribution at policy, strategic, political, and international level (p. 7).*

Working alongside women, midwives exercise what has been referred to as 'skilled companionship' (Dierckx de Casterlé 2015) as they journey 'with women' through the birth and postnatally. Through this concept, midwives integrate skills and companionship and bring together the scientific and moral aspects of care. This requires midwives to be committed to provide an empathic presence during childbirth events. Women thus feel accompanied and supported. However, ethical challenges may arise should women make choices which are considered detrimental to the health of themselves, their baby or the midwife (Jenkinson et al. 2017). In such situations, midwives may experience ethical uncertainty or, perhaps, unpreparedness to respond ethically to women's needs and preferences. There may, for example, be a conflict of principles between respect for autonomy and beneficence/non-maleficence and justice. The midwife should use her advocacy role by taking the lead to facilitate making decisions for the woman and meeting her holistic needs and interests through empathetic, intuitive and sensitive support and 'companionship'.

Empathy, Intuition and Sensitivity

A definition of empathy is the action of understanding, being aware of, being sensitive to and vicariously experiencing the feelings, thoughts and experience of another (Medical Dictionary 2019). Both empathy and intuitive knowledge are integral components of what is perceived by experts as creating competence and is expressed through touch and physical closeness or emotionally through spiritual oneness 'with woman'. Facilitative or cathartic interventions enable emotional and supportive approaches to acknowledge the woman's worth and demonstrate mutual respect. Sensitivity to women's needs is another aspect of the 'with woman' concept and is illustrated below. In addition, a midwife who makes an effort to be compassionate demonstrates empathy and intuition as spiritual care (Linhares 2012, Crowther and Hall 2015), as documented by Moloney and Gair (2015).

Observation that the nature of midwifery practice changes in an environment in which the midwife is engaged in being 'with woman' rather than doing, concurs with Brown's (2012) findings of watching and waiting and not just doing. Leap's publication in 2000 remains at the centre of this midwifery philosophy and was perceptive in suggesting that midwives give when they do less (Leap 2000). A key element of ensuring midwives and healthcare professionals are 'with woman' in their daily contact with childbearing women is well-developed communication skills. In this respect, Gibbons (2010) suggests that communication goes beyond just words into the environment which is created in order to encourage comfort and privacy and promote unspoken dialogue. Positive first impressions created by midwives influence the quality of rapport and the relationship that is grown between woman and midwife (NHS England 2016). Raynor and England (2010) suggest that attitudes of acceptance and warmth, sharing a genuineness of transparent thoughts and feelings demonstrated in empathetic understanding by the midwife placing herself in the woman's position, are a humanistic approach to therapeutic verbal and non-verbal communication.

The 'Good' Midwife

The concept of being a 'good midwife', as explored in systematic reviews by both Nicholls and Webb (2006) and Byrom and Downe (2010), identifies well-developed communication skills, compassion, kindness, knowledge and midwifery skills as key elements. Attitudes and feelings together with midwifery knowledge create clinical competence to fulfil being 'with woman' (Carolan 2011). Halldorsdottir and Karlsdottir (2011) debate the primacy of the midwife's professionalism as central to the role of the 'good midwife' and identify essential key elements of professionalism, wisdom, competence, interprofessional competence and personal and professional self-development as supporting attributes. A 'good midwife' is perceived by women to be able to provide them with information and is competent in fulfilling their needs whilst they feel listened to (Overgaard et al. 2014). In addition, women want to be individuals cared for by a midwife who provides 'presence' and makes them feel safe and cared for through their attitude and behaviour (Dahlberg et al. 2016).

One aspect which develops skills and knowledge essential to the 'with woman' competence is the reflective process: both internal as a reflective process and shared through discussion or story-telling. Johns and Freshwater's (1998) interpretation of reflection, although now dated, is still relevant in that practitioners' experience informs embodied knowledge translated into clinical decisions to become intuitive knowledge. The relationship between a midwife's practice experiences and self-development through reflection transforms perceptions and beliefs and ultimately results in skilled empathetic midwifery practice and competence. One paper from Australia explores the issues surrounding the situation when a woman declines recommended care (Jenkinson et al. 2017). The authors examine, from a feminist perspective, how the woman's and the midwife's autonomy may be upheld with specific guidance from clinicians providing care in this situation and suggest that models of care which support reflexive practice may enable midwives to advocate the right of refusal and maintain the 'with woman' concept empathetically.

Table 2.1 summarises the literature in relation to 'with woman' concept from an ethical perspective for both women and midwives. Rodgers' framework (1989) underpins the analysis in terms of antecedents, attributes and consequences.

Conclusion

Rodgers's framework (1989) suggests that related concepts exist as part of a network of concepts that provide significance to the concept of interest. In the analysis, related concepts were identified related to the continuity of carer, the ritual companion and the 'good' midwife in examining the literature. The impact of the continuity of carer concept suggests attributes of confidence to offer choices of sound judgement by midwives in their relationship 'with woman'. The consequences are respect for 'women' autonomy, empowerment to make the right decisions, fulfilling women's expectations and preserving safe midwifery care. These attributes are explored further in Chapter 3.

Ethical issues related to fulfilling the 'with woman' concept, which examine the impact of moral and practice dilemmas on delivery of current midwifery practice, underpin the consequences of this and related concepts. Midwives' and women's perspectives of ethical practice, embedded in shared knowledge, power and trust, have highlighted the challenges faced in making decisions to ensure safe and positive birth experiences; this is within the remit of relational autonomy and codes of professional midwifery practice. The stories that follow

Table 2.1 Concept Analysis of the ethical perspective of being 'with woman'.

'With woman' antecedents	Evidence	Attributes (A) and consequences (C)
Continuity of carer	Taylor et al. (2018) and Yoshida and Sandall (2013) raised issues practical barriers to C of C role	Confidence (A) Safety (A) Need for training (C) Adequate staffing (C) Sound leadership and Management (C)
Decision making	Katz Rothman (2013) Challenges to making decisions as a social process based on bioethics Chadwick (2015) importance of safety	Mother–midwife relationship (A) Respect for autonomy (A) Promoting professionalism and trust (A) Preserving safety (C) prioritising people (C) Effective practice (C)
Care and responsibility	MacLellan (2014) The role of care and responsibility through ethics of care Newnham and Kirkham (2019) Dodwell and Newburn (2010) explore relational support	Actions and judgement (A) Interpersonal relationship (C) Valued social relationship (C) Balance of care and responsibility (A) Compassion (C) Non-maleficence and accountability (C) Offering choices and fulfilling women's expectations (A) Control (C) Empowerment (C)
Choices	Jefford and Jomeen (2015) impact on midwives' working practices Hastings-Tolsma and Nolte (2014) 'failure to rescue' Griffiths (2011) law of negligence Smith (2016), Jefford and Fahy (2015) intuitive humanistic theory. Daemers et al. (2017) sharing decision making Newnham et al. (2017) lack of choices. Borelli et al. (2017) influencing factors on the expectations of the midwife's role	Legal and professional accountability (A) Autonomous practice (C) Professional vulnerability (C) Defensive practice (C) 'Safe' practice (A) Interventions in childbirth (C) Right not to be harmed (A) Midwifery evidence and logical rationale (C) Intuitive practice to include knowledge, experience and attitudes (C) Fulfilling women's wishes (C) Centres the woman (C) Organisational & resource limitations (A) Biased and not true informed consent (C) May impact their place of birth choices (C) Need for safety and fulfilling experience (C)

(Continued)

Table 2.1 (Continued)

'With woman' antecedents	Evidence	Attributes (A) and consequences (C)
Relational autonomy	Christman (2015) dynamics of deliberation and reasoning Nieuwenhuijze et al. (2014) Thompson (2013) women's awareness of constraining factors Morad et al. (2013) trusting relationships. Noseworthy et al. (2013) relational autonomy Hall et al. (2018) women's dynamic experience of birth Meadow (2014) Social context of relational model and Lewis (2019) principle of respect. Dahlberg and Aune (2013) quality and content of care	Informed choices (A) Shared knowledge (C) Negotiation (C) Shifting power between woman and midwife (C) Professional self-esteem & self-respect(C) Women's dignity (A) Mutual trust & sympathetic understanding (C) Caring and nurturing environment (A) 'Being with others' (C) Women's autonomy fulfilled (A) Confidence and self-belief in the body's ability to give birth (C) Creating a space to develop skills (A) Self-confidence and self-esteem for women (C) Holistic care through presence and emotional support by MWs (C) Importance of positive birth experience(A) MW as advocate & companion (C)
Ritual companion	Reed et al. (2016) 'Rites of passage' Pembroke and Pembroke (2008) women at centre of care Brown (2012) 'with woman' Moloney & Gair (2015) compassion Raynor and England (2010) transparency and therapeutic communication Dierckx de Casterlé (2015) ethical perspectives of the skilled companion	Rites of protection (A) Relationship that is enabling and empowering (C) Caring presence (C) Environment of security and trust (A) Spirituality (A) Responsiveness and availability (C) Perceptiveness (A) Responsive to needs and values (C) Empathy and intuition (A) Warmth and acceptance (C) A fulfilling birth experience (C) Empathetic presence (A) Women feel accompanied and supported (C)
'The good midwife'	Nicholls and Webb (2006) Byrom and Downe (2010) key elements of the good midwife Overgaard et al. (2014) Dahlberg et al. (2016) attitudes and behaviour	Clinical competence (A) Well-developed skills of compassion, kindness, knowledge and skills (C) Women provided with information and listened to (C) Fulfil women's needs (C) Feel safe and cared for (C)

illustrate how midwives fulfil and deliver compassionate, empathetic and ethical 'with woman' care and how one woman challenged routine care and opted for an unconventional delivery to achieve the transformative and life-changing experience of birthing her baby.

A Midwife's Story

Anna's Story

In 2012, I conducted a study exploring how midwives learn, develop and demonstrate communication to embrace elements of empathy, intuition and sensitivity when 'with woman' at the point of birth. The purpose of this study was to develop a better understanding of 'hidden' skills that midwives perceive they need to draw upon to truly be 'with woman'. The findings suggest that midwives fulfil the 'with woman' concept in different ways and identify several attributes which describe the interplay between woman and her midwife during the time of birth.

The perceived therapeutic relationship between women and midwives is one attribute of this concept which a midwife perceived as building *'a relationship with them [women] and understanding what they want'. 'Identifying their needs without them having to ask you.' 'Being in tune with their [women's] emotional state'* and *'being trusted'. 'Having a good interpersonal relationship.' 'If you don't have that empathy you don't build up that rapport with women . . . pick up cues from the women'.* Another attribute of the 'with woman' concept is being able to identify and support women's needs and was seen by midwives as *'being perceptive to their needs'* and *'responding to things that she [the woman] says, by nodding to acknowledge you've heard what she said'* and 'it's about what her [woman's] body is doing and what your body is doing in response', *'. . . and being sensitive to when some parents don't want you with them'.*

Another interesting attribute of the 'with woman' concept became apparent in this study (Brown 2012). This was demonstrated through compassion, by giving women time to adjust during their pregnancy and in labour played out through watching and waiting. A midwife said, *'You can show presence, a supportive presence, its watching and waiting, it's not just doing.'* Another midwife said, *'You just need the women to get used to their surroundings, and to me, they just need to get used to my voice.' 'Kindness is so hard to measure, and it is a sixth sense . . . and I think it's sensitivity – there is something there that you cannot explain but you have a feeling'* and *'reading the situation'* and *'knowing when you should shut up and when you shouldn't', 'the language you use because you have to adapt to their [the women's] ability to understand the language you are using'*

(Continued)

and '*tone of voice*'; '*recognising when it is good not to say anything*' and '*recognising silence*'.

Findings from this study (Brown 2012) suggest a resulting consequence of the above 'with woman' attributes which was a positive birthing experience overall. One participant said, it is '*not just being there, but exploring everything that will make labour time and delivery bring pleasure to them, something they will always remember*' and '*make her [the woman] feel empowered*' whilst '*being an advocate for her*' and '*just keeping her the focus*'. A midwife succinctly explained that, '*part of it is your own personality . . . an innate thing . . . your own belief . . . a self-awareness*', whilst another midwife sums up the learning from being 'with woman' in terms of, '*By just being there I am able to instil autonomy and confidence*.' One midwife concludes, '*A good midwife achieves an awful lot by doing nothing and that is what it's all about.*' '*Women are great teachers and so always use them as a resource as well, be good listeners and if you listen to women, then very often they're very, very intuitive to their own bodies so they can teach us a lot and we can learn a lot from them.*'

Donna's Stories

Rosie*'s Story

Being a community-based midwife, means that our contact with women is on a one-to-one basis, outside of the hospital environment. Often in GP surgeries, clinics or women's homes. As such, we have the opportunity to bond with the women in our care and provide them with not only clinical care but continuity, friendship and support in a way that is less possible within a busy hospital-based setting.

I have found that having had the opportunity to build relationships with women during their pregnancy, they will seek my support more willingly than other healthcare professionals as there is a level of trust that has been built.

I recently saw Rosie for her antenatal check. I could tell the moment she came into my room that she was distressed, as was her partner John. They had received the news that their baby was very likely to have a life-limiting condition. They had attended a number of scans to confirm this, and only a matter of days before hand, had the confirmed diagnosis. Although they had been given the clinical outlook from the medical professionals they had seen, in their words: 'no-one had given them the space to understand what this would mean for them, and what their choices were'.

This is not normally a conversation held in a community setting, as there are specialist healthcare professionals that are trained in this field; but they wanted my support. From a deeply personal perspective as a mother I was desperately upset for them, while also knowing the clinic appointments are only 20 minutes long, and I knew that this was not going to be a quick chat and I had a busy clinic. I was worried that I wouldn't have all the answers, but I gave them the space to talk about everything that had happened. Rosie cried, and John just held his head in his hands. Sometimes all the clinical training in the world can't give you the words for a time like this. I held Rosie's hand and asked how I could help. She needed someone to talk to her in 'lay' terms; simply to discuss what their options were.

I gave the couple what information I was able to and then made phone calls to the relevant support teams to get advice. There were no decisions made in the room at that point, but I assured Rosie she had my support in whatever decision she made. They left with a clear idea of what their options were, and in circumstances like this, that is whether to continue the pregnancy or not.

I have to be honest that when I started my midwifery journey, I had 'rose coloured spectacles' about the role of a midwife, bringing new life into the world. I still have a great belief that all birth is sacred, but there are times when my personal and professional beliefs are challenged. No textbook or hospital policy can give you the insight needed to deal with deeply emotional situations such as talking to a woman about whether or not to continue her pregnancy. I could only support Rosie in the right choice for her. I told her she was a brave woman who would make the right decision for her and her baby and family.

Forty-five minutes later the couple left the clinic, and I cried on my own. There were now two women in the waiting room, eagerly waiting for my care and attention to discuss their continuing pregnancies. I composed myself and carried on with clinic, apologising to everyone for the rest of the clinic about being late, but assuring them that they would have my care attention for however long they need it.

Being a midwife is a privilege, walking 'with women' at every point during their pregnancy, birth and beyond and is often full of pure joy and the wonder of new life, yet can be interspersed with tragic and ethically challenging moments where the support of a midwife is second to none.

Lois*'s Story

Whilst working on labour ward, I cared for a woman who had her first baby. Our shifts are 12.5 hours long, so we spent a good amount of time with Lois and Jake,

(Continued)

her birth partner. I got to know them well and at the end of the shift I left and wished them well.

Three weeks later I came onto shift and Lois's name was on the board as having just arrived in triage. I offered to go and see her as I already knew her. Upon greeting the couple, Jake was holding the baby, who was well and settled. However, Lois had been suffering with her mental health since birth, despite good family and community midwife support. Jake stated that overnight Lois had been having psychotic episodes and had come to triage.

Lois remembered me and embraced me when I entered the room, so very happy to see someone she knew. She was very lucid, and I was able to take her observations and talk to her about her baby. She had struggled with breastfeeding over the last few weeks but was now feeling like it was going much better. I helped her get comfortable and she breastfed her baby beautifully and calmly.

I stayed with her the whole day and was present when all the relevant medics and psychiatrists reviewed her. She was veering between being lucid and experiencing psychotic episodes all day. The first line decision was for Lois to be medicated initially; however, this would mean stopping breastfeeding as the drug would pass through the breastmilk to her baby. She was adamant that she would not stop breastfeeding as it was the only thing she was doing well for her baby.

Lois's capacity was limited, and as her midwife I needed to advocate for her. I knew how much breastfeeding meant to her, and there is very good evidence that links breastfeeding and emotional wellbeing of a new mother. The psychiatrists were adamant that Lois would need to stop immediately and take the medications. I stayed until she was lucid enough to ensure that she had an understanding that for her benefit and of her baby, the medication was the best option for now. However, this wouldn't mean stopping breastfeeding altogether. I got a breast pump for her, with a view to keeping up her milk supply whilst on the medication.

Jake was bereft and felt unable to help, so I arranged for a nursery nurse to show the couple how to correctly make up a formula feed and to sterilise the feeding equipment.

As a midwife I would always support breastfeeding continuation for the benefits of both mother and baby, but ethically at this time, stopping breastfeeding was the only option to try and help with Lois's psychosis. But keeping her milk supply established, using a pump, would give her the option to return to breastfeeding once the medication was stopped.

A Woman's Story

Emily's Story

I see birth as a huge part of my life experience, something that is completely trans-formative, in every aspect of life. When I became pregnant with my first child, I actively sought out and became informed about how I was more likely to achieve a positive experience. This led to the knowledge that having a known care pro-vider throughout my experience is more likely to lead to positive feelings, even if things don't go as expected. My babies were all born at home, I saw making this decision as me being in control and more likely to have the experience I wanted. However, I did have the constant worry that a midwife would not be available to attend my births due to shortages.

I was fortunate to see the same midwife for my first and second pregnancies. In fact, I swapped my maternity care to a different GP practice (we had moved to a new house) to see the midwife I 'clicked' the most with. However, it turns out I didn't receive any midwifery support during my first and second births. The first was because I didn't realise I was in active labour and so we did not call in time (I birth quickly!); the second, despite phoning in time, there wasn't enough staff to send out to me due to other home births happening in the area.

I decided to stay at home when this was stated as I instinctively knew my son would be born soon and I really didn't want to birth at the roadside! His birth was straightforward as expected and paramedics were on standby but did not interfere (as there was no need), but I felt like I had to fight with the midwives over the phone and justify my decisions, something that I really did not want to deal with during labour, nor should have to. I had made an informed decision, which was not taken lightly. For me, the risks of transferring outweighed staying at home at this point. I felt a huge pressure to comply even though what the midwives were sug-gesting was not the safest option for me and my baby at that time. I feel like because we were unknown to the hospital staff on the phone, they did not under-stand my decision making or know anything about us. Perhaps if it had been a known midwife we would have been able to work together easier as the relation-ship would have already been established.

This experience unfortunately led to an unnecessary backlash in the immediate few weeks with my baby, a time where we should have been resting and bonding following what should have been a positive straightforward labour at home. I felt very low even though the hospital immediately apologised. I had an overwhelming urge to prevent this from happening to another woman, I wanted to understand why women's basic human rights in labour were not respected or understood.

(Continued)

I had several meetings to address this, but it led to me feeling a complete mistrust in the system as they really weren't 'with woman' when I needed them to be; it felt like they were 'against woman unless you comply', so when I became pregnant with my third child, I actively sought out continuity of care elsewhere.

I did my research and I was fortunate at this moment in our lives to budget for an independent midwife. Myself and my husband are not well-off people, but with some savings and inheritance money we were able to prioritise the care that I needed emotionally during this time. This was to be our last baby and her entrance to the world mattered for her, but also for me as a parent. I needed to emotionally heal after the experience around my second birth. I needed the time to build up a relationship with my midwife and I needed to trust them completely. I can honestly say this was money well spent!

My independent midwife, Rachel, came to my home for mutually convenient appointments. My husband and children got to know her; she was there for us as a family. I felt able to contact her whenever I wanted/needed, and she would provide me with sound evidence and support. I felt my choices and decisions were respected, heard and unjudged. But I think the most important thing was that I felt comfortable and at ease emotionally! This was somebody that was going to be attending my birth, which is so intimate, so this was important to me. Also, having that reassurance throughout my pregnancy that she was more likely to be able to attend my birth was worth paying for! Rachel provided six weeks postpartum care and I knew that if I needed to speak to/see her in between visits I could.

For me, continuity of care brings back midwives to be more 'with woman'. I am aware there are NHS pilot schemes in our area to bring back this model; I'm sure this will bring many benefits to the women it will support. I hope that in turn the system can be more 'with midwife' to support them to be 'with woman'.

Lessons Learnt

The literature at the start of this chapter identified the many issues that challenge midwifery practice in fulfilling women's expectations and wishes to achieve the childbearing experience that they want. As illustrated in the stories above, physical and intuitive emotional effort is required of midwives to ensure positive experiences for every woman, but they are sometimes ethically challenged by events. Women, on the other hand, suggest that they perceive a need to push the boundaries of conventional maternity care to achieve childbirth expectations, steered by an instinctive need to preserve their rights to be in control throughout these events to achieve a 'normal' childbearing experience.

Acknowledgement

Thanks to Ann Gallagher (Professor of Ethics) for her valuable contribution to the content of this chapter.

References

Beauchamp, T.L. and Childress, J.F. (2013). *Principles of Biomedical Ethics*, 7e. New York: Oxford University Press.

Birthplace in England Collaborative Group (2011). Perinatal and maternal outcomes by planned place of birth for healthy women with low risk pregnancies: the birthplace in England national prospective cohort study. *British Medical Journal* 343: d7400.

Borelli, S.E., Walsh, D., and Spiby, H. (2017). First-time mothers' choice of birthplace: influencing factors, expectations of midwife's role and perceived safety. *Journal of Advanced Nursing* 73 (8): 1937–1946. Wiley.

Boyle, S., Thomas, H., and Brooks, F. (2016). Women's views on partnership working with midwives during pregnancy and childbirth. *Midwifery* 32: 21–29.

Brown, A.M. (2012). Assessment strategies for teaching empathy, intuition and sensitivity on the labour ward. *Evidence Based Midwifery* 10 (2): 64–70.

Brown, A.M. and Gallagher, A. (2015). Ethical aspects of current challenges to women's choice of planned place of birth. *MIDIRS Midwifery Digest* 25 (4): 419–423.

Brown, S.L. and Salmon, P. (2018). Reconciling the theory and reality of shared decision-making: a matching approach to practitioner leadership. *Health Expectations* 22: 275–283.

Byrom, S. and Downe, S. (2010). "She sort of shine": Midwives' accounts of "good" midwifery and "good" leadership. *Midwifery* 26: 126–137.

Care Quality Commission (2013). National findings from the 2013 survey of women's experiences of maternity care. https://www.cqc.org.uk/sites/default/files/documents/maternity_report_for_publication.pdf (accessed 13 September 2019).

Carolan, M. (2011). The good midwife: commencing students' views. *Midwifery* 27 (4): 503–508.

Chadwick, R. (2015). The ethical importance of safety. *Bioethics* 29 (4): ii.

Cheyne, H., McCourt, C., and Semple, K. (2013). Mother knows best: developing a consumer led evidence informed research agenda for maternity care. *Midwifery* 29 (6): 705–712.

Christman, J. (2015). Autonomy in moral and political philosophy. In: *The Stanford Encyclopaedia of Philosophy* (ed. E.N. Zalta). Stanford, CA: Stanford University. http://plato.stanford.edu/archives/spr2015/entroies/autonomy-moral (accessed 30 July 2019).

Cole, C., Wellard, S., and Mummery, J. (2014). Problematising autonomy and advocacy in nursing? *Nursing Ethics* 21 (5): 576–582.

Crowther, S. and Hall, J. (2015). Spirituality and spiritual care in and around childbirth. *Women and Birth* 28: 173–178.

Daemers, D.O., van Limbeek, E.B., Wijnen, H.A. et al. (2017). Factors influencing the clinical decision-making of midwives: a qualitative study. *BMC Pregnancy & Childbirth* 17: 1–12.

Dahlberg, U. and Aune, I. (2013). The woman's birth experience- the effect of interpersonal relationships and continuity of care. *Midwifery* 29: 407–415.

Dahlberg, U., Persen, J., Skogas, A.K. et al. (2016). How can midwives promote a normal birth and a positive birth experience? The experience of first-time Norwegian mothers. *Sexual and Reproductive Healthcare* 7: 2–7.

Dann, L. (2007). Grace's story: an analysis of ethical issues in a case of informed consent. *British Journal of Midwifery* 15 (10): 634–639.

Davis, D. and Walker, K. (2010). The corporeal, the social and the space/place: exploring intersections from a midwifery perspective in New Zealand. *A Journal of Feminist Geography: Gender, Place & Culture* 17 (3): 377–391.

Dierckx de Casterlé, B. (2015). Realising skilled companionship in nursing: a utopian idea or difficult challenge. *Journal of Clinical Nursing* 24 (21–22): 3327–3335.

Dodwell, M. and Newburn, M. (2010). *Normal Birth as a Measure of Quality Care: Evidence on Safety, Effectiveness and Women's Experiences*. London: NCT.

Dunkley-Bent, J. (2018). A year of opportunity: continuity of carer. *Midwives Spring*: 68–69.

Foster, I.R. and Lasser, J. (2011). *Professional Ethics in Midwifery Practice*. London: Jones & Bartlett Publishers.

Gallagher, A. (2017). Care ethics & nursing practice. In: *Key Concepts & Issues in Nursing Ethics* (ed. A. Scott), 55–68. Springer International Publications.

Gibbons, K. (2010). It's more than just talking. *Midwives* 13 (1): 36–37.

Griffiths, R. (2011). Key concepts in human rights and midwifery practice. *British Journal of Midwifery* 19 (11): 748–749.

Halfdansdottir, B., Wilson, M.E., Hildingsson, I. et al. (2015). Autonomy in place of birth: a concept analysis. *Medicine, Health Care and Philosophy* 18: 591–600.

Hall, P.J., Whitman Foster, J., Yount, K.M. et al. (2018). Keeping it together and falling apart: women's dynamic experience of birth. *Midwifery* 58: 130–136.

Halldorsdottir, S. and Karlsdottir, S.I. (2011). The primacy of the good midwife in midwifery services: an evolving theory of professionalism in midwifery. *Scandinavian Journal of Caring Sciences* 25 (4): 806–817.

Hastings-Tolsma, M. and Nolte, A.G. (2014). Reconceptualising failure to rescue in midwifery: a concept analysis. *Midwifery* 30 (6): 585–594.

Hermansson, E. and Martensson, L. (2011). Empowerment in the midwifery context- a concept analysis. *Midwifery* 27: 811–816.

Janssen, B.K. and Wiegers, T.A. (2006). Strengths and weaknesses of midwifery care from the perspective of women. *Evidence Based Midwifery* 4 (2): 53–59.

Jefford, E. and Fahy, K. (2015). Midwives' clinical reasoning during second stage of labour: report on an interpretive study. *Midwifery* 31 (5): 519–525.

Jefford, E. and Jomeen, J. (2015). Midwifery abdication: a finding from an interpretive study. *International Journal of Childbirth* 5 (3): 116–125.

Jefford, E., Fahy, K., and Sundin, D. (2010). Decision-making theories and their usefulness to the midwifery profession both in terms of midwifery practice and the education of midwives. *International Journal of Nursing Practice* 17: 246–253.

Jenkinson, B., Krushe, S., and Kildea, S. (2017). The experience of women, midwives and obstetricians when women decline recommended maternity care: the feminist thematic perspective. *Midwifery* 52: 1–10.

Jepsen, I., Mark, E., Nohr, E.A. et al. (2016). A qualitiative study of how caseload midwifery is constituted and experienced by Danish midwives. *Midwifery* 36: 61–69.

Johns, C. and Freshwater, D. (1998). *Transforming Nursing through Reflective Practice*. Oxford: Blackwell Science.

Katz Rothman, B. (2013). Caught between autonomy and caring: still struggling towards an ethics of midwifery. *MIDIRS Midwifery Digest* 23 (2): 143–150.

Leap, N. (2000). The less we do, the more we give. In: *The Midwife-Mother Relationship* (ed. M. Kirkam). Basingstoke: Macmillan Press.

Lewis, J. (2019). Does shared decision making respect a patient's relational autonomy? *Journal of Evaluation in Clinical Practice* 25 (6): 1063–1069.

Linhares, C.H. (2012). The lived experience of midwives with spirituality in childbirth. *Journal of Midwifery & Women's Health* 57 (2): 165–171.

MacLellan, J. (2014). Claiming an ethics of care for midwives. *Nursing Ethics* 21 (7): 803–811.

McCormick, T.R. (2013). *Principles of Bioethics. Ethics in Medicine*. University of Washington, School of Medicine.

McCourt, C. and Stevens, T. (2009). Relationships and reciprocity in caseload midwifery. In: *Emotions in Midwifery & Reproduction* (eds. B. Hunter and R. Deery). Basingstoke: Palgrave Macmillan.

Meadow, S. (2014). Defining the doula's role: fostering relational autonomy. *Health Expectations* 18: 3057–3068.

Medical Dictionary (2019). Empathy and Relexivity. In: The Free Dictionary https://medical-dictionary.thefreedictionary.com/empathy/reflexivity (accessed 2 August 2019).

Midwifery (2020). *Programme (2010) in Association with Department of Health & Social Care Midwifery 2020: Delivering Expectations*. Cambridge: Jill Rogers Associates.

Moloney, S. and Gair, S. (2015). Empathy and spiritual carein midwifery practice: contributing to women's enhanced birth experiences. *Women & Birth* 28 (4): 323–328. https://doi.org/10.1016/j.wombi.2015.04.009.

Morad, S., Parry-Smith, W., and McSherry, W. (2013). Dignity in maternity care. *Evidence Based Midwifery* 11 (2): 67–70.

Newnham, E. and Kirkham, M. (2019). Beyond autonomy: care ethics for midwifery and the humanisation of birth. *Nursing Ethics* 26 (7–8): 2147–2157.

Newnham, E., McKellar, L., and Pincombe, J. (2017). "It's your body, but . . ." Mixed messages to childbirth education: findings from a hospital ethnography. *Midwifery* 55: 53–59.

NHS England (2016). *Better Births: Improving Outcomes of Maternity Services in England: A Five Year Forward for Better Maternity Care*. NHS England.

NHS England (2017). Implementing Better Births: Continuity of carer. https://www.england.nhs.uk/wp-content/uploads/2017/12/implementing-better-births.pdf (accessed 23 January 2019).

Nicholls, L. and Webb, C. (2006). What makes a good miwife? An integrative reviw of methodologically-diverse research. *Journal of Advanced Nursing* 56 (4): 414–429.

Nieuwenhuijze, M.J., Korstjens, I., de Jonge, A. et al. (2014). On speaking terms: a Delphi study on shared decision-making in maternity care. *BMC Pregnancy and Childbirth* 14: 223.

NMC (2018). *Code of Professional Conduct*. London: The Nursing and Midwifery Council Publications.

Noseworthy, D.A., Phibbs, R.A., and Benn, C.A. (2013). Towards a relational model of decision-making in midwifery care. *Midwifery* 29 (7): e42–e48.

Overgaard, C., Fenger-Gron, M., and Sandall, J. (2014). The impact of birthplace on women's birth experiences and perceptions of care. *Social Science & Medicine* 74 (7): 973–981.

Pembroke, N.F. and Pembroke, J.J. (2008). The spirituality of presence in midwifery care. *Midwifery* 24: 321–327.

Prainsack, B. and Buyx, A. (2011). *Solodarity: Reflections on an Emerging Concept in Bioethics*. London: Nuffield Council on Bioethics.

Raynor, M. and England, C. (2010). *Psychology for Midwives: Pregnancy, Birth and Puerperium*. London: Open University press.

Reed, R., Rowe, J., and Barnes, M. (2016). Midwifery practice during birth: ritual companionship. *Women and Birth* 29: 269–278.

Renfew, M.J., Dyson, L., Herbet, G. et al. (2008). Developing evidence based recommendations in public health: incorporating the views of practitioners, service users and user representatives. *Health Expectations* 11 (1): 3–15.

Rodgers, B.L. (1989). Concepts, analysis and the development of nursing knowledge: the evolutionary cycle. *Journal of Advanced Nursing* 14: 330–335.

Ross-Davie, M. and Cheyne, H. (2014). Intrapartum support: what do women want? A literature review. *Evidence Based Midwifery* 12 (2): 52–58.

Royal College of Midwives (2017). Can continuity work for us? A resource for midwives. London: Royal College of Midwives Publication.

Sandall, J. (2017). *The Contribution of Continuity of Midwifery Care to High Quality Maternity Care*. London: Royal College of Midwives.

Sandall, J., Soltani, H., Gate, S. et al. (2015). Midwife-led continuity models versus other models of care for childbearing. *The Cochrane Database of Systematic Reviews* (8). https://doi.org/10.1002/14651858.CD004667.pub5 (Accessed 14 September 2019).

Smith, J. (2016). Decision making in midwifery: a tripartite clinical decision. *British Journal of Midwifery* 24 (8): 574–580.

Smith, E., Ross, F., Donovan, S. et al. (2008). Service user involvement in nursing, midwifery and health visiting research: a review of the evidence and practice. *International Journal of Nursing Studies* 45 (2): 298–315.

Taylor, B., Cross-Sudworth, F., and MacArthur, C. (2018). *Better Births and Continuity: Midwife Survey Results*. Institute of Applied Health Research, University of Birmingham.

Thompson, F.E. (2005). The emotional impact on mothers and midwives of conflict between workplace and personal/professional ethics. *Australian Midwifery* 18 (3): 17–21.

Thompson, A. (2013). Midwives' experiences of caring fro women whose requests are not within policies and guidelines. *British Journal of Midwifery* 21 (8): 564–570.

Thompson, S.M., Nieuwenhuize, M.J., Kane Low, L., and de Vries, R. (2016). Exploring Dutch midwives' attitudes to promoting physiological childbirth: a qualitative study. *Midwifery* 42: 67–73.

Walsh, D. and Devane, D. (2012). A metasynthesis of midwife-led care. *Qualitative Health Research* 22 (7): 897.

Weltens, M., de Nooijer, J., and Nieuwenhuijze, M. (2019). Influencing factors in midwives' decision making during childbirth: a qualitiative study in the Netherlands. *Women & Birth* 32 (2): e197–e203.

Whitburn, L.Y., Jones, L.E., Davey, M.A., and McDonald, S. (2019). The nature of labour pain: an updated review of the literature. *Women & Birth* 32: 28–38.

Yoshida, Y. and Sandall, J. (2013). Occupational burnout and work factors in community and hospital midwives: a survey analysis. *Midwifery* 29 (8): 921–926.

3

'With Woman' in 'Normal Birth'

Anna M. Brown; Laura Pagden, Rhiannon Brown, Donna Hunt (midwives); and Sarah, Helen, and Lissie (women)

Introduction

The birth of a baby remains a life-changing event, which has been shrouded in mystery and tradition throughout the history of womankind. Childbirth is a rite of passage for the neonate, the mother and her significant others and has evolved with time dependant on influencing factors such as cultural norms and spiritual rituals. Equally, women's position and the part they play during this event has transformed over the years. Childbirth, as a normal life occurrence, was viewed as part of a community's events – and was supported by local midwives and female relatives and friends. It was empowering for the women giving birth and those that closely protected and supported her in the true sense of being 'with woman'. Sadly, the art of midwifery, in this natural and spiritual event, has been transformed into a controlled and frequently scientifically managed intervention. The childbearing woman in this event is no longer centre stage but has become objectified as a medical procedure.

The traditions, environment and artefacts that surround childbirth have changed throughout history depending on the position of women in society, its politics, culture and religion. Some of these changes and effects on childbearing practices have been discussed in Chapter 1. However, the essence of being 'with woman', in the spiritual and physical context, remains a thread throughout the ages despite changing influences. It is this phenomenon that is teased out in the literature review of each chapter, and illustrated by narrative from midwives, practitioners and women. Hunter (2006) suggests that the concept of being 'with woman' enables a therapeutic space to be created through which both midwives and women are empowered. The concept of being 'with woman' is the

Better Births: The Midwife 'with Woman', First Edition. Edited by Anna M. Brown.
© 2021 John Wiley & Sons Ltd. Published 2021 by John Wiley & Sons Ltd.

foundation of midwifery practice today and evolves with each relationship that is forged between woman and midwife. Therefore, it is distressing to hear and read women's stories that seem to reflect a distancing of the very heart of midwifery practices and skills, resulting in negative and extremely disappointing birth experiences for women. This is illustrated in the previous chapter through Emily's story.

The philosophy of midwifery practice strives to enrich the birthing event. However, women's childbirth experiences suggest that the profession has erred towards a medical approach, rather than a celebration of a natural and spiritual event (Fahy 1998). A 'with woman' concept is more in tune with midwifery philosophy, in terms of emergence of midwifery knowledge and skills, to complement intuition and empathy – so essential to core midwifery values (Brown 2012). Being 'with woman' is a celebration of women's dignity and empowerment in childbirth, far removed from the medicalised concept of managing labour and childbirth inherent in midwifery practice in the not so distant past. In this chapter, the midwife's perspective of the 'with woman' concept is explored further.

Defining Normality

What is normality in the childbirth experience? This is a concept that is difficult to define but it is a philosophy which is promoted by midwives in a woman's life process, during pregnancy and childbirth. It does not always follow that a midwife's management of care towards normality necessarily results in a normal outcome. Experienced midwives learn to recognise the normal and 'know' when things become abnormal, so that they can adjust care accordingly. It is difficult for midwives to articulate what '*normal*' means but understanding the relationship between midwifery practices and achieving a '*normal*' outcome, for mother and neonate, is some way towards gaining this understanding.

Literature documents the concepts of normalising birth and the experiences of midwives in promoting normal births in a number of settings (Powell Kennedy et al. 2010; Meyer 2012; Mapute and Donavon 2013; Thompson et al. 2016; Aune et al. 2017; Neerland 2018). Most concepts align with the 'with woman' concept in terms of a midwife's knowledge and skills, '*waiting on nature*' in the physiological normality of childbirth, a woman's physiological ability and self-belief to give birth, the midwife and woman '*therapeutic relation*' and the birth environment (Davis 2010). Contemporary midwifery practice facilitates physiological birth and labour, underpinned by scientific knowledge and well-developed midwifery skills, which can become interventionist when abnormalities develop in the childbearing process. Hunter (2008: 410) suggests that a midwife's 'self-knowledge' is '*a midwife's belief in what she knows, knowing what she believes and acting upon those beliefs'*. Hunter (2009) also believes that a midwife can achieve such self-knowledge by being 'with woman' and being a '*positive presence'*, aided by the midwife's continuous and intuitive assessment of the unfolding birth.

The concept of normality in childbirth is reinforced by mutual sensitivity to the birth environment and a '*dynamic'* and '*therapeutic'* relationship between the woman and the midwife (Davis 2010). Developing trust is based on the midwife's philosophy and values of normality, and respect for the woman's individuality and autonomy in making safe decisions sensitively and responsibly supported by the midwife (Duff 2016). The environment of birth is also influential in birth outcomes. Results of a normalising philosophy of childbirth are the woman's satisfaction with an optimal birth outcome (Powell Kennedy et al. 2010) and being in a safe, non-interventionist environment. Natural ways of giving birth, such as in water, and supportive strategies to cope with pain, such as hypnobirthing, enhance the journey towards a positive birth outcome. A midwife's ability to support women through labour pain is based on the relationship built on an understanding of a woman's needs, through listening and observing unfolding birth processes and acting appropriately to these needs. Through this approach women are trusted to make choices most suited to their needs and safeguarded by midwives through their '*knowing presence'*.

As suggested, the birth environment can have an impact on the birth process and outcomes. A woman feels safest in her own home environment and, thus, a midwifery philosophy to promote normality in childbirth is encouraged in a home birth setting. However, not all women are necessarily safe in a home birth if their circumstances of health and wellbeing are deemed to be 'high risk'. The notion of risk needs to be explored to gain an understanding of how this impacts birth outcomes. Midwives, as protectors of normal birth, give ownership to women and where necessary advocate for them, especially when it comes to choices for place of birth. The study by Aune et al. (2017) examines the experiences of midwives promoting normal birth in a home birth setting in Norway and concludes that a midwife's fundamental beliefs and attitudes, when shared in a trusting partnership with women, are essential to avoid birth interventions. The attribute of patience, whilst not disturbing the birth process, is seen as an attitude promoted in a safe home environment and supported by a familiar midwife, and as a good foundation for normal birth. The authors suggest that confidence and believing in the normal birth process, establishing relational continuity and being sensitive to women's needs through communicative listening are some of the attributes necessary in promoting a home-like environment in which to give birth. In addition, previous literature by Huber and Sandall (2009) implied that the association between relational continuity and creating calm in a birthing environment may be linked to positive care outcomes. Familiarity of a known midwife, in a continuity of carer model, can foster confidence and a feeling of safety and reassurance in which the woman can retreat into an undisturbed and calm environment. Equally, some researchers (Davis and Homer 2016) suggest that a conducive environment to birth has been found to be conducive to safe midwifery practice.

Defining Risk

Risk is defined as a situation that could be dangerous or have a bad outcome Oxford English Dictionary (2002). In terms of childbearing, a 'high-risk' woman is one that has increased adverse outcomes due to maternal age, lifestyle, medical or health issues, either pre-existing or as a result of pregnancy and childbirth.

The notion of risk within maternity care is attributed to a population of child-bearing women who are becoming increasingly at risk due to a number of factors. Economic and sociological pressures mean that women are having their first child at an older age and therefore an increase in health and age related conditions – such as obesity, diabetes and other medical conditions – combined with birth abnormalities are prevalent in a higher risk maternity population (Healy et al. 2017). In addition to this, increased interventions in maternity care and childbirth are also attributed to a 'risk and blame' culture in maternity services in which birth is increasingly seen as abnormal. Healthcare professionals err from a grounded, naturalistic midwifery philosophy in favour of preventative measures from adverse abnormal birth outcomes – and consequently litigious implications.

A recent MBRRACE-UK (2019) report asserts that there is a non-statistically significant increase in the number of direct maternal deaths in the period from 2015 to 2017, with 209 women dying in pregnancy and up to six weeks postnatally. That is equivalent to about nine women dying in every 100000. However, the overall indication is a rise in the number of older and heavier women who have more complex physical and mental health issues. These predisposing conditions result in co-morbidities. The leading cause of maternal deaths in the UK is cardio-vascular disease and related causes of thrombosis and thromboembolism resulting in cardiac arrest, epilepsy and stroke. Sepsis (10%), psychiatric conditions – such as depression leading to suicide (10%) – and cancer (4%) are still also listed as direct causes of maternal deaths. The report recommends improving the care of vulnerable women, especially black, mixed ethnicity and Asian women. Black women have a five times higher risk of dying in pregnancy than white women; those from mixed ethnicity are three times as likely to die and Asians are twice as likely to die than white women. Therefore, midwives need to broaden their knowledge and understanding of abnormal related conditions in childbearing to be able to recognise these and act accordingly. However, Healy et al. (2017) suggest that increased medicalisation of the birth process is contributing to the lack of responsibility by midwives in supporting and championing normality in childbirth. The midwife's autonomy and ability to advocate for women will affect future midwifery practices and skills and undermine the true philosophy of being 'with woman'. Organisational influences and lack of resources are also a contributing factor in undervaluing midwifery-led care, and focus on managing risk rather than enhancing evidence-based care (Lothian 2012) and the empowerment of the woman–midwife partnership in the birth event.

So, what is acceptable risk? This depends on the woman's perspective as opposed to that of the health professional – such as the obstetrician, the midwife and the provider or organisation providing maternity care. A pregnant woman is generally led to believe, either through the media or through hearsay, that she is at risk unless her care is managed by professionals and the maternity care services available. Her autonomy and decision-making skills are diminished and professionals control maternity care provision outcomes, generally instigated due to the limited availability of resources of staff and technology. A woman's innate ability to give birth, a belief in her own capabilities and autonomy in making the right decisions for herself are undermined by fear of birth disasters and outcomes. Lack of trust between woman and midwife fuels risk factors and sets off a cascade of interventions and loss of faith in the normal birth process. Walsh and Devane's (2012) meta synthesis of midwifery care models confirms that there is a relationship between risk and the discourse of medicalised maternity care on hospital labour wards, reinforcing a culture of behaviour and practices to 'process' the childbearing event, dominated by organisational care priorities and institutional pressures. This results in dehumanising the woman and dissociates both woman and midwife from the labour experience.

Sandall (2011) suggests that it is the risk in the provider/maternity care system that needs to be managed and not women's birth experiences. The author implies that the focus should be on safety and moving away from risk reduction towards women-centred and evidence-based birth care outcomes, where women make informed decisions about what is the safest option for them. Childbirth education provides both knowledge and support in making these decisions confidently and with relevance to individual women's needs. Midwives can instigate this 'with woman' journey through information and evidence-based skills to ensure a mutually satisfactory outcome for each and every birth.

Woman-Centred Care

The philosophy of woman-centred care is that a midwife *'focuses on a woman's health needs, her expectations and her aspirations'* to ensure both the physical and emotional health of mother and baby, built on a relationship of compassion, warmth and attention to ensure safety (ANMCM 2010: 7). However, in current

UK models there is a conflict between a commitment to being 'with woman' and advocacy towards a woman-centred philosophy by autonomous midwives, and the restraints and reality of the organisational management of maternity care provision. The concept of women-centred care has been explored in the last few years (Fahy 2012, Mapute and Donavon 2013) and more recently in an integrative review of the associated literature (Brady et al. 2019). This literature highlights that interpretation of the concept can vary when discussed in light of health policy documents and frameworks to inform clinical practice, maternity services and education. The authors determined that essential attributes of the 'woman-centred care' concept were mutual participation and responsibility sharing between woman and midwife, information sharing and, therefore, empowerment and autonomy to facilitate participation in decision making, communication, respect and listening and accommodative midwifery actions through a continuous presence and/or continuity of care.

There are three aspects of the continuity of care model, which includes the professional (either the midwife and/or the obstetrician), midwifery care models – such as continuity of care through team midwifery and case loading, and the geographical continuity of the birth environment in which maternity care is placed – such as a woman's home, midwifery-led units, birth centres or clinics and maternity units in hospitals.

Continuity of Care

Continuity of care requires radical changes in midwives' care models to accommodate more flexible working patterns, making additional demands on maternity services, and, as previously discussed, may impact the midwife's life–work balance. Evidence suggests that models of continuity of care and carer have beneficial and satisfactory birth outcomes for both mother and midwife. In fulfilling the 'with woman' philosophy in this therapeutic relationship, midwives need to take up responsibility, autonomy and advocacy as mantles towards safer nurturing and positive birth outcomes. However, a recent survey suggests that many midwives are not able or willing to provide maternity care through continuity models, unless working patterns are organised to accommodate greater choices and autonomy in midwives' roles (Taylor et al. 2019).

Midwife-Led Care

A meta synthesis of midwife-led care (Walsh and Devane 2012) suggests that this model of care results in lower rates of intervention in the birth process, increasing midwives' and women's autonomy and the experience of more empathetic care. The woman–midwife relationship enhanced compassionate, sensitive and nurturing care and instigated a feeling of equality and empowerment in women. Perriman et al. (2018) found that the midwife–woman relationship is central to the development of trust, personalised care and empowerment. Midwives through this relationship are able to reassure, reduce anxiety and stress through their 'continuing' presence, are able to detect deviations from normal birth and make early decisions with the women about appropriate care (Sandall 2017).

Soltani, Fair and Duxbury (2015) carried out a systemic review from a different perspective to explore women's awareness of midwifery-led continuity models of care and concluded that there is a need to better inform women about their maternity care options. Such models provide a level of safety and benefits for women and neonates as compared to other models of maternity care, and make a difference to birth outcomes (Hatem et al. 2008, Houghton et al. 2008, Sandall et al. 2010, Sandall et al. 2015). Sandall (2017) also indicate that when women are supported through midwifery-led continuity of care from a known midwife or companion, women in labour require fewer epidurals and there is less need for an episiotomy or instrumental delivery.

Case Loading and Team Midwifery

In the UK, there is a move to implement the Better Births recommendations of 2016 (NHS England) through published strategies by NHS England (2017), encouraging a review of maternity care provision and models of care. Many maternity units have piloted team midwifery and case loading with varying degrees of success. Previous studies from Australia have indicated that caseload midwifery, as compared to standard maternity care, is safe and cost effective for women of any risk and ensures continuity of carer in labour (Tracy et al. 2013). In addition, this care approach appears to reduce caesarean section rates of low obstetric risk in early pregnancy (McLachlan et al. 2012a). More recent evidence (Gidaszewski et al. 2019) also suggests that caseload midwifery increases rates of normal vaginal births managed through a restructuring of the workforce and reallocation of resources. Women are more likely to use water immersion as a pain-relieving method during labour and are less likely to have the interventions and complications of assisted deliveries than women receiving midwifery-led care. In the case loading model, midwives also continued to provide care even when women developed complications in pregnancy, which did not result in increased number of neonatal complications at birth, despite the women's risk status (Forster et al. 2016) A study in Australia (Williams et al. 2010) supports these findings, from women's perspectives, and suggests that a case loading model resulted in an associated relationship between maternal satisfaction and continuity of care.

In addition, previous literature (Fontein 2010) explored the impact of team midwifery and team sizes in midwifery practice on birth outcomes and birth experiences of low-risk women. The author concluded that teams with a maximum of two midwives resulted in better birth experiences for the women as they were more likely to know their midwife and experienced fewer interventions during the birth. Larger midwifery teams appear to reduce the continuity of carer element and reduce midwives' and women's satisfaction with birth outcomes.

Recently, from an opposing perspective, the unknown midwife (UM) model was explored from midwives' experiences working in this model in Australia (Bradfield et al. 2019). Elsewhere, previous literature examining outcomes from the UM model suggests that women were more likely to have a caesarean section, the uptake of epidural increases, episiotomies and instrumental birth rates increase whilst women's satisfaction with the birth process decreases (Tracy et al. 2013, McLachlan et al. 2012b, Sandall et al. 2015). However, the findings from Bradfield et al.'s (2019) descriptive phenomenological study presented new insight on how the 'with woman' concept can be achieved and facilitated in an UM model in which the woman, in most cases, has never met the midwife supporting her in labour. Through an adaptive process gained from experience, the midwives displayed characteristics of resilience and self-awareness and identified the need to build a connection and rapport with the woman and her partner as a key essential element to foster women-centred care and improve birth outcomes. Despite interventions, such as assisted labour and the use of Syntocinon and epidurals, the midwives suggested that an attitude of flexibility and adapting how they were 'with woman' overcame challenges to accommodate the woman's needs (Hunter et al. 2017), to be connected with her and enhanced the effectiveness of resilient midwifery practice through self-awareness and reflexibility (Feeley et al. 2019).

The acute problem of lack of resources and shortage of midwifery staff has instigated an exploration into alternatives of maternity care provision other than solely by a midwife for low-risk women wanting to give birth in their home (Taylor et al. 2018a, 2018b). Issues of role redesign are explored through the midwife–maternity support worker (MSW) model to shift pressure away from midwives and enable more women to experience home births, supported by a MSW in addition to a sole midwife. Some would argue that this shifting of responsibility away from the role of the midwife would make women vulnerable and subject to risk. However, the authors conclude that when considering the diminishing number of practising midwives and women's need to normalise their birth experience in a home environment, then through careful recruitment, training and support the MSW may have a role to play in promoting this model of care and may accommodate more home births.

Place of Birth

Finally, Cochrane reviews comparing the effectiveness of patterns of care indicate that women and their newborns have more beneficial outcomes when cared for by midwives in a low-risk environment such as a home birth, a birth centre or a midwifery-led unit (Hodnett et al. 2011, Sandall et al. 2015). When comparing birth outcomes which took place in a low-risk setting against those that occurred in a hospital labour ward, there appears to be a reduced uptake of pain relief and greater mobility during labour, decreased need for augmentation and fewer operative interventions at delivery. Most importantly, women experienced a greater satisfaction with their birth experience (Hodnett et al. 2011). More recently, a study by Hunter et al. (2018) suggests that being confident is fundamental to midwives in providing care in labour in a community or freestanding/standalone midwifery unit. Interestingly, in addition, a study by Hammond et al. (2013) explored the relationship between the space and place in which midwives work, and the authors suggest that the thoughts, feelings and responses of the midwives that interact with the birth environment are stimulated by oxytocin release that contributes to the attributes of a 'good midwife' in building social trusting relationships with the woman. This results in provision of emotional sensitive care which reduces stress and increases empathetic midwifery support.

In a bid to organise safe and effective care for women, alongside midwifery units (AMUs) have also been considered, in the birthplace study, as a hybrid organisational form of providing maternity care (Birthplace in England Collaborative Group 2011). An exploration of outcomes and effectiveness of care provision in AMUs suggests that only about a third of women who are eligible to give birth outside an obstetric unit are accessing these services (McCourt et al. 2018) due to inadequate information and challenges on admission in early labour (Rayment et al. 2019). Staff training and development to support physiological birth in therapeutic environments was still lacking, continuity-based models were still facing challenges, and AMU services were still marginal rather than core services. The findings suggest that an integrated service between obstetric units and midwifery-led units, whatever their location as either AMUs or standalone/freestanding units, was challenged due to intraprofessional tensions, and a lack of communication, mutual trust and understanding amongst midwives working in different environments of hospital- and community-based services. Some hospital-based midwives reported that lack of confidence in supporting women to achieve a physiological birth had an impact on the development of midwifery-led care. However, AMUs are seen to be a cost-effective and a positive environment in which midwives can develop confidence and competence in midwifery-led care and improve quality of care and birth experiences for women.

Despite these findings, a recent study by Bradfield et al. (2018) suggest that the 'with woman' philosophy and concept can also be fulfilled within an obstetric model of care, but is dependent on the relationship between the woman, the midwife and the obstetrician to enable fulfilment of birth aspirations and expectations with positive outcomes. Equally, research from the Netherlands (de Jonge et al. 2014) implies that continuity of care during labour, contributing to a feeling of safety, is more important to women than place of birth. Women were flexible about place of birth should the need from home to hospital transfer be required during labour, and the evidence suggests a fluid concept rather than a dichotomous choice for place of birth would be acceptable to women as long as the midwife stayed with them during the labour. These views concur with findings by Hadjigourgiou et al. (2012) and Fawsitt et al. (2017) when exploring preferences for models of maternity care in pregnant women (Table 3.1).

The Birthplace's cost-effectiveness study (Schroeder et al. 2011) identified key findings which suggest that, for a second and subsequent baby, the most cost-effective place of birth is at home. This is also true for women having a first baby, although there is a higher risk of poor outcomes for the baby in this group (Wax et al. 2010). This is in contrast to more recent studies and a meta-analysis (Scarf et al. 2018) which suggest that that there are no statistically significant differences in infant mortality by planned place of birth. Other findings in this review also suggest that women experience severe perineal trauma or haemorrhage at a lower rate in a planned home birth as opposed to birth in an obstetric unit. In addition, they are more likely to experience a normal vaginal delivery when giving birth at home.

As with previous chapters, the literature is examined through Rodgers' Conceptual Analysis framework.

Conclusion

This chapter has explored the evidence of how midwives, midwifery practices and services can fulfil the 'with woman' concept. Many issues include the reality of sustainable and continuing support by midwives at a cost to their work–life balance. Other studies explored the implications for maternity services and the impact, in terms of cost and childbirth outcomes, this has on women and their partners' birth experiences.

The literature identifies some of the related antecedents to the 'with woman' concept. The home-like birth environment, or a woman's home as a place of birth, enables midwives and women to achieve a relationship that fulfils the 'with woman' concept. Attributes of trust and patience are demonstrated in this

Table 3.1 Analysis of the midwife's perspective of 'with woman' concept.

'With woman' antecedents	Evidence	Attributes (A) & Consequences (C)
Normality	Powell Kennedy et al. (2010) Meyer (2012) Mapute and Donavon (2013) Thompson et al. (2016) Aune et al. (2017) Neerland (2018) normalising birth	Normal physiology of birth (A) 'Waiting on nature' (C) Continuous and intuitive assessment (A) 'positive presence' (C) Women's physiological ability to birth (A) Self-belief (C) Facilitating physiological birth and labour (A) 'Dynamic and therapeutic relationship' (C)
Birth environment	Davis (2010), Duff (2016), Powell Kennedy et al. (2010) midwifery philosophy and value of normality Aune et al. (2017) home birth Huber and Sandall (2009) relational continuity Davis and Homer (2016) conducive environment	Trust (A) Respect for woman's individuality and autonomy (C) Making safe decisions (A) Sensitive and responsible support by MW (C) Avoiding intervention (A) Optimal birth outcome (C) Women's satisfaction (C) Patience (A) Undisturbed birth process (C) Communicative listening (A) Creating calm in a birth environment (A) Foster confidence, safety and reassurance (C) Positive care outcomes (C) Conducive to safe midwifery practice (C)
Risk	Healy et al. (2017) defining high-risk birth conditions Lothian (2012) evidence-based care	High-risk midwifery (A) 'Risk and blame' culture (C) Birth seen as abnormal (C) Litigious implications (C) Increased medicalisation (A) Lack of responsibility by MWs to champion women(C) Organisational influences and lack of resources (A) Managing risk (C) Disempowerment of woman–midwife relationship (C)
Midwifery care models	Walsh and Devane (2012) meta synthesis of care models Sandall (2011) managing risk	Relationship of risk and medicalised maternity care discourse (A) Reinforced cultural behaviour to 'process' birth (C) Cascade of intervention (C) Dehumanising of women (C) Dissociates women and MWs from the birth experience (C) Focus on safety (A) Move away from risk reduction (C) Women-centred and evidence-based care (C)

Table 3.1 (Continued)

'With woman' antecedents	Evidence	Attributes (A) & Consequences (C)
Woman centred care	Fahy (2012), Mapute and Donavon (2013), Brady et al. (2019) women-centred concept	Linked to health policy documents (A) Mutual & responsible participation (C) Information sharing (C) Empowerment & autonomy in decision-making (C) Respect & listening (C)
Continuity of Care	Soltani, Fair and Duxbury (2015) Midwife-led care perspectives Hatem et al. (2008), Houghton et al. (2008), Sandall et al. (2010), Sandall et al. (2013, 2017) midwifery-led continuity of care Tracy et al. (2013), McLachlan et al. (2012a, 2012b), Case loading effect Bradfield et al. (2019) 'with woman' from unknown MW	Women uninformed about different models (A) Information would provide better safety and benefits (C) Care from a known midwife or companion (A) Women in labour required fewer interventions (C) Continuity of carer through mode (A) Maternal satisfaction and continuity of care (C) Resilience and self-awareness (A) Flexibility and need to build rapport (C)
Place of birth	Hodnett et al. (2011), Sandall et al. (2016), Hunter et al. (2018) home birth, birth centre and standalone midwifery unit Hammond et al. (2013) interaction with the birth environment	Reduced interventions (A) Greater satisfaction with birth experience (C) Relationship between space and place (A) 'Good midwife' attributes (A) Build trusting relationships (C) Emotional sensitive care (C) Reduces stress and increases empathy (C)

relationship to make safe decisions and reduce intervention during labour, through communicative listening in a calm birth environment. The consequences are respect for women's individuality and autonomy through sensitive and responsible support by midwives resulting in a safe, undisturbed and stress-free birth process and optimal birth outcomes.

The antecedents of normality, reducing risk through midwifery care models, which engender continuity of care and women-centred care, reflect a 'with woman' concept. Attributes which focus on maintaining the natural physiology of birth, through continuous and intuitive assessment by the midwives, encourage women's self-belief in their innate ability to give birth. A dynamic and therapeutic relationship between the woman and the midwife is the resulting consequence. Midwives' and women's stories illustrate these findings.

Midwives' Stories

Laura's Story

When looking after Lily* in the birth centre, I felt that I was able to truly be 'with woman'. I had met Lily in a previous pregnancy and had been able to look after her in the postnatal period before. When she attended in labour in this pregnancy, I was able to see that she was very anxious about the prospect of being sent home if not in established labour. We discussed the rationale for being at home in latent phase but on further discussion I sensed this would not be appropriate for her.

I admitted Lily to the birth centre and set the room up accordingly. Lily's contractions were very irregular, so I suggested doing some aromatherapy to try and relax and stimulate contractions. I then went on to provide Lily with a lower back massage for 20 minutes which Lily enjoyed. Whilst I was in the room with Lily she began to relax, and it became apparent that her labour was progressing. I ran the pool for her as she wanted a water birth as she had been unable to do so with her first delivery. It was at this point that Lily informed me she had to have a manual removal of her placenta first time. I explained that we would recommend an active third stage because of this. Lily was very against this as she felt the drug made her very sick and impacted on her initial bonding with her baby. I made Lily aware of the potential for another retained placenta and we discussed risks and benefits and I explained to Lily that if she wanted to try a physiological third stage then she could if that's what she wanted. We agreed that if the placenta hadn't been delivered in 15 minutes then she would consent to an active third stage.

Lily went on to have a lovely water birth in the birth centre an hour later and delivered her placenta naturally with baby breastfeeding five minutes after delivery. The cord remained attached to the placenta in a 'lotus birth'. I was able to facilitate cord ties rather than a cord clamp as Lily wished. Following delivery, Lily told me how different this experience was to her first labour and delivery and how she felt grateful that I listened to her wishes and although what she wanted was outside of normal guidelines, I was able to facilitate this for her. I felt as though I made a difference for her and her birth experience.

Rhiannon's Story

Nancy*, a low-risk para two, came into the birthing centre in spontaneous labour. Her membranes were still intact, and she was contracting 4 in 10 minutes. I did not feel it was necessary to examine at this stage as her contractions were strong on palpation and lasting around 60 seconds.

While she breathed through the contractions with her partner's help, I prepared one of the birthing suites, running the birthing pool and dimming the lights so that it was a relaxing environment. When in the room I took time to discuss Nancy's birthing plan with her and her partner between contractions. I wanted to ensure that I was addressing all Nancy's individual needs and wishes to ensure she had the birthing experience that she wanted.

Nancy explained that she wanted to use the birthing pool as a form of pain relief in addition to breathing techniques. At first, I sat in front of Nancy, talking her through the breathing techniques. Although Nancy had not specified that she felt in control of her breathing now, Nancy communicated this through body language, which I was able to pick up on and allowed her partner to take over supporting. She did not need a lot of encouragement and help but instead just wanted my reassurances from a distance that she was doing well and that her baby's heartbeat was within normal range every 15 minutes. I ensured that clinically everything was ok and aided the partner in supporting Nancy through her labour.

I took on board Nancy's wishes from her birth plan and helped her out of the pool just before delivery. During my time of being in the room with Nancy and her partner, a sense of trust had been built as I ensured that everything was explained fully. At delivery, Nancy listened to my guidance when delivering the baby's head which helped to ensure an intact perineum. A baby girl was born in a very calm, relaxed environment, which had been tailored to Nancy's wishes.

Donna's Story

After the rather fast yet traumatic birth of my first son that involved forceps and a stay in NICU, I was rather anxious about my second birth. When my second labour started, I knew with my history that I would need to get to hospital ASAP. When I arrived, triage was very busy, and I was hastily seen by a midwife who examined me and said I was 6 cm dilated and needed to go to labour ward ASAP. She got me a wheelchair and transferred me; I wanted to walk but was told I had to be transferred in a chair. Labour pains were worse sitting, so I was beginning to not cope. When we arrived onto the labour ward the midwife left me in a corridor and went to find a room and midwife to hand over to. The pain was getting worse and I was getting distressed, and it felt like I had been there for ages, that was when an angel appeared! Her name was Ann* she came out of a room at the other end of the corridor and saw me, although busy herself she came straight over to me. She bent down and smiled and introduced herself to me and asked my name. She then kindly asked 'may I put my hands on your shoulders?', I nodded, she placed warm and loving hands onto my shoulders and relaxed them down away from my ears!

(Continued)

She was calm and reassuring, she asked who was looking after me, I said I didn't know. She immediately said that in that case she would look after me, turned to the room we were outside of and showed me in.

She said that she would need to go and inform the team leader she was caring for me and would be right back. She ensured I was comfortable and had given me gas and air to help cope with my contractions. I was worried she wouldn't come back, but as good as her word she did. I tried to get onto the bed, so she could examine me, and she said that she didn't need to. She trusted her colleague and could see I was labouring well so didn't need to intervene. She got me pillows, water and a floor mat so I could change positions. She radiated positivity and kindness and assured me I was OK. She was also very reassuring to my husband, keeping him involved. My labour was progressing quickly, and my waters went mid contraction, I started to become distressed and was asking for intervention as that was how I expected my birth to be. She came close, nose to nose with me and looked me in the eyes and said 'You don't need me. You've got this!' I had a moment of clarity where this wonderful midwife believed in me, she believed I could have my baby without intervention, so I had no other option than to believe her too!

As soon as my mindset changed, with her and my husband's encouragement and support, 20 minutes later my beautiful 8 lb 15 oz baby boy was born! I had no intervention and no need for stitches! She encouraged my husband to cut the cord, which he had not done before and helped me skin to skin and to breastfeed in what seemed like moments after birth! She very quickly tidied us up and got us tea and toast!

From meeting her in the corridor to being bathed and in bed with baby, tea and toast was just over an hour! She popped back in to check on us in her own clothes as she was going home. It turned out we had arrived at shift handover, she had worked over her shift to stay and support me through my birth. She explained she was a community midwife who had come in to help as the unit was busy, her husband had been waiting outside to pick her up all this time! Not once had she rushed us or made us feel like a bother, or even handed my care over to another midwife.

She was, and still is, an inspiration to me. I left the hospital eight years ago, saying I needed to do what she does. The way she believed in me and my ability to have a baby and the love she showed me was very special, her actions changed my life. When my son was six weeks old I started my application process to become a midwife and have been qualified now for nearly two years. I still work with the wonderful Ann and can't help but hug and kiss her every time I see her! As a midwife she practises the true meaning of 'with woman'.

Women's Stories

Sarah's Story

I was five days past my baby's estimated due date (this whole concept bothers me; everyone should have a 'due month' like members of the Royal Family!). Despite trying not to focus on this, I was going completely insane with waiting for some labour signs to appear. I'd been listening to the birth affirmations mp3 (my favourite track) every single morning since the course. The phrases would often pop into my mind throughout the day, and by this point I strongly believed them. I'd also spent a lot of time since the course (bus journeys, before bed etc.) listening to the other tracks and music.

The choice to have a home birth was originally based on wanting the guarantee of access to a water pool but was later boosted by wanting to feel in as safe and familiar an environment as possible; for me this was not hospital or even a midwife-led unit. I had had severe symphysis pubis dysfunction for months and also have a visual impairment which worsens in stressful/unfamiliar situations, so the thought of having to navigate around a hospital room etc. made me feel uneasy.

After the fantastic hypnobirthing course my partner Matt and I had completed, I had gained so much more confidence in my body's natural abilities and knew to trust my instincts about where I'd be most calm and relaxed.

We also felt prepared for the potential that things might not go to plan and how to stay in the zone should things change and I did need to be transferred into hospital.

When my waters finally did break at 6 p.m. I was SO excited that my baby was finally on its way – I literally couldn't stop grinning! The living room was already all set up with pool, oil burner, low lighting, towels, gym ball and snacks, so after a giant fish and chips takeaway I was excited to go in there and finally be putting it all to use for real!

__Understanding my choices:__ We had to really stand our ground about not going into hospital for an assessment, as the team were so short-staffed that evening they didn't currently have any midwives they could send out.

I was adamant not to go in, but things progressed quite quickly, and for many hours of intensifying surges we were on our own not knowing if any midwives would be available later, or if Matt would be delivering the baby solo! He was very brave at this point having to explain to triage that I was refusing to go into hospital because being at home was right for us, and them telling him that we had no choice but to go in. This was one part I know we would have been very panicked

(Continued)

about had we not been taught how dads (or other birth partners) can take charge of being the contact with medical staff to take this job away from the mum so she can focus solely on the job in hand.

After the phone calls, Matt would return to reading bits from the birth partners' script, reminding me I was safe and doing well and to go to my relaxing place. Eventually some midwives did become available and there was someone with us from about 3 a.m. onwards. Some weren't usually part of the community midwife team, but they were all just AMAZING. They gave us both constant reassurance and space. Matt gave them chocolate cake.

Water magic: *To start with Matt's light touch massage was enough to help with the surges. But while he was filling the pool I started using the TENS machine. After a while though, this made me go very cold and shivery. So, at that point I got into the pool which felt great. Throughout we played the hypnobirthing tracks and used the breathing techniques, without which I wouldn't have got half as far without any medical pain relief. It didn't feel like there was long between surges to go back to my relaxing place, but I tried to fit in as many 'easy breathing' breaths before beginning the surge breathing/ mountain/breathing again (I used counting up and counting down alongside visualising the rolling waves).*

I later asked for gas and air and had one dose of diamorphine as I was worried about how tired I was becoming from being awake and labouring all night. Although neither was part of my original birth plan, I knew I didn't need to see this as any sort of failure, and they really helped at that stage. I tried not to focus on how much time was passing or how long might be left, but this was something I struggled with at times. For a while we lay in the dark in bed with a midwife popping in every 15 minutes to check on baby. I actually liked this as I knew that each time they crept in we were 15 minutes closer.

One of the best moments was as the sun was rising was finding out that our wonderful midwife Natasha that we had seen exclusively antenatally was starting her day shift and would be coming to take over and would be the one delivering baby – it was the icing on the cake of being able to stay at home.

Passive pushing: *She arrived and about 8 a.m. announced I was fully dilated (happy days!!) so I got straight back in the pool once it was warm enough again. There was an hour of 'passive pushing' or in more hypnobirthing type words, nudging baby gently down, not rushing it and waiting until it felt totally ready to let my body 'push'.*

I think by this point I was a bit delirious with all sorts of mixed emotions and tiredness that I was talking a fair bit of nonsense to the midwives and Matt (I don't remember!). Matt's hand truly took a bashing with how hard I squeezed it at times!

Something I do remember is having a few spoonfuls of honey just in the final stages, and it gave such a hit of energy!

Baby Noah was delivered in the pool at 10.01 a.m. by Natasha, and I had the amazing first cuddle. We really wanted to ensure optimal cord clamping, so we waited the full time before the cord turned white before Daddy cut it and had some skin on skin cuddles of his own. Natasha helped dress Noah, started us off breastfeeding and stayed at our house for a fair while afterwards, which was lovely. (We did have some breastfeeding struggles, and I'd recommend to all new mamas to check out the Breastfeeding Network to find a local peer supporter.)

It was for me the perfect birth experience. I'm so glad we were stubborn on the day about staying at home despite lots of efforts to talk us out of it. Being super prepared with all the stuff that I may or may not have needed during labour all carefully organised and on hand meant I felt comfortable that there was no need to go anywhere else. We are so, so glad that we did the hypnobirthing; so much of how well the birth went was down to what we'd learnt and practised, and the calm and positivity that filled the room throughout.

Helen's Story

I have had five children, the first in September 2013 and my most recent in June 2019. My first four children were born in very similar circumstances: I have fast labours (less than 1 hr in each case) and find my accounts of previous labours are often doubted. As such, my first four children were born respectively in a car park, a bath tub, a delivery room (yay!) and an unused delivery room which was being used as a storage area. In each birth I have suffered second degree tears and have also lost varying amounts of blood, with three of them being quantified as post-partum haemorrhage (PPH) and the planned delivery room birth having been the only time that my bleeding was within normal limits.

As I entered my fifth pregnancy, I was very aware of the factors which had, and could, influence my birth story. I asked at my booking appointment to be referred to the consultant midwife so that I could discuss a birth plan to induce me, at 40 weeks or as soon as possible thereafter, through the method of breaking my waters, the same process I had requested with my third baby and which had protected me from PPH. I entered the room prepared to fight my corner. I wanted access to a birthing pool, which I am always denied because of my history of PPH, I wanted a birth photographer in the room, I wanted a darkened room with my choice of music playing, and I wanted all these things in place before my waters were broken. The midwife I met with could not have been more open to my requests. I explained that I wanted to maximise the opportunities for natural

(Continued)

oxytocin production in the hope of avoiding another haemorrhage. The midwife identified herself as an aromatherapist outside of her NHS job and suggested various oils I could use in massage or in baths to help my body to prepare for a 40-week induction. She gave me a document describing several massage techniques I could use for relaxation throughout the pregnancy and more specifically the ones I could use in the final weeks to help my body to prepare. A plan was put in place for us to discuss my birth plan later in the pregnancy once the anomaly scan had been performed.

Unfortunately, my anomaly scan revealed marginal placenta previa and several follow up scans were performed throughout the rest of the pregnancy, during which the placenta previa failed to resolve. Ultimately, I was booked to undergo a caesarean birth, but the consultant listened to my appeals to make this as late as possible, and given my history of always reaching my EDD, was happy to delay my caesarean as late as possible, to 39+5 weeks. It was agreed I would have one final scan in case the placenta previa had resolved, and to my delight it was found to have done so at 38+5 weeks, so I was able to return to my original plan of being induced at 40 weeks.

Alongside all of this, and rather unusually, I had become involved in a BBC2 documentary looking at families welcoming a new arrival into the family. They wanted to film my baby's birth. The hospital allowed this and so, on my due date, my husband and I arrived on the delivery suite with my birth photographer and a BBC film crew in tow. I was met on the ward by a midwife who greeted me with a cuddle and said the room with the birthing pool was available. She took me through to the delivery room and allowed me to set up everything just as I wanted. I set up my battery-operated candles and my music, made the room darker, and the midwife agreed to fill the pool before breaking my waters as I knew my labour was likely to progress very quickly once it started. My birth photographer was able to discuss with the midwife how the two of them could each do their jobs without getting in each other's way, and the midwife could not have been more accommodating in all the requests and needs of myself, the birth photographer and the filming crew.

Ahead of breaking my waters, the midwife checked the position of the baby and was unsure whether the baby might be breech – this had been an issue on and off towards the end of the pregnancy. I asked whether this would cause any problems as I was keen to have a vaginal birth and the midwife assured me we would continue with a vaginal birth anyway, she just wanted to be prepared if the baby was breech. She fetched an ultrasound and checked the baby but was able to confirm it was head down and ready to be born.

My waters were broken and we all waited for labour to begin. With my third baby (also induced through artificial rupture of membranes (ARM)), labour started within 10 minutes of my waters being broken and my daughter was born within half an hour. I had expected a similar timeline but two hours after breaking my waters, I was still waiting for labour to begin. The midwife was so lovely, suggesting walks and stairs and even leaving my husband and I alone (as did the TV crew) to help me to relax as much as possible. Three hours after my waters were broken, the midwife came to explain to me that if nothing had started by the four-hour mark, I would have to decide whether to accept a hormone drip or to go home and wait for labour to start there. Although this may sound a little pressured, she was so gentle in her explanation and covered the options I had: to stay there where a drip would be needed; or to go home where I would have to take my chances on how the birth then unfolded. As luck would have it, labour started just minutes later and within 20 minutes I was in an established pattern of contracting every two minutes for a minute at a time. The midwife re-filled the birthing pool with hot water as soon as the contractions started up and she agreed with me that the 20 minutes of contractions had settled into a pattern. I got into the water and felt immediate relief when the next contraction came. I was in the water for 20 minutes in total, and that contraction was the only one I had. The water had stopped my labour. I looked up at the midwife and said I thought I had stopped labour. She nodded and said she was thinking the same thing. She suggested leaving the pool for a bit and was keen to point out that I could always get back in if needed later. As I stepped out of the bath, I immediately went into transition contractions. I had asked the midwife to remind me not to push as I know from my previous labours that the baby will come anyway, and that pushing too hard with my third and fourth children had caused them both to be born with head injuries. I became aware of the midwife at my side whispering to me that this was the time to just trust my body and to not push. It made such a difference to me as I was just in that moment where pushing felt like the only way to help the pain. Moments later, without pushing, my daughter was born.

The end of the story is less special. Despite avoiding blood loss in the birth, I then lost a litre during attempts to repair a second-degree tear. Even then, the midwife was so careful to keep me included in things. She explained that every time she attempted to stitch, I was bleeding from the needle entry point. I asked if I was bleeding 'too much' and she said yes. A doctor was called in to stitch me and I was transferred up to the labour ward which I found far less positive, as with previous births.

My fifth birth was such a positive experience – in part this was because I was so prescriptive in my plans for the birth, but above all I credit my amazing midwife

(Continued)

with helping me to achieve everything I wanted. I still didn't get my water birth, but that was down to my body and nothing else. She was so accommodating and supportive and attentive to not only my needs but my requests, and all under the watchful eyes of TV cameras which can't have been easy. None of my births have gone the way I had hoped, and none of them have felt negative, but my fifth birth was absolutely my most positive experience to date and it's all down to two amazing midwives: one who listened to me in pregnancy and one who listened to me in the moment of birth.

Lissie's Story

I can't believe that just one short week ago I gave birth to this little poppet. As she rests her eyes, I thought I would share my story in the hope that others might gain a bit of reassurance from it, should they decide to go for a home birth. I spent much of my pregnancy reading up on positive home birth stories and it gave me hope that I could still have the birth I had dreamed of.

My first child was born nine years ago after a very long labour which had me transferred from a birthing clinic to the hospital. I was in such a state of exhaustion that in the end I opted for pethidine and an epidural and, due to meconium in my waters and fetal distress, he was eventually delivered by ventouse. My second child was induced at two weeks overdue and, again, I struggled with the hospital birth experience as my partner was not allowed to stay with me and I felt very self-conscious about showing pain in front of strangers. Another long labour resulted in the pethidine/epidural cocktail and a ventouse delivery. With each I had second-degree tears which left me unable to sit or walk comfortably for weeks. Not the worst births, I know, but each validated the belief that my body just wasn't good at giving birth.

Right from the beginning of this pregnancy I decided that I wanted to do things differently. I wanted to be prepared both mentally and physically for the birth and not fear it. It helped massively that a dear friend of mine had had a successful home birth and introduced me to the Surrey Hills Team and home birth Facebook group. I felt very strongly that the difficulty of my two previous births was due having epidurals and pushing whilst on my back. I wanted to put everything in place in an attempt not to go there again. Once more, I had a pretty smooth pregnancy and planned to keep working within a couple of days of my due date. I assumed that I would be overdue for a third time. By this point, I felt completely relaxed about what was to come and was actually looking forward to going into labour.

In the weeks leading up to the birth I had a few nights of false labour and experienced mild contractions from the moment I went to bed and into the early hours of the morning. Frustratingly, they were regular and painful enough that I couldn't sleep through them, but they disappeared when I got up and moved around. I hadn't had this with the other two pregnancies but felt reassured that it was just the baby engaging. I continued using the birthing ball in the evenings as much as possible and I credit this for getting the baby into a good position.

A couple of days before my last day at work I woke feeling a bit more crampy than usual. After lunch,

I noticed I had had a bloody show and within about half an hour I was having mild contractions every 15–20 min. I decided to wait and see if they continued, and a couple of hours later, I was pretty sure that things were kicking off so let my boss know that I was heading home. When I got back my partner and I set about getting the kids fed and into bed and making sure we had everything we needed in place. The contractions were steadily getting more uncomfortable and closer together, so I connected the TENS machine and took some paracetamol. Around 10 p.m., my partner turned in for the night and I thought I might be able to get a few hours' sleep too but as it turned out it was just too uncomfortable.

During this time, I was in contact with two close friends: one who had had a home birth and had offered support should I need it; and another who would go around and look after the first friend's three children as her husband is a policeman and on nights. What amazing women I have around me!! I kept saying that I was fine but by 11:30 p.m. the contractions were becoming more intense. I self-examined and I thought I was still only about 1–2 cm dilated. At this point I was feeling a little stressed about how slowly things were progressing so gladly accepted my friend's offer, who then came armed with brownies! From this point I felt like I could relax and just let things happen. My friend turned off the tv and main lights, leaving just the fairy lights and candles to light the room, put on some relaxation music and got me to drink some water. At this time, we also inflated the birthing pool. For the next 5–6 hours we chatted away, and I changed positions every so often depending on how I felt. Did I mention how brilliant my friend is! I found that when I was sat astride the birthing ball, or on my knees, belly bent over a pillow, that the contractions were coming every 3–5 minutes. When I needed a rest, I would lie on my side with a pillow between my knees or slightly reclined with my legs propped up. This would cause the contractions to slow to every 10–12 minutes and gave me a chance to catch my breath and rest. I had never used a TENS machine before but found it very effective! I contacted the midwife around 2 a.m. to let her know that I was in labour but coping.

My partner got up around 5 a.m. to see how we were getting on. After a rest, I decided that I needed to get things moving again, even though the contractions whilst sitting on the ball were becoming very intense. My son rose around 6 a.m.

(Continued)

and was a brilliant help, chatting away and timing the contractions while the adults went about the process of filling up the pool and getting our daughter ready for school. This period of time is a bit of a haze, but I recall that I was becoming a lot more vocal with each contraction. I was also feeling a lot of pressure in my lower back/tailbone which I hadn't experienced before. My previous labours were felt around the front. The TENS machine was turned up high and having someone push hard into my lower spine really helped with the pain. I went to the toilet and found that more of the plug had come away. Now, the contractions really stepped up a gear and were coming every three minutes. My waters were slowly trickling out too.

My partner took the kids to school and arrived back just after 8:30 a.m. I felt overwhelmed (transition?) and decided to lie down on my side but experienced two very intense contractions where my body involuntarily pushed at the end. This had me in a state of panic (I must admit I started screaming!) as I didn't know whether I was 'ready' or not. The midwives were due to arrive any minute. My partner rang the midwife and she instructed him to get me into the pool. As soon as I got into the water, I had another strong contraction and felt the baby's head move down and crown. I felt the top of her fuzzy head and a sense of relief washed over me. One more contraction and push later and her body slipped into the water, caught and passed through to me by my amazing friend. I absolutely could not believe it and the look of bafflement was caught brilliantly in a couple of photos. The two midwives arrived shortly afterwards and set about checking us over. Another beautiful daughter, born at 8: 41 a.m.! The placenta came out 20 minutes later with no issue. And amazingly, no tears to repair, only very slight grazing!

As I look back over the last nine months, I can't help but feeling totally blessed and thankful. The midwives from the Home Birth Team were brilliant, as was having the appointments in a home setting. I always felt in safe hands. I have no doubts that being in my own home, surrounded and supported by my loved ones, contributed greatly to the ease of this birth. I look now at my daughter sleeping and feel overwhelmingly that I made the right decision. This was such a special moment in time and one I will feel most proud of for years to come.

Lessons Learnt

Women have different perceptions of their birth experiences, as is illustrated in these stories. However, the main constant is the kindness and support to fulfil needs and wishes which women remember far more clearly than an unpleasant or traumatic event that they experience. Women want to be listened to empathetically, supported in their belief to give birth normally. They want a satisfactory birth outcome, aided by the 'positive presence' of a known midwife or companion to foster confidence, safety and reassurance.

References

Aune, I., Hoston, M.A., Kolshus, N.J., and Larsen, C.E.G. (2017). Nature works best when allowed to run its course. The experience of midwives promoting normal birth in a home birth setting. *Midwifery* 50: 21–26.

Australian Nursing & Midwifery Council (2010). Standards and Criteria for the Accreditation of Nursing and Midwifery Courses Leading to Registration, Enrolment, Endorsement and Authorisation in Australia— with Evidence Guide. www.anmc.org.au

Birthplace in England Collaborative Group (2011). Perinatal and maternal outcomes by planned place of birth for healthy women with low risk pregnancies: the birthplace in England national prospective cohort study. *British Medical Journal* 343: d7400.

Bradfield, Z., Kelly, M., Hauck, Y., and Duggan, R. (2018). Midwives "with woman" in the private obstetric model: where divergent philosophies meet. *Women and Birth*. https://doi.org/10.1016/j.wombi.2018.07.013.

Bradfield, Z., Hauck, Y., Kelly, M., and Duggan, R. (2019). Midwives' experiences of being "with woman" in a model where midwives are unknown. *Midwifery* 69: 150–157.

Brady, S., Lee, N., Gibbons, K., and Bogossian, F. (2019). Women-centred care: an integrative review of the empirical literature. *International Journal of Nursing Studies* 94: 107–119.

Brown, A.M. (2012). Assessment strategies for teaching empathy, intuition and sensitivity on the labour ward. *Evidence Based Midwifery* 10 (2): 64–70.

Davis, J.A.P. (2010). Midwives and Normalcy in childbirth: a phenomenologic concept development study. *Journal of Midwifery and Women's Health* 55 (3): 206–215.

Davis, D.L. and Homer, C.S. (2016). Birthplace as the midwife's work place: how does place of birth impct on midwives? *Women and Birth* 29: 407–415.

De Jonge, A., Stuijt, R., Eijke, I., and Westerman, M. (2014). Continuity of care: what matters to women when they are referred from primary to secondary care during labour? A qualitative interview study in the Netherlands. *BMC Pregnancy and Childbirth* 14: 103.

Duff, E. (2016). Better births: moving from "failure to progress" to "rhetoric into reality"? *MIDIRS Midwifery Digest* 26 (3): 290–294.

Fahy, K. (1998). Being a midwife or doing midwifery? *Australian College of Midwives Incorporated Journal* 11 (2): 11–16.

Fahy, K. (2012). What is woman-centered care and what does it matter? *Woman and Birth: Journal of the Australian College of Midwives* 25 (4): 149–151.

Fawsitt, C.G., Bourke, J., Lutomski, E. et al. (2017). What women want: exploring pregnant women's preferences for alternative models of maternity care. *Health Policy* 121 (1): 66–74.

Feeley, C., Thomson, G., and Downe, S. (2019). Caring for women making unconventional birth choices: a meta-ethnography exploring views, attitudes and experiences of midwives. *Midwifery* 72: 50–59.

Fontein, Y. (2010). The comparison of birth outcomes and birth experiences of low risk women in different sized midwifery practices in the Netherlands. *Women and Birth* 23: 103–110.

Forster, D.A., McLachlan, H.L., Davey, M.A. et al. (2016). Continuity of care by a primary midwife (caseload midwifery) increases women's satisfaction with antenatal, intrapartum and postpartum care: results from the COSMOS randomised control trial. *BMC Pregnancy and Childbirth* 16: 28. https://doi.org/10.1186/s12884-016-0798-y.

Gidaszewski, B., Khajehei, M., Gibbs, E., and Chai Chua, S. (2019). Comparison of the effect of caseload midwifery program and standard midwifery-led care on pimiparous birth outcomes: a retrospective cohort matching study. *Midwifery* 69: 10–16.

Hadjigourgiou, E., Konta, C., Papastavrou, E. et al. (2012). Women's perceptions of their right to choose the place of childbirth: A qualitative study. *International Journal of Childbirth* 2(4): DOI: 10.1891/0886-6708.2.4.230.

Hammond, A., Foureur, M., Homer, C.S., and Davis, D. (2013). Space, place and the midwife: exploring the relationship between the birth environment, neurobiology and midwifery practice. *Women and Birth* 26: 277–281.

Hatem, M., Sandall, J., DeVane, D. et al. (2008). Midwife-led versus other models of care for childbearing women. *Cochran Database Systematic Reviews* 4 (Art. No.: CD004667).

Healy, S., Humphreys, E., and Kennedy, C. (2017). A qualitative exploration of how midwives' and obstetricians' perception of risk affects care practices for low-risk women and normal birth. *Women and Birth* 30: 367–375.

Hodnett, E.D., Downe, S., and Walsh, D. (2011). Alternative versus conventional institutional settings for birth. *The Cochrane Database of Systematic Reviews* 8.

Houghton, G., Bedwell, C., Forsey, M. et al. (2008). Factors influencing choice in birth place- an exploration of the views of women, their partners and professionals. *Evidence Based Midwifery* 6 (2): 59–64.

Huber, U.S. and Sandall, J. (2009). A qualitative exploration of the creation of calm in a continuity of carer model of maternity care in London. *Midwifery* 25: 613–621.

Hunter, B. (2006). The importance of reciprocity in relationships between community-based midwives and mothers. *Midwifery* 22: 308–322.

Hunter, L.P. (2008). A hermeneutic phenomenological analysis of midwives' ways of knowing during childbirth. *Midwifery* 24: 405–415.

Hunter, L.P. (2009). A descriptive study of "being with woman" during labour and birth. *Journal of Midwifery and Women's Health* 54: 111–118.

Hunter, B., Henley, J., Fenwick, J. et al. (2017). *Work, Health and Emotional Life of Midwives in the United Kingdom: The UK WHELM Study*. Cardiff University and Queensland University commissioned by The Royal College of Midwives.

Hunter, M., Smythe, E., and Spence, D. (2018). Confidence: fundamental to midwives providing labour care in freestanding midwifery-led units. *Midwifery* 66: 176–181.

Lothian, J.A. (2012). Risk, safety and choice in childbirth. *The Journal of Perinatal Education* 21 (1): 45–47.

Mapute, M.S. and Donavon, H. (2013). Women-centred care in childbirth: a concept analysis (part 1). *Curationis* 36 (1): 49–57.

MBRRACE-UK (2019). Saving lives, improving mothers' care: Lessons learned to inform maternity care from the UK and Ireland Confidential Enquiries into Maternal Deaths and Morbidity 2015–2017. Confidential Enquiries into Maternal Deaths and Morbidity 2015–2017. Oxford Perinatal Epidemiology Unit, University of Oxford.

McCourt, C., Rance, S., Rayment, J. et al. (2018). Organising safe and sustainable care in alongside midwifery units: Findings from an organisational ethnographic case study. *Midwifery* 65: 26–34.

McLachlan, H.L., Foster, D.A., Davey, M.A. et al. (2012a). Effects of continuity of care by a primary midwife (caseload midwifery) on caesarean section rates in women of low obstetric risk: the COSMOS randomised controlled trial. *BJOG : An International Journal of Obstetrics and Gynaecology*. https://doi.org/10.1111/j.1471-0528.2012.03446.x.

McLachlan, H.L., Foster, D.A., Davey, M.A. et al. (2012b). The effects of primary midwife-led care on women's experience of childbirth: results from the COSMOS randomised control trial. *BJOG* 123: 465–474.

Meyer, S. (2012). Control in childbirth: a concept analysis and synthesis. *Journal of Advanced Nursing* 69 (1): 218–228.

Neerland, C.E. (2018). Maternal confidence in physiologic childbirth: a concept analysis. *Journal of Midwifery & Women's Health* 63 (4): 425–435.

NHS England (2016). Better Births: Improving outcomes of maternity services in England: A five year forward for better maternity care. NHS England.

NHS England (2017). Implementing Better Births: Continuity of carer. https://www.england.nhs.uk/wp-content/uploads/2017/12/implementing-better-births.pdf (accessed 23 January 2019).

Oxford University (2002). *The Oxford English Dictionary*. Oxford: Oxford University Press.

Perriman, N.M., Davis, D.L., and Ferguson, S. (2018). What women value in the midwifery continuity of care model: a systematic review with meta-analysis. *Midwifery* 62: 220–229.

Powell Kennedy, H., Walton, C., Shaw-Battista, J., and Sandall, J. (2010). Normalizing birth in England: a qualitative study. *Journal of Midwifery and Women's Health* 55 (3): 262–269.

Rayment, J., Rance, S., McCourt, C. et al. (2019). Barriers to women's access to alongside midwifery units in England. *Midwifery* 77: 78–85.

Sandall J. (2011). Re-framing safety: Risky health systems and safer childbearing. Presentation at Fear and Loathing in Maternity Care: Imagining, Managing and Creating Risk in Pregnancy and Childbirth symposium. 26 May 2011, University of Maastricht, School of Midwifery Science, Maastricht, The Netherlands.

Sandall, J. (2017). *The Contribution of Continuity of Midwifery Care to High Quality Maternity Care*. London: Royal College of Midwives.

Sandall, J., Devane, D., Hatem, M., and Gate, S. (2010). Improving quality and safety in maternity care: the contribution of midwifery-led care. *Journal of Midwifery and Women's Health* 55 (3): 255–261.

Sandall, J., Soltani, H., Gates, S. et al. (2013). Midwifery-led continuity models versus other models of care for childbearing women. *Cochrane Database Syst. Rev.* 8: CD004667.

Sandall, J., Soltani, H., Gate, S. et al. (2015). Midwife-led continuity models versus other models of care for childbearing. *The Cochrane Database of Systematic Reviews* (8).

Sandall, J., Soltani, H., Gates, S. et al. (2016). Midwife-led continuity models of care compared to other models of care for wome during pregnancy, birth and early parenting. 8: CD004667

Scarf, V.L., Rossiter, C., Vedam, S. et al. (2018). Maternal and perinatal outcomes by planned place of birth amongst women with low-risk pregnancies in high-income countries: a systematic review and meta-analysis. *Midwifery* 62: 240–255.

Schroeder, E., Petrou, S., Patel, N., et al. (2011). Birthplace cost-effectiveness analysis of planned place of birth: individual level analysis Birthplace in England Research Programme: final report Part 5. Oxford: NEPU.

Soltani, H., Fair, F., and Duxbury, A. (2015). Exploring health professionals' and womens' awareness of maternity care evidence. *British Journal of Midwifery* 23 (1): 22–31.

Taylor, B., Cross-Sudworth, F. and MacArthur, C. (2018a). Better Births and continuity: Midwife survey results. Institute of Applied Health Research, University of Birmingham.

Taylor, B., Henshall, C., Goodwin, L., and Kenyon, S. (2018b). Task shifting midwifery support workers as the second health worker at a home birth in the UK: a qualitative study. *Midwifery* 62: 109–115.

Taylor, B., Cross-Sudworth, F., Goodwin, L. et al. (2019). Midwives' perspectives of continuity based working in the UK: a cross-sectional survey. *Midwifery* 75: 127–137.

Thompson, S.M., Nieuwenhuize, M.J., Kane Low, L., and de Vries, R. (2016). Exploring Dutch midwives' attitudes to promoting physiological childbirth: a qualitative study. *Midwifery* 42: 67–73.

Tracy, S.K., Hartz, D.L., Tracy, M.B. et al. (2013). Caselaod midwifery care versus standard maternity care for women of any risk: M@NGO, a randomised controlled trial. *The Lancet* 23 (382): 1723–1732.

Walsh, D. and Devane, D. (2012). A metasynthesis of midwife-led care. *Qualitative Health Research* 22 (7): 897.

Wax, J.R., Lucas, F.L., Lamont, M. et al. (2010). Maternal and newborn outcomes in planned home birth vs planned hospital births: a meta-analysis. *American Journal of Obstetrics and Gynaecology* 243: e1–e7.

Williams, K., Lago, L., Lainchbury, A., and Eagar, K. (2010). Mothers' views of caseload midwifery and the value of continuity of care at an Australian regional hospital. *Midwifery* 26: 615–621.

4

'With Woman' in Screening and Fetal Medicine

Angie Bowles (Independent Midwife); Anna M. Brown; and Hannah (woman)

Introduction

This chapter explores issues around the compromised fetus and will address related psychosocial and ethical factors from both women's and midwives' perspectives. How midwives offer screening services and the implications of medical intervention and midwifery support on compromised pregnancies, will be discussed.

Screening and Fetal Medicine

All pregnant women receiving National Health Service (NHS) care are offered routine antenatal care which includes screening for fetal anomaly. Information is offered to women as to the nature of the screening offered, to help childbearing women and their families to make the choices that are right for them. An audit undertaken in one large NHS Trust, however, found that at the point of first trimester screening, only 40% of women said that they recognised an image of the standard NHS screening information leaflet, whilst 100% of them had signed a form saying that they had *'read the information in the leaflet provided'* (Angie Bowles in 2017 private correspondence).

The NHS screening pathway describes opportunities for women to discuss the implications and impact of screening choices and outcomes. This is expected to form part of the initial 'booking' consultation, enabling informed consent prior to the blood sampling or ultrasound scans. As a result, it could be assumed that most women are now generally well informed about their developing infant and can request detailed information about risks of tests and associated procedures, which may impact on their choices and decisions about pregnancy and childbirth (Lennon 2016). However, some women tend to accept the tests and examinations on offer without considering preparedness of adverse findings. Earlier research suggests that effective provision of information by healthcare providers, prior to consent, can be difficult (Lalor and Begley 2006).

Several screening programmes are available to detect fetal anomalies. The first trimester scan is offered with additional screening for the three most common chromosomal conditions in pregnancies which progress to term. These are trisomy 21 (Down's syndrome), trisomy 18 (Edward's syndrome) and trisomy 13 (Patau's syndrome). Until recently, results for these tests were referred to as high or low *risk*; there has been an acceptance that this could be perceived to be a value laden expression and so there has been a national drive to change the language to refer to high and low *chance* results.

A combined test giving a 'high chance' result leads to the offer of further, more detailed testing. The definition of high chance is set by the national screening committee at 1 in 150 or greater chance. The way in which individuals perceive chance means that a woman with a 1 in 5 chance may perceive that is only a 20% chance and so in her mind that is a low-ish chance; whereas another woman with a 1 in 5000 result may feel that to be very high chance compared to her friend's 1 in 50000 chance. Discussion of these results challenges the midwife to provide very individualised care and to explore the meaning and impact for the individual woman.

At the time of writing, there is a wide and passionate national debate underway regarding this screening programme, around both the ethical implications and the actual tests used. This debate is beyond the scope of this single chapter and readers are encouraged to explore the issues more widely and to ascertain the national position at the time of reading this chapter.

Currently, the national screening programme requires Trusts to offer those with high chance screening a diagnostic test, such as chorionic villus sampling (CVS) or amniocentesis. This offer has to be made with acknowledgment of the increased rate of miscarriage in women who have had invasive tests. This is not to say that invasive tests *cause* miscarriage. There is a higher rate in those women who have them (currently stated nationally as 1 in 100 chance) but it must be remembered that most invasive tests are done when there are already concerns regarding fetal development.

Over the last 10 years, non-invasive prenatal testing (NIPT) has become widely available in the UK. However, it is not yet an accepted part of the national screening programme. Trusts have had to make individual decisions about procuring and offering such tests, which has created a situation commonly referred to as a 'postcode lottery'. This alternative method of screening for chromosomal anomalies looks at fetal DNA in a maternal venous blood sample. The sensitivity and specificity of these tests is very much greater than the nationally offered combined or quad tests, but at far greater financial cost. There are many issues arising from this which cannot be explored here and are part of a fast-moving debate at present. These include arguments regarding eugenics (does offering a test imply that the condition is undesirable, frightening or 'bad'?). If the tests are more accurate, fewer babies will remain unidentified in pregnancy and so will this mean that fewer people will be born with such conditions (currently most confirmed diagnoses lead to termination)? Would better information pre-test mean that fewer women would undergo testing? Is it ethical that women in some areas are offered, at NHS expense, a test which increases the chance of miscarriage but are not offered an enhanced screening test without such a risk – in many cases telling them that they can go to the (unregulated) private sector for this? It is worth noting that the cost to the NHS of invasive and non-invasive testing are very similar – both very much more than the current combined or quad screening tests.

Further anomaly scanning takes place at 20 weeks of pregnancy to detect fetal structural abnormalities (Rydberg and Tuton 2016). Midwives need to ensure that women are aware of the purpose of this scan – that it is an anomaly scan. There is a widespread misunderstanding about this scan, with many referring to it as 'the gender scan'. Many specialist midwives can recount a great many situations where women are desperately angry and upset when an anomaly is identified at this scan, saying that 'they said everything was alright at the last scan' Women cannot truly give informed consent if they do not understand the purpose of the anomaly scan.

Benefits and Costs of Prenatal Screening

Ethical implications related to the broader application of NIPT need to be considered. Testing can be done from 10 weeks gestation. Early, easy and miscarriage risk free prediction of aneuploidies makes this approach acceptable and desirable to many women, in theory decreasing the risks of diagnostic tests. It is argued that this approach can provide early reassurances of a normal pregnancy or, alternatively, enables space for decision making in the case of a higher-chance result. It is vital to remember that, at the start of 2020, NIPT is only validated as a reliable screening test for trisomy 21, 18 and 13. This has not stopped various providers in the unregulated industry offering 'expanded testing' or 'platinum services' where the report offers an estimate of chance for other, much rarer, conditions. The Nuffield Council on Bioethics have been monitoring and reporting on this situation (https://www.nuffieldbioethics.org/publications/non-invasive-prenatal-testing).

Equally, NIPT may become available for predictors of a range of disorders which will be manifest in the unborn fetus's adult life. Currently, NHS genetic testing does not offer prenatal testing for adult onset conditions, but outside the NHS there is little effective regulation. Issues are therefore raised about the child's right not to be informed about predicted diseases in their life through broadening NIPT (de Jong et al. 2010).

It has been shown that NIPT is a highly sensitive and effective predictor for three specific fetal anomalies and can improve choices for women, quality of care and be cost effective overall (Chitty et al. 2016; Le Conte et al. 2017). The test, it is argued, can be useful in providing women with information and time for preparation should a woman prefer to continue her pregnancy in the understanding of fetal difference. Early use of the test could also provide a much-needed space in which midwives and clinicians can provide support and counselling (after effective training), to women and their families, towards prenatal psychosocial adaptation to parenthood (Hui Choi et al. 2012). Healthcare providers, in collaboration with sociologist and ethicists, must develop appropriate guidelines to address the needs of families and ethical challenges resulting from NIPT (Horn and Parker 2018). Evidence has suggested, however, that screening for trisomy anomalies, such as Down's syndrome, is still presented as a routine test by midwives, rather than an option where users can consider the information and are supported by providers to make individualised choices that meet their needs (Ukohor et al. 2017). Early aneuploidy screening tests may create uncertainty with decision making that could impact the informed consent process (Farrell et al. 2011), and some evidence suggests that choices should only be made through rigorous and appropriately supported processes to enable autonomous informed consent and procedures (Deans and Newson 2011). Equally, professional training to provide the support and guidance for women, prior to informed consent for fetal screening, must be effectively implemented (Silcock et al. 2014).

Healthcare Professionals' Experiences of Fetal Screening

Midwives who spend more time asking psychosocial questions of women undertaking fetal anomaly screening encourage effective communication with women which may ease and facilitate decision making (Martin et al. 2016). On the other hand, evidence suggests that women expressed dissatisfaction on how and what information is provided regarding prenatal screening (Asplin et al. 2012). It has been suggested that women would benefit from easy and frequent access to health professionals, who could deliver transparent information to support them in making decisions that reflect their values and beliefs (Aune and Moller 2012).

The views of midwives in relation to ultrasound during pregnancy have been examined in a study from Australia. Findings suggest that using ultrasound as a routine scanning tool has far reaching consequences and can influence women's decision making. Ultrasound scanning has become routine and normalised and therefore is unquestioned by women and can impact negatively on informed consent processes. As a result of routine screening, women may view the fetus as a person and subsequently put the health of the fetus before their own, leading to ethical and professional challenges for midwives, and which has implications for women's rights and the autonomy to make informed decisions in pregnancy and childbirth (Edvardsson et al. 2015, 2016). However, evidence suggests that women have differing views on informed consent and although they wish to be autonomous in their decisions, they seek and value advice from midwives (Ahmed et al. 2012). Midwives, however, perceive their roles to vary as facilitators of informed choice in antenatal screening, but seek clinical guidance on how to actively facilitate choices without compromising women's autonomy (Ahmed et al. 2013).

Women's Views of Fetal Screening

Women's views of fetal screening are explored in this section, due to the increased uptake of testing as women want to be informed about the possible risk of fetal abnormalities (Miltoft et al. 2018; Maiz et al. 2016; Lewis et al. 2014). However, many women expressed the view that extensive information about tests and possible results causes anxiety and worry (Lalor and Begley 2006) and places a burden of information on them which detracts from decision making about screening. Timely information, provided during individualised discussion, should be delivered by knowledgeable health professionals through pre-test counselling to aid informed decision making (Barr and Skirton 2013). More recently, Ledward (2017) suggested that greater emphasis should be placed on *'striking a balance'* to tailor individual maternal information needs and a better understanding of their preferences through adaptive communication skills by midwives. These findings concur with an earlier study by Carroll et al. (2012), which indicates that future research is required about the nature, form and means through which information is provided for parents to make decisions about fetal screening.

Women undergoing NIPT generally have positive experiences of this prenatal testing. However, there is a need for pre- and post-test counselling to ensure informed consent (Bowman-Smart et al. 2019). Brett et al. (2015) stress the importance of informed knowledge and understanding of some of the fetal abnormalities that could be identified, before women/parents make decisions, especially about conditions that could be life threatening for the fetus. Consequently, healthcare professionals have an ethical duty to continue to improve their clinical practice and develop theoretical knowledge to ensure that appropriate and timely information is available to women making difficult decisions about fetal screening (Howe 2014).

An interesting study from Iceland explored women's reflections on positive fetal screening and suggested that those women who continued with their pregnancy were still experiencing anxiety and concerns more than year after the birth and remembered in detail how results were presented and their feelings at the time. The women suggested that face-to-face news and extended knowledge about the test results was conducive to working through mixed feelings, especially if supported by a named midwife (Kristjansdottir and Gottfredsdottir 2014). Of equal importance is the role played by partners during fetal screening and the decisions made post results. It is suggested that midwives need to give more consideration to the fathers' views to ensure participation in the screening process (Reed 2009), and to ensure that informed decision making also involves the partner (Farrell et al. 2019). Communication training for midwives could improve care delivery and truly fulfil the concept of 'with woman', not just from the woman's perspective but 'with' men or partners too to improve relationships (Dheensa et al. 2013, 2015).

Termination After Diagnosis

Some women unfortunately need to make difficult decisions to terminate a pregnancy after diagnosis of a fetal anomaly. The information and support provided by healthcare professionals, and specifically midwives, can have an impact on how women and their families deal with fetal loss (Lipp 2008). The needs of the partner and how compassionate care was delivered are also considered (Andersson et al. 2014). In addition, literature also describes how midwives deal with preparing women for the termination and how they emotionally and physically support women, encouraging them to use adaptive coping strategies (Lafarge et al. 2013). It was equally important that psychological care, continuity of care and follow up care were provided by midwives (Asplin et al. 2014; Fisher and Lafarge 2015). However, little support or debriefing was immediately available to these professionals after they provided care for women at this very difficult time (Armour et al. 2018).

Women's experiences of a termination for fetal abnormalities resulted at times in dissociating themselves from the procedure, but ultimately wanting to attribute meaning to the birth experience despite the outcome (Hurt et al. 2008; Lafarge et al. 2013). Women described how they sought to acknowledge the baby and create memories that would validate their experience. They also commented on the quality of care and the kindness and compassion of healthcare staff who offered support through their presence (Andersson et al. 2014). Women need to make choices about viewing the fetus after termination and being cared for by experienced staff who provide empathetic care (Carlsson et al. 2016). Bereaved women are known to experience feelings of isolation and loss, but a period of reflection and quiet helped towards coming to terms with the ending of their pregnancy (Lotto et al. 2016). Further research is required to understand and acknowledge women's experiences during the labour and birth leading to a termination of a pregnancy for fetal abnormalities and indicate that there is still a need to prioritise women- centred care in these difficult and sensitive situations (Jones et al. 2017).

The literature was examined to identify how fetal screening and medicine impacts on the pregnant woman and her family and the views of health professionals in supporting women experiencing antenatal screening testing. Studies on women's views about fetal anomaly screening are also explored and analysed through Rodgers' framework of analysis, as in Table 4.1.

Conclusion

It is likely that there will be advancements and developments in NIPT in the future and therefore it is important that midwives can keep up with the changes and new information that is emerging. This will enable them to share information and support women and their partners with making decisions to meet needs and expectations. It is also important that they understand the type of information that could be shared and how this is delivered ethically, and with confidence, to ensure that the best care is delivered to fulfil the concept of 'with woman' and her family. Therefore, there is still a need for development of a range of multi-professional courses and resources to support rapidly changing knowledge and procedures in fetal medicine and screening (Patch et al. 2019). A competency framework, developed through expert knowledge, is being developed to assist healthcare professionals (HCPs) in their role to support women experiencing fetal screening processes and the consequent outcomes for them and their neonate.

The stories below illustrate the literature discussed earlier in this chapter.

Table 4.1 Concept analysis of 'with woman' in screening and fetal medicine.

Antecedents	Evidence	Attributes (A) and Consequences (C)
Benefits and cost of prenatal screening	Chitty et al. (2016) implementation of NIPT	Uptake of test (A) Choices for women (A) Informed decision making (C) Improved quality of care (C)
	Hui Choi et al. (2012) social support in prenatal psychosocial adaptation	Guidance for clinicians and MWs (A) MWs should receive adequate training to provide psychosocial assessment (C)
	Horn and Parker (2018) MWs understanding of genome techniques	Model of good ethical practice (A) Address needs and concerns of parents (C)
	Ukohor et al. (2017) organisation and delivery of fetal anomaly screening	A social model of care (A) Empowers service users and less tension for providers (C) Decision making uncertainty (A) Mechanisms to facilitate decision making (C)
	Farrell et al. (2011) early 1st trimester aneuploidy screening	Rigorous and appropriately supported processes (A) Enable autonomous informed consent and procedures (C)
	Deans and Newson (2011) choices on early screening	Professional and training programmes and practice guidelines (A) Prioritise informed consent and views/needs of service users (C)
	Silcock et al. (2014) effect of introduction of NIPT	
Healthcare professionals' experience	Martin et al. (2016) verbal and non-verbal communication during prenatal counselling	More psychosocial questions asked by MWs (A) Higher psychosocial communication by women (C)
	Asplin et al. (2012) needs and preferences regarding information after screening	Needs to improve care givers' methods for giving information(A) Improve women's satisfaction (C)
	Edvardsson et al. (2015, 2016) influence and use of ultrasound for screening	Unnecessary medicalisation of pregnancy (A) Protects women's rights to informed decision making and autonomy (C)
	Ahmed et al. (2012, 2013) perception of MWs' role as facilitators of informed choice in screening	Discussion rather than provide information through guidelines (A) Checking women's understanding of information given without compromising their autonomy (C)
	Aune and Moller (2012) making choices after risk assessment through prenatal screening	Improved distribution of information and frequent contact with healthcare professionals (A) Stress-free and easy access to transparent information to support informed choices to suit values and beliefs (C)

(Continued)

Table 4.1 (Continued)

Antecedents	Evidence	Attributes (A) and Consequences (C)
Women's views of fetal screening	Miltoft et al. (2018) uptake of follow up testing cfDNA	Need to avoid routine screening (A) Improved uptake of test without corresponding rise of termination (C)
	Maiz et al. (2016) maternal attitudes towards screening	Characteristics of women are maternal age, gestational age and attitude towards termination (A) Women prefer to be informed of results even in minor or suspected abnormalities (C)
		Balancing information with less detailed information in low-risk pregnancies (A) To reduce anxiety and worry in women (C)
	Lalor and Begley (2006) what do women want to know about fetal anomaly screening?	Overload of information detracts from decision making (A) Not sufficiently informed on screening (A) Appropriate timing, personal discussion by knowledgeable HCP will ensure informed decisions made (C)
	Barr and Skirton (2013) informed decision making about antenatal screening	Pre- and post-test counselling before informed consent (A) Generally positive experiences with NIPT (C)
	Ledward (2017) Lewis et al. (2014) Bowman-Smart et al. (2019) Women's experience with NIPT	Need for knowledge and understanding, clear and written information (A) Structured follow up programme with continued and easy access to HCPs (C)
	Brett et al. (2015) parent's experiences of counselling	Need for bad news to be delivered face to face, extended information and help to sort out feelings (A) Support from a named MW (C)
	Kristjansdottir and Gottfredsdottir (2014) Adjustment to positive screening	Consideration to the fathers' views (A) Ensure participation in the screening process (C) Ensures that informed decision making involves the partner (C) Communication training for midwives (A) Improves care delivery and truly fulfils the concept of 'with woman' and improves relationships with partners (C)
	Reed (2009), Farrell et al. (2019), and Dheensa et al. (2015) fathers' needs and involvement in decision making in prenatal screening	

Table 4.1 (Continued)

Antecedents	Evidence	Attributes (A) and Consequences (C)
Termination of pregnancy	Lipp (2008) healthcare professionals	Impact of information and support (A) Women and families dealing with fetal loss (C)
	Andersson et al. (2014) needs of partners	
	Lafarge et al. (2013) MWs preparing women	Compassionate care (A) Support for partners (C) Presence of MWs (C)
	Asplin et al. (2014)	Emotional and physical support of women (A) Encourages adaptive coping strategies (C)
	Fisher and Lafarge (2015) MW's care	
Women's experiences	Armour et al. (2018) MW's wellbeing	Continuity and follow up care (A) impact on psychological wellbeing (C)
	Hurt et al. (2008)	Support and debriefing (A) Need for organisational strategies to support MWs (C)
	Carlsson et al. (2016)	Isolation (A) Need to validate the birth (C)
	Lotto et al. (2016)	Need to make choices (A) Viewing the fetus (A) Cared for by experienced staff (A) Empathetic care (C)
	Jones et al. (2017)	Isolation and loss (A) Given time for reflection and quiet (C)
		Further research (A) Understand and acknowledge women's experiences (C)
		Prioritising women-centred care (C)

The Specialist Midwife's Stories

Angie's Story

Almost every expectant parent asks the question 'Is my baby ok?'. The NHS offers screening tests to all women to try to identify babies affected by a range of conditions. Many issues are raised by the offer of screening, including misunderstanding of the purpose of screening, ethical issues about the desirability of prenatal identification of conditions such as trisomy 21 (Downs syndrome) and the impact of a screen positive result on a woman.

The role of the specialist midwife for screening and fetal medicine is broad and complex. One of the most important aspects is working with women on an individualised basis. This also includes a discussion as to whether to have screening at all. It is widely assumed by healthcare workers that screening will

(Continued)

be accepted by all. It is frequently reported that the offer of screening (an option within the care pathway) has been presented as 'we'll just do ..', as though the woman had either already consented or did not have an option. If the woman's moral or spiritual beliefs are such that she would not consider termination of pregnancy, some will conclude that they may be better not to have the information provided through screening, preferring to wait to meet their baby before gaining information about any health issues. The author has worked with several women who know that they have a one in four chance that their baby being affected by a very serious inherited condition which is likely to be fatal, where it is possible to identify the conditions prenatally. Their individual decisions about when and if they want testing have been wide ranging, based on their life circumstances, religious beliefs, previous experience and so on.

Inaya*'s Story

A secretary in the maternity ultrasound department contacted the specialist midwife concerned that Inaya had phoned to decline the offered first trimester scan. It is widely assumed that 'everyone' wants and has scans in pregnancy. Inaya had simply stated that she didn't want any scans at all and had not appeared willing to discuss this.

When the specialist midwife contacted Inaya, she explained that she respected Inaya's right to accept or decline the offer of scans but wanted the opportunity to check if she required any information or if there were any special circumstances which she would like the team to be aware of. Inaya explained that this was her third pregnancy. Both her previous children had died within days of birth due to an inherited condition, the effects of which can readily be seen on ultrasound scans. She told the midwife 'I just can't live through this pregnancy if I know that I will watch this child die too. My religion means that I have no choice but to continue with the pregnancy, so the best thing for me is simply not to know – that way I can continue to hope.'

An issue in this situation was that declining scans meant that other, possibly important, information would not be available. Understandably, her focus was on information that she did not want to know; however, the potential benefits of placental location, confirmation of gestational age and identification of other (potentially treatable) health issues affecting the baby needed to be explained and discussed, ensuring that Inaya was making a truly informed decision. After a great deal of discussion, the agreement was made that no scan appointments would be made, but if at any stage Inaya felt that she was ready for and wanted a scan, the team would attempt to fit her in on that day.

At 26 weeks, Inaya phoned the midwife, saying that she felt 'as ready as I will ever be', and asking that the midwife should accompany her. A senior sonographer, understanding the sensitivity of this situation, agreed to give up her lunch break to undertake the scan. At the start of the scan Inaya asked not to see the scan image. Focusing immediately on the potential concern, the sonographer was able to tell Inaya that the initial appearance was that her baby was growing and developing entirely normally. The midwife and sonographer felt hugely privileged to share this experience with Inaya. Many happy and relieved tears were shed that day.

Individualised care may be perceived to take greater effort and to require caregivers and 'the system' to work flexibly, but experiencing positive outcomes, such as the midwife and sonographer shared with Inaya, provide rich reward. Often there are multiple factors which affect decision making. The impact of religious teaching can be powerful, even in cases where the woman says that she does not have a faith. Religious teachings are shared with children in many ways, often simply as one point of view being 'right' and another 'wrong' within that society. The author has learned to explore the woman's broad social, cultural and religious background when negotiating complicated decision making. At times of crisis, a basic human need to is to seek direction from principles we have learned earlier in life. It is important to acknowledge these principles, but it can also be important to offer appropriate challenge to clarify the relevance of such inculcated beliefs to the individual at this moment in their life. This requires skill and experience. Midwives facing working in complex areas such as this should consider the need to undertake formal counselling training, or to refer on to appropriately qualified colleagues.

Midwives need to develop cultural and religious awareness. It is appropriate to ask about faith issues in the context of decision making. This can show both awareness and respect. It can feel daunting to ask a question when you may not understand the implications of the answer. However, asking is the first step. If the woman refers to a cultural or faith tradition which you are not familiar with, acknowledging this is both honest and potentially powerful. The woman may be willing and able to share information with you, alternatively you may need to seek advice and guidance from a faith leader. Hospital chaplains are well placed to support both patients as well as care providers in such situations.

Tess*'s Story

At her first scan (12 weeks) Tess was given the news that her baby had anencephaly. Anencephaly affects 1 in 2000 pregnancies in the UK. It is usually seen at the 12-week scan and is a clear diagnosis. There is no treatment possible and babies with this condition will usually die before birth or very soon afterwards (Moore 2010).

(Continued)

The sonographer explained her findings to Tess and advised that because this is a lethal anomaly a termination would be arranged in the next few days. The specialist midwife was asked to see Tess to explain the termination arrangements. As a midwife, Liz started the conversation by acknowledging that there had been unexpected news at the scan, and asked what Tess felt about what she had been told. She was therefore starting with the principle of being 'with woman'. To do this we have to ask; we cannot and must not assume.

Tess was clearly dealing with very complex emotions and appeared initially to be unwilling to discuss the situation. Using gentle, open ended questions, Liz gathered the information that for Tess, the idea of a termination was contrary to the religious beliefs and moral code she had grown up with. She felt that the sonographer's approach and assumption had disrespected her belief system and so had caused Tess to question the reasoning and motivation behind the advice being offered. Liz was clear in her explanation that, as a midwife, her role was to help Tess reach the decision which was right for her, whether that was to continue the pregnancy or to bring it to an end. Liz would be there to support her and arrange ongoing care. It was agreed that Tess needed some time to reflect on the news and she agreed to meet with Liz again the following day. Liz provided information about various support groups and information sources that Tess could access, if she wished.

On her return, it was clear that Tess was experiencing major dissonance between her religious beliefs and her understanding of the facts of the situation which faced her child. Tess accepted Liz's offer to involve the Roman Catholic chaplain at the hospital, who was able to offer spiritual guidance. Over the following two weeks, Tess had two appointments to commence termination, but on both occasions decided that she could not go ahead. On both occasions, Liz spent time with her and acted as her advocate. Thus, Tess made the decision to carry her baby to term. She understood that this might mean that her baby would die before birth, and if liveborn her baby would probably die very soon.

Liz became her named midwife, providing all her antenatal care and initiating discussions with other members of the healthcare team to negotiate care which Tess found acceptable and supportive. She attended scans and other appointments with Tess, working to ensure that everyone involved in Tess's care was respectful of her decision to continue the pregnancy. At 20 weeks, it was identified that Tess's baby was a girl. She named her Ava.

The neonatal team were involved very early, working to agree a plan with Tess about how to best care for Ava after birth. There is little recent experience in the UK of caring for babies with anencephaly because it is so readily identified and in almost every case termination is agreed. It was agreed with Tess that we would follow a parallel planning approach, preparing for both the best and the worst outcomes. Liz suggested referral to the local children's hospice and Tess felt that this respected the reality of Ava's life; even if it would only be very short, it should be the very best it could be. Tess was clear that because no medical intervention would help Ava, she should not be admitted to the neonatal unit. The principles of care were to be maximising Ava's time with her mum and ensuring that it was as peaceful and uninterrupted as it could be. At each scan or antenatal check, the team focused on celebrating Ava's presence at that moment and Liz and Tess shared several very poignant times. Palpating and auscultation can be a task, or it can become an opportunity for communication between midwife and mother, mother and baby and indeed between midwife and baby. Although it was known that Ava's brain was being damaged because it lacked the protection of the skull, she reacted to palpation on almost every occasion.

Liz discussed the situation with the neonatal team, and Tess was able to meet with one of the neonatal consultants to discuss her wishes for Ava's care after birth. It was agreed that as no active treatment was possible to prolong Ava's life, she should stay with Tess for whatever time she had after birth. Advice was sought from the tissue viability specialist nurse to ensure that appropriate dressings were available to cover Ava's brain. Ava was not able to present in the usual cephalic position because of her incomplete skull. As is reported in most cases of anencephaly, there was a degree of polyhydramnios and so a risk of cord prolapsed existed. After several discussions, it was agreed that if Ava was alive at 39 weeks, elective caesarean section was appropriate, both to avoid the potential risks of emergency caesarean but also to maximise the chance of live birth.

Approaching the birth, Tess was troubled by the idea that Ava might die after birth, before it was possible for her to be baptised. Liz discussed this with members of the multi-disciplinary team, including the catholic chaplain, and it was agreed that the chaplain would be present outside the operating theatre in case emergency baptism was required. As it so happened this was the case and Ava was baptised in theatre. Her heart continued to beat, and she took intermittent gasping breaths over the next three hours but remained in skin to skin contact with Tess throughout this time. Liz remained with Tess and Ava, providing both routine post-operative, post-delivery care and emotional support. During this time Tess's parish priest attended and conducted a full baptism.

Liz provided postnatal care for Tess and attended Ava's funeral, during which time it was evident that Tess, although naturally grieving for her daughter, was at peace with her decision to carry Ava to term and believed that she had done her best for her daughter.

(Continued)

Cultural identity and social expectations are powerful influences on humans. A sense of belonging has been recognised to be a fundamental human need (Maslow 1954). For the parent of a baby who dies, there is often a sense that life should be recognised by society in some way. A baby born before 24 weeks gestation is not recognised as a person in British law, with no formal certification of life or death being available. The stillbirth and neonatal death charity SANDS recommends that parents should be offered some form of certification as a tangible recognition of their baby's existence. Being 'with woman', entering her experience of the world, can sometimes raise issues of belonging that are more challenging.

A Woman's Story

Hannah's Story

I discovered I was pregnant for the first time in the summer of 2014; this happy surprise was quickly followed by the onset of hyperemesis gravidarum . . . in the weeks that followed my partner and I daydreamed about what parenthood might be like, we wondered if the baby might have my blonde hair, or James' hazel eyes; we debated if we would bring them up as a Liverpool or an Arsenal Fan . . . Between asking all of these 'important' questions I was being relentlessly sick; whilst anti-emetics and fluid therapy provided some relief, not a day went by without pregnancy and sickness at the forefront of my mind. An ultrasound scan at seven weeks showed a heartbeat and James and I fell head over heels for the grainy blob on the screen; our baby was growing, and everything was wonderful, however terrible I might have felt we knew our baby would be worth it.

I reached my 12-week dating scan over a stone lighter than my pre-pregnancy weight, my vomit now blood-stained from the damage to my throat: yet my stomach beginning to swell into the cutest little bump. I felt as though my body was working so hard for my baby – and James and I were so excited to see how our little one had grown, having already heard a healthy heartbeat and with such strong pregnancy symptoms we felt reassured all would be well and the scan would be a positive bonding experience. We bought our scan picture frames from the antenatal reception – it was hospital policy to pay for a scan picture prior to your appointment – and sat down in a waiting room with other excitable expectant parents.

There were two sonographers in our room, Janine and her student. The scan began as with any other – we declined the combined screening and then watched eagerly as the image of our baby flickered onto the screen. I saw my 'baby' and I instantly began to panic, I felt like I couldn't breathe and began to cry – I couldn't find my words but managed to say 'that's not right!' James tried to calm me; he had never seen a dating scan before and pointed out the movements that in his eyes meant this was still all normal. Janine looked panicked too; her student held onto my hand tightly. I finally managed to ask if what I was seeing was conjoined twins – Janine said she believed it was but needed to continue the scan, I became strangely calm at this point as James and I continued to watch the scan on the screen – as if with new eyes – we could see our two babies! Beautiful twins, hearts beating, legs kicking and despite everything perfect to us – a fierce love and protectivity swept over me and I knew I would do anything to keep my babies safe. Janine left the scan to speak with a consultant and her student helped me to clean my face and calm my breathing before I left. The atmosphere in the waiting area had changed – perhaps they had heard my cries or seen the mascara staining my cheeks, or our empty picture frames – it was silent and solemn; I kept my head down as we were escorted to the quiet room to meet with our consultant.

Our consultant Miss R was able to scan us again later that afternoon; the more we saw of our babies the more we fell in love. It was difficult to determine at this stage whether the babies had one or two hearts between them – making it impossible to know what their chances of survival might be. As much as Miss R tried to explain that a poor outcome was very likely, I was determined to continue with the pregnancy and was already dreaming about leaving the hospital with our separated medical miracle babies in a few months' time. We were referred for an urgent review with a fetal cardiologist at St Georges the next morning – so we went home praying for a miracle.

St Georges was a horrible experience; everyone we met was perfectly pleasant, however it is difficult to feel warmly to people who are telling you things you just don't want to hear. After an hour of scanning in silence we were given the diagnosis of thoracophagus conjoined twins. We were told in no uncertain terms that our babies would die. The twins shared a single complex heart which was already beginning to fail leading to hydrops in both babies. We were told our twins would likely die at some point during my pregnancy; if they did survive to term they would need to be delivered by classical caesarean section, they would not be resuscitated. There was no chance of separation.

I was told that I was young and that I should 'save my uterus'; that I would have another baby and that this would not happen again. None of this made me feel any better. I felt like my world had ended; our last shreds of hope had been stolen from us and it was so unfair.

(Continued)

We were faced with an impossible choice.

I could continue with my pregnancy as long as it may last – eventually delivering my dead or dying twins by caesarean section; or I could interrupt my pregnancy – delivering my dead babies naturally but in turn taking on a lifetime of guilt, pain, and what-ifs . . . Essentially our final decision was one of love; as I believe all decisions regarding termination of pregnancy for abnormalities are. Our babies were suffering; they were in heart failure – for them birth would bring so much pain. This way we could let them go whilst all they would ever know was my warmth and my love.

Our care was returned to the bereavement team at my local hospital, Miss R cried with us as we discussed the termination. The antenatal screening midwives answered my questions as best they could, the bereavement specialist midwife sat with us as we discussed our wishes and helped to devise a 'birth plan' of sorts; part of this was an additional scan – performed by Miss R – which allowed our parents to see our babies, their first grandchildren, wriggling and kicking on the screen. We were shown nothing but compassion and support, we were given the time we needed and chose the date for admission ourselves – allowing 'family time' and vital access to counselling in the interim. Gentle support and guidance carried us from the abyss of a lethal diagnosis to a place where we were ready to meet our babies.

I was eventually induced at 14 weeks, cared for in the specialist forget-me-not suite on the labour ward. My labour was straightforward – around six hours of mild back ache and cramping, my midwives remained present enough to make me feel safe but also respected our privacy and grief by giving us space. My waters broke, and I began to panic, huge quantities of blood-stained liquor spilled onto the floor, staining my legs and feet. Two midwives were instantly at my side, a sudden fear that my babies would be delivered into all this mess overwhelmed me. My midwife Aimee changed the bedding and washed my shaking legs and feet when I was too scared to stand for myself; 20 minutes later at 15:30 on the 29 September 2014 she handed me my baby boys.

Jude and Henry were absolutely gorgeous and perfect to us, despite their early gestation we marvelled at their detailed beauty. We held and loved them for hours. Jude and Henry were beautifully wrapped and respectfully cared for by our midwives, who also provided a memory box with footprints and photographs. The hospital chaplain performed a blessing for our boys and Miss R our consultant visited us on the ward, she cleaned the bed and I felt humbled that she would find time in her day to be with us.

We left the hospital the next day with a memory box and broken hearts – we continued to be supported at home by our bereavement midwife Sheryl – including practical advice with funeral arrangements. We also received vital support from the SANDs helpline and counselling services through my university. By the time we reached our six-week postnatal appointment at the hospital we were grieving healthily and coping well – something I attribute to the exceptional care we received from the time of our 12-week scan to the funeral of our babies. I felt as if our midwives and the wider obstetric team had walked with us through the darkest days and supported us to a healthier place. We were given a number to call for when I next became pregnant – at which point the seamless support began again – this time resulting in the birth of our rainbow baby, Alfie.

Providing sensitive and compassionate care can make a real difference to parents like me and James, and we are eternally grateful for all the wonderful care that we, Jude and Henry received.

Lessons Learnt

As has been discussed in this chapter, being 'with woman' has broad implications, not all of which are addressed in the usual midwifery curriculum. As midwives work with women and families, their understanding of the variety of human experience should develop. Cultural, religious and social awareness is fundamental towards efforts to be 'with woman'.

In being 'with woman', midwives achieve greatly enhanced satisfaction in the care provided (for both the woman and the midwife), but also open themselves to issues of dissonance and emotional conflict. If healthcare professionals are committed to this style of working, it is important that midwifery education programmes and employers recognise and support emotional growth and wellbeing. Above all, however, midwives must take responsibility for developing their skills and knowledge but also for their continued emotional wellbeing. This means addressing work–life balance, identifying sources of support and being willing to talk about this often-invisible part of midwifery work and the impact and cost to their lives.

Finally, the compassion displayed and support offered by healthcare professionals is forever remembered by women who tragically have to opt for a termination. Hannah's story highlights the moments during which acts of kindness by a midwife and consultant are portraited and perceived as steps towards the healing process. As Hannah says, 'sensitive and compassionate care can make a real difference'.

References

Ahmed, S., Bryant, L.D., Tizro, Z. et al. (2012). Interpretations of informed choice in antenatal screening: a cross-cultural Q-methodology study. *Social Science & Medicine* 74: 997–1004.

Ahmed, S., Bryant, L.D., and Cole, P. (2013). Midwives' perceptions of their role as facilitators of informed choice in antenatal screening. *Midwifery* 29: 745–750.

Andersson, L.M., Christensson, K., and Gemzell-Danielsson, K. (2014). Experiences, feelings and thoughts of women undergoing second trimester medical termination of pregnancy. *PLoS One* 9: 29. https://doi.org/10.1371/journal.pone.0115957.

Armour, S., Gilkison, A., and Hunter, M. (2018). The lived experience of midwives caring for women facing termination of pregnancy in the late second and third trimester. *Women and Birth* 31 (Supp 1): S14.

Asplin, N., Wessel, H., Marions, L. et al. (2012). Pregnant women's experiences, needs and preferences regarding information about malformations detected by ultrasound scan. *Sexual & Reproductive Health* 3: 73–78.

Asplin, N., Wessel, H., Marions, L. et al. (2014). Pregnancy termination due to fetal anomaly: women's reactions, satisfaction & experiences of care. *Midwifery* 30: 620–627.

Aune, I. and Moller, A. (2012). "I want a choice, but I don't want to decide"- a qualitative study of pregnant women's experiences regarding early ultrasound risk assessment for chromosomal abnormalities. *Midwifery* 28: 14–23.

Barr, O. and Skirton, H. (2013). Informed decision making regarding antenatal screening for fetal abnormality in the United Kingdom: a qualitative study of parents and professionals. *Nursing and Health Sciences* 15: 318–325.

Bowman-Smart, H., Savulescu, J., Mand, C. et al. (2019). Small cost to pay for peace of mind: women's experiences with non-invasive prenatal testing. *Australian and New Zealand Journal of Obstetrics and Gynaecology* 59: 649–655.

Brett, E.L., Jarvholm, S., Ekman-Joelsson, B.M. et al. (2015). Parents' experience of counselling and their need for support following a prenatal diagnosis of congenital heart disease- a qualitative study in a Swedish context. *BMC Pregnancy and Childbirth* 15: 171. https://doi.org/10.1186/s12884-015-0610-4.

Carlsson, T., Bergman, G., Karlsson, A.M. et al. (2016). Experiences of termination of pregnancy for a fetal anomaly: a qualitative study of virtual community messages. *Midwifery* 41: 54–60.

Carroll, E., Owen-Smith, A., Shaw, A. et al. (2012). A qualitative investigation of the decision-making process of couples considering prenatal screening for Down syndrome. *Prenatal Diagnosis* 32: 57–63.

Chitty, L.S., Wright, D., Hill, M. et al. (2016). Uptake, outcomes and costs of implementing non-invasive prenatal testing for Down's syndrome into NHS maternity care: prospective cohort study in eight diverse maternity units. *British Medical Journal* 354: i3426. https://doi.org/10.1136/bmj.i3426.

De Jong, A., Dondorp, W.J., de Die-Smulders, C. et al. (2010). Non-invasive prenatal testing: ethical issues explored. *European Journal of Human Genetics* 18: 272–277.

Deans, Z. and Newson, A.J. (2011). Should non-invasiveness change informed consent procedures for prenatal diagnosis? *Health Care Analysis* 19 (2): 122–132.

Dheensa, S., Metcalfe, A., and Williams, R.A. (2013). Men's experiences of antenatal screening: a meta synthesis of the qualitative research. *International Journal of Nursing Studies* 50: 121–133.

Dheensa, S., Metcalfe, A., and Williams, R.A. (2015). What do men want from antenatal screening? Findings from an interview study in England. *Midwifery* 31: 208–214.

Edvardsson, K., Mogren, I., Lalos, A. et al. (2015). A routine tool with far-reaching influence: Australian midwives' views on the use of ultrasound during pregnancy. *BMC Pregnancy and Childbirth* 15: 195. https://doi.org/10.1186/s12884-015-0632-y.

Edvardsson, K., Lalos, A., Ahman, A. et al. (2016). Increasing possibilities- increasing dilemmas: a qualitative study of Swedish midwives' experiences of ultrasound use in pregnancy. *Midwifery* 42: 46–53.

Farrell, R.M., Dolgin, N., Flocke, S.A. et al. (2011). Risk and uncertainty: shifting decision making for aneuploidy screening to the first trimester of pregnancy. *Genetics in Medicine* 13 (5): 429–436.

Farrell, R.M., Mercer, M.B., Agatisa, P.K. et al. (2019). Balancing needs and autonomy: the involvement of partners of pregnant women's partners in decisions about cfDNA. *Qualitative Health Research* 29 (2): 211–221.

Fisher, J. and Lafarge, C. (2015). Women's experience of care when undergoing termination of pregnancyfor fetal anomaly in England. *Journal of Reproduction & Infant Psychology* 33 (1): 69–87.

Horn, R. and Parker, M. (2018). Health professionals' and researchers' perspectives on prenatal whole genome. and exome sequencing: "we can't shut the door now, the genie's out, we need to refine it". *PLoS One* 13 (9): e0204158. https://doi.org/10.10371/journal.pone.0204158.

Howe, D. (2014). Ethics of prenatal ultrasound. *Best Practice & Research: Clinical Obstetrics & Gynaecology* 28: 443–451.

Hui Choi, W.H., Lee, G.L., Chan, C.H.Y. et al. (2012). The relationship of social support, uncertainty, self-efficacy and commitment to prenatal psychosocial adaptation. *Journal of Advanced Nursing* 68 (12): 2633–2645.

Hurt, K., France, E., and Ziebland, S. (2008). "My brain couldn't move from planning a birth to planning a funeral": a qualitative study of parent's experiences of decisions after ending a pregnancy for fetal abnormalities. *International Journal of Nursing Studies* 46 (8): 1111–1121.

Jones, K., Baird, K., and Fenwick, J. (2017). Women's experiences of labour and birth when having a termination of pregnancy for fetal abnormality in the second trimester of pregnancy: a qualitative meta-synthesis. *Midwifery* 50: 42–54.

Kristjansdottir, H. and Gottfredsdottir, H. (2014). Making sense of the situation: women's reflection of positive fetal screening 11-21 months after giving birth. *Midwifery* 30: 643–649.

Lafarge, C., Mitchell, K., and Fox, P. (2013). Women's experiences of coping with pregnancy termination for fetal abnormality. *Qualitative Health Research* 23: 924–936.

Lalor, J. and Begley, C. (2006). Fetal anomaly screening: what do women want to know? *Journal of Advanced Nursing* 55 (1): 11–19.

Le Conte, G., Letourneau, A., Jani, J. et al. (2017). Cell-free fetal DNA analysis in maternal plasma as screening test for trisomies 21, 18 and 13 in twin pregnancies. *Ultrasound in Obstetrics & Gynecology* 52: 318–324.

Ledward, A. (2017). Pregnat women's experiences of screening for fetal abnormalities according to NICE guidelines: how should midwives communicate information? *Evidence Based Midwifery* 15 (4): 112–119.

Lennon, S.L. (2016). Risk perception in pregnancy: a concept analysis. *Journal of Advanced Nursing* 72 (9): 2016–2029.

Lewis, C., Hill, M., Silcock, C. et al. (2014). Non-invasive prenatal testing for trisomy 21: a cross-sectional survey for service users' views and likely uptake. *BJOG* 121: 582–594.

Lipp, A. (2008). A woman centred service in termination of pregnancy: a grounded theory study. *Contemporary Nurse* 31: 9–19.

Lotto, R., Armstrong, N., and Smith, L.K. (2016). Care provision during termination of pregnancy following diagnosis of a severe congenital anomaly: a qualitative study of what is important to parents. *Midwifery* 43: 14–20. https://doi.org/10.1016/j.midw.2016.10.003.

Maiz, N., Burgos, J., Barbazan, M.J. et al. (2016). Maternal attitude towards first trimester screening for fetal abnormalities. *Prenatal Diagnosis* 36: 449–455.

Martin, L., der Wal, J.J., Gitsels-van, T. et al. (2016). Clients' psychosocial communication and midwives' verbal and nonverbal communication during prenatal counselling for anomaly screening. *Patient Education and Counselling* 99 (1): 85–91.

Maslow, A.H. (1954). *Motivation and Personality*. New York: Harper & Row.

Miltoft, C.B., Rode, L., and Tabor, A. (2018). Positive view and increased likely uptake of follow-up testing with analysis of cell-free fetal DNA as alternative to invasive testing among Danish pregnant women. *Acta Obstetricia et Gynecologica Scandinavica* 97: 577–586.

Moore, L. (2010). Anencephaly. *Journal of Diagnostic Medical Sonography* 26 (6): 286–289.

Patch, C., Hill, S., Sigsworth, J. et al. (2019). Advances in genomics translate into clinical practice nowhere more significant than in maternity care. *Midwives* 22: 42–46.

Reed, K. (2009). Fathers' involvement in antenatal screening: midwives' views. *British Journal of Midwifery* 17 (4): 218–222.

Rydberg, C. and Tuton, K. (2016). Detection of fetal abnormalities by second – trimester ultrasound screening in a non-selected population. *Acta Obstetricia et Gynecologica Scandinavica* 96: 176–182.

Silcock, C., Liao, L.M., Hill, M. et al. (2014). Will the introduction of non-invasive prenatal testing for Down's syndrome undermine informed choice? *Health Expectations* 18: 1658–1671.

Ukohor, H.O., Hirst, J., Closs, S.J. et al. (2017). A framework for describing the influence of service organisation and delivery on participation in fetal anomaly screening in England. *Journal of Pregnancy* 2017: 4975091. https://doi.org/10.1155/2017/4975091.

5

'With the High-Risk Woman and Neonate'

Anna M. Brown, Leontia Pillay, Kath Lawton, Ann Robinson;
Kerry-Anne Horne, Rhiannon Brown, Victoria Walker,
Julia Derrick, Amy Duncan, Olivia Boswell, Jo Willard (midwives); and
Katrina (woman) and Angela* (woman)

Introduction

This chapter explores the 'with woman' concept for the high-risk woman. Whilst putting together the content for this chapter, COVID-19 became a global pandemic and pregnant women were placed in a 'vulnerable' category.

The Royal College of Obstetricians & Gynaecologists (RCOG) together with the Royal College of Midwives (RCM), Royal College of Paediatricians & Child Health (RCPCH), Public Health England (PHE) and Public Health Scotland (PHS) issued information and guidance regarding maternity services and care by healthcare professionals to ensure prevention and reduce viral transmission and the provision of safe care for pregnant women suspected or confirmed with COVID-19 (RCOG 2020a). The virus is relatively new and therefore there is a dearth of evidence which is being updated on a weekly basis as more information and data about COVID-19 is collated and analysed. To date, little is known about the effects of the virus on vulnerable groups such as pregnant women and their fetuses and the risks to women and neonates during labour and postpartum (UKOSS 2020).

Some very recent publications emerging from China suggest that pregnant women are no more likely than the general population to succumb to COVID-19, although it is known that pregnancy alters the immune system and its response to infections (Mor and Cardenas 2010). However, it is not yet known if vertical transmission from mother to neonate in utero or intrapartum is probable, and the number of pregnancies that have been affected with significance to the infant is not yet determined (Chen et al. 2020a; Chen et al. 2020b; Li et al. 2020).

Global evidence to date suggests that although pregnant women may display symptoms of COVID-19, these are usual mild to moderate and most women make a full recovery with little or no morbidity (PHE 2020). However, all pregnant women with other risk factors and long-term conditions – such as cystic fibrosis, asthma, cancer and other rare diseases such as sickle cell anaemia – are more vulnerable, and advice and guidance from the Department of Health encourages self-isolation and social distancing to avoid the virus.

During the time when lockdown was enforced, pregnancy care continued with midwifery teams and a known midwife, although this was carried out in a virtual capacity, either through telephone consultation or available apps (RCOG 2020a). Face-to-face contact for physical assessments (a minimum of six visits: WHO 2020) and scanning was carried out in a designated maternity unit or pre-planned location, should complications develop such as hypertension or pre-eclampsia. This is to ensure minimal contact with healthcare professionals and risk to both woman and midwife (RCOG 2020b). Other advice and guidance for both expectant women and health professionals during the intrapartum period and then postnatally was updated on a regular basis as and when new evidence emerged (RCOG 2020a). Despite the lack of published evidence, stories from women and midwives during the pandemic illustrate how supportive care could demonstrate 'with woman' compassion and empathy by many frontline healthcare professionals who placed their own lives at risk during these unprecedented times.

A Midwife's Experience

Kerry – Being 'with Woman' during a Global Pandemic

It's interesting to think about how a global pandemic can have such an impact on the ways in which midwives care for women. For many women, the role of their midwife has taken on a greater importance than ever. Restrictions on visitors may mean that women feel more alone and isolated than they would have expected when admitted to antenatal or postnatal wards, and for some women, difficulties such as arranging childcare may mean that they cannot have a birth partner other than their midwife. This has caused anxiety and upset for many women, but the feedback we have received would seem to show that they feel grateful for the care and support they have received from their midwives (and other maternity staff) and that it has still been possible to be a positive experience for them. However, I don't believe this means that there has been a change in how we care for them; we have always been 'with woman' – caring for and supporting them by journeying together with their hands in ours – however, by removing or reducing other forms of support, our role has been brought into the forefront and its importance highlighted.

The difference that I have noticed, though, which has made me think more carefully about how I offer that support, is the barriers which have been put up between midwives and the women we care for; physical barriers such as the wearing of masks and aprons even for routine contact such as antenatal appointments, and barriers of distance as we change our practice to provide care remotely when possible, over the telephone. Can you truly be 'with' someone if you can't read their facial expressions and body language, or they yours? Simple things, such as a reassuring smile that all is well whilst I silently count the fetal heart rate, cannot be seen as easily. Supporting a woman whose mental health may be deteriorating can be more difficult when you cannot see the visual cues that may contradict her words. Even face-to-face support can be made difficult by feeling unable to offer a reassuring touch to the arm or hand. There may also be emotional barriers; concern for our own welfare and that of our families and how our work may put us at risk of exposure could have an impact on how open we are able to be to the concerns of our women. Having to pause on the way to answering a call bell, even an emergency one, to put on our PPE, again puts a barrier in between us and the women, and feels like we are putting ourselves ahead of them, which may be something we are not used to feeling.

However, do these barriers adversely affect the care we give? I don't believe so, I certainly haven't found that women feel less supported, or that they find the precautions we are having to take off-putting. Perhaps the wearing of masks and gloves, and the caution to place physical distance between ourselves and others, has become so commonplace that they don't notice it as much as we would otherwise expect – or maybe they do notice and simply find it reassuring in a time of worry and uncertainty. Will this pandemic have a long-term effect on how we are 'with woman'? Possibly, but I believe this will be for the better; forcing us to reflect on why and how we do things, and to find different ways to communicate and care.

High-Risk Pregnancies and Birth

Raised BMI, Pregnancy Induced Hypertension, Postpartum Haemorrhage and Multiple Pregnancy

The rest of this chapter will focus on the impact of high-risk pregnancies on the 'with woman' concept and how conditions in pregnancy – such as pregnancy induced hypertension, obesity and multiple pregnancies – can affect the outcome for women and neonates in both a physical and a psychological sense (Bothamley & Boyle 2009). The literature is now examined from both the women's and health professional's perspective and how they perceive 'with woman' was fulfilled in these at-risk pregnancies.

Midwives' Perspectives

Midwives may find it difficult to accommodate a woman's expectations and wishes when faced with difficult decisions related to high-risk pregnancies and birth. However, midwives must provide maternity care that will minimise risk and give a positive outcome for both the mother and her baby, thus ensuring that care given is both sensitive and respectful and tailored to individual women's circumstances (Lee 2014).

An interesting study from Japan sought to find out the views of midwives on how they could humanise birth in high-risk pregnancies and concluded that professionals perceived a barrier to normalising birth. They felt that their responsibilities to ensure a safe outcome for both mother and baby involved medical intervention and a fear of potential legal repercussions if maternal and fetal morbidity and mortality resulted. Women were also seen to lack active involvement in the decision-making process and reported a lack of confidence and competence by midwives in providing high-risk care. The authors suggested that improved communication and a trusting relationship between mother and healthcare professionals would facilitate shared decision making, continued care and reduced stress for both mother and midwife (Behruzi et al. 2010).

It has been found that the behaviours and attitudes of senior midwifery and neonatal staff play a significant role in enhancing the performance of the more junior workforce in providing safe and quality maternity care (Sinni et al. 2014,). The findings in Sinni et al.'s 2014 study suggest that enhanced performance by senior midwives through role modelling and training for less experienced staff would ensure the development in confidence and competence, especially in high-risk perinatal care. In addition, a robust and clear clinical governance framework, a sound knowledge of organisational policies and procedures and a dominant role of midwives amongst junior staff strongly influenced the quality of care provision and outcomes (Sinni et al. 2014). Nippita et al.'s (2017) findings reiterate the importance of experience and knowledge, the care relationship between woman and professionals, involving women in decision making and the resources available to ensure improved outcomes and reduced interventions in high-risk pregnancies. In an effort to minimise risk over-estimation, a trusting relationship between provider and women could be effective in encouraging the development of self-efficacy in these women (Robinson et al. 2011). It is imperative that all healthcare professionals caring for childbearing women are skilled in recognising the signs and symptoms of pregnancy related complications in pre and post-delivery maternity care (Lowe 2019).

Women's Perspectives

Women experiencing high-risk pregnancy may not perceive associated risks in the same way as they are viewed by midwives and other healthcare professionals. This may affect women's attitude towards maternity care and services. They may view advice and information provided by midwives as not reflecting their own expectations and needs in the best interest of their baby and the visualised outcome of their pregnancy (Lee et al. 2012, 2013; Lee 2014).

Bibeau (2014) suggests that the manner in which interventions in high-risk pregnancies was explained and facilitated impacted greatly on women's experience. Those women whose expectations matched those of the professional in managing interventions during childbirth were more likely to have a positive experience in relation to how they expressed apprehension about the information and clinical care required for the interventions. However, generally, women were ambivalent or confused about the need for interventions during pregnancy and childbirth. Reed et al. (2017) support this description by women who experienced childbirth trauma because midwives' and obstetricians' actions and interaction with them impacted on their psychosocial outcomes. Other research suggests that the impact of a high-risk pregnancy is that women struggle to attain maternal roles due to the fear of the pregnancy outcome and future pregnancies (Badakhsh et al. 2020).

Recent research suggests that women, after a traumatic childbirth experience, perceived that they were mis/uninformed by maternity healthcare workers, felt disrespected and objectified and mentioned lack of support in making decisions about the interventions required (Roderiquez-Almagro et al. 2019). The literature suggests that maternity services need to develop a service that prioritises both the physical and emotional needs of women experiencing high-risk care (Reed et al. 2017).

The literature on high-risk pregnancies has been analysed through Rodgers' framework and presented in Table 5.1

Hypertension in Pregnancy

One of the conditions that affects about 10% of women in pregnancy is pregnancy induced hypertension, also known as pre-eclampsia (Tucker et al. 2017). In the latest MBBRACE (Knight et al. 2019) report, six women died in the period 2015–2017 as a direct result of hypertensive disorders in pregnancy. NICE (2019) provide guidance as to what constitutes a raised blood pressure (BP) reading. Hypertension in pregnancy is defined as two readings of 140/90 mmHG taken at least four hours apart or one diastolic reading of >110 mmHG. BP readings above these levels results in increased perinatal mortality. However, BP readings are often measured inaccurately due to incorrect size and positioning of the syphgmanometer cuff and the position of the woman during blood pressure reading (Reinders et al. 2005).

The aetiology of hypertension in pregnancy depends on whether this is a chronic or gestational condition. Chronic hypertension predates a pregnancy or appears prior to 20 weeks of gestation, may be superimposed or secondary to another

Table 5.1 Concept analysis of 'with the high-risk woman and neonate'.

Antecedents	Evidence	Attributes (A) and Consequences (C)
Minimising risk	Lee (2014) minimising risk in complicated pregnancy and birth	Individual women's circumstances (A) Sensitive and respectful care (A) Positive outcomes for mother and baby (C)
Midwives' perspective	Behruzi et al. (2010) perceiving barriers to normalising birth	Ensuring safe outcome, need for intervention and fear of legal repercussions (A) Women's lack of involvement in decision making (A) Lack of confidence and competence by MWs of high-risk care (C)
	Sinni et al. (2014) role modelling	Experienced midwives and staff provided training and role modelling (A) Enhanced performance and confidence of junior staff (C)
	Nippita et al. (2017), Lowe (2019) staff experience and skills	Experience and knowledge of staff (A) Recognising signs and symptoms of pregnancy related complications (A) Care relationship between woman and
	Robinson et al. (2011) trusting relationships	professionals (A) Involving women in decision making (A) Improved outcomes and reduced interventions in high-risk pregnancies (C) Trusting relationships between provider and women (A) Encourages development of self-efficacy in these women (C)
Women's perspective	Lee et al. (2012, 2013) Lee (2014) Different perceptions of associated risk	Women may not perceive associated risks in the same way as viewed by MWs (A) May affect women's attitude towards maternity care and services (C) View advice and information as not reflecting their own expectations and needs (C) Different visualised outcome of their pregnancy (C)
	Bibeau (2014) managing expectations	Explanation and facilitation of information by MWs (A) Matching expectations and interventions results in positive experience (C)
	Reed et al. (2017) Roderiquez-Almagro et al. (2019) MWs and obstetricians' action and interaction	Women felt disrespected and objectified (A) Impact on psychosocial outcomes (C)

medical condition, but is at an increased risk of developing into pre-eclampsia. Gestational hypertension or pregnancy induced hypertension is hypertension which is new in pregnancy, appears after 20 weeks of gestation with no accompanying proteinuria and usually resolves within six weeks of delivery of the fetus.

Hypertensive disorders in pregnancy can worsen as the pregnancy progresses, resulting in a pre-eclampsia when hypertension new to the pregnancy manifesting after 20 weeks of gestation is associated with a new onset of proteinuria and a BP ranging from 140/90 to 150/109 mmHG. Severe pre-eclampsia is diagnosed if a systolic BP is greater than 160 mmHG and a diastolic BP is a 110 mmHG or greater (NICE 2019). Pre-eclampsia can evolve in weeks or even hours and increases the risk of hypertension or cardiovascular disease in later life. A convulsive condition or fit could result when the BP is raised above these levels and can affect 2–8% of primigravid women with pregnancy induced hypertension, culminating in widespread endothelial cell damage secondary to an ischaemic placenta (NICE 2019). The implications for the mother are serious, resulting in intracranial haemorrhage (which is a leading cause of maternal death), placental abruption, HELLP syndrome, disseminated intravascular coagulation (DIC), renal failure, pulmonary oedema and acute respiratory distress syndrome. Implications for the fetus are equally severe resulting in fetal growth restriction, oligohydramnios, hypoxia from placental insufficiency, placental abruption and premature delivery (Jordan and Gabzdyl 2019).

Care in Pregnancy, Labour and Postpartum

Several risk factors are associated with pregnancy induced hypertension leading to pre-eclampsia, and midwives can minimise these risks through a careful risk assessment of those women that fall in these categories. These include hypertensive disease in previous pregnancy, chronic renal disease, autoimmune diseases, Type 1 or Type 2 diabetics, those women over 40 years of age – especially with a first pregnancy, pregnancy interval of more than 10 years, a Body Mass Index (BMI) of over 35 kg/m^2 and multiple pregnancies (ACOG 2014; Jordan and Gabzdyl 2019). In addition, some research suggests that recurrent hypertensive diseases in pregnancy may lead to long-term mortality risk and impact on life expectancy (Theilen et al. 2018).

The treatment of choice at the first risk assessment is aspirin, which is an antiplatelet agent taken from 12 weeks gestation until the birth of the baby, which statistically significantly reduces the risk of pre-eclampsia in moderate to high risk women . When conditions worsen, the antihypertensive drugs of choice are labetalol, nifedipine or hydralazine (Dudley et al. 2010).

Some of the symptoms which should alert healthcare professions to deteriorating condition in a woman with hypertension are new or significant hypertension and/or proteinuria, maternal symptoms of headache and blurred vision, epigastric pain or vomiting, reduced fetal movements or small for gestational age fetus or sudden and marked oedema in face, hands and feet occurring in approximately 80% of these women (Robson and Waugh 2013). If the systolic or diastolic are raised above 140/90 mmHG on two occasions in labour or immediately after birth, then a transfer to a consultant unit with special care baby unit facilities should be considered (Narayan 2015).

In cases when the blood pressure continues to rise, the prevention of seizures is managed through a magnesium sulphate infusion and maintaining basic life support of airways, breathing and circulation in the case of a seizure occurring (Magpie Trial Collaborative Group 2002).

A Midwife's Story

Victoria's Story

Whilst working on labour ward I cared for a woman in labour with moderate pre-eclampsia. Jane* was 39 weeks pregnant and had been admitted through triage with her first episode of high blood pressure and proteinuria.

Bloods were sent for analysis and moderate pre-eclampsia was diagnosed. Anti-hypertensives had been given and an obstetric decision was made to induce her labour.

Prior to this episode, Jane had a low-risk pregnancy and had been planning to deliver in the midwife-led birthing unit. As I introduced myself, I could tell that she was unhappy about being on labour ward. She voiced to me that she felt disappointed as she had done a hypnobirthing course and wanted a water birth.

I spent time asking about her birth preferences and talked through her birth plan with her and Jane's partner. I explained that once she was in active labour, she needed to have continuous monitoring and was unable to use the water as a form of pain relief. However, I encouraged her to use the bath in the latent phase of her labour. I also turned the lights down in the room and her partner put on calming music. She began listening to her music and hypnobirthing meditations and said that she felt much more relaxed.

Shortly after the start of Jane's induction process, she began contracting and getting herself into labour. As I handed over care to the midwife on the night shift, I emphasised Jane's birth preferences. Although being admitted to labour ward had deviated from her birth plan, it was important in this situation to work 'with woman' to find a compromise whereby we could give Jane appropriate care whilst allowing her the agency to make decisions about her birth experience.

A Woman's Story

Katrina's Story

I have had pre-eclampsia twice. My son was born in 2015 by emergency c-section and my daughter in 2019 also by emergency c-section.

My pregnancy with my son was very straightforward. There was a midwife at my GP surgery, so I always saw the same person – which I liked because we built a rapport and she knew me, I didn't have to answer the same questions each time. With two weeks to go to my due date, protein was found in my urine and my blood pressure was extremely high. It was so high I was at risk of having a stroke. Unfortunately, this wasn't explained to me at the time and I was sent home to carry on towards my due date. A week later my waters broke but labour failed to progress, and my blood pressure was just getting higher, so I was taken in for a c-section.

The two midwives who looked after me during the labour process were amazing, they rarely left my side and really put me at ease. After my son was born, I stayed in hospital for a week but I didn't see my two midwives again. I began to feel like a burden, I was depressed, and I just wanted to take my baby home. I saw so many different midwives, doctors and consultants then and it was overwhelming. They all had different opinions and advised different plans, I didn't know whether I was coming or going and there was no continuity of care. After I was allowed home, I saw one midwife and that was it, the care had ended, and I felt cut off. It didn't seem as though there was any compassion for me as a woman, as a new mum or for my mental or physical health. I was diagnosed with postnatal depression and things improved once I was put onto medication.

My pregnancy with my daughter was totally different. I had morning sickness throughout the entire pregnancy, and I was apprehensive due to my previous experience. The midwife service had changed by this point, so I could no longer go to my GP, I had to go to a Sure Start centre instead. I saw three different midwives until I was switched to a new trial designed to improve continuity of care. The idea was that I would see just one midwife and she would come to my home. This worked really well, I liked being in the comfort of my own home as it felt more like a friend coming over instead of someone to look after me. My midwife was always honest with me. She went through everything I could possibly think of with birth options and plans for monitoring my blood pressure, which I found reassuring knowing she was so on top of things.

> *My blood pressure once again was high, and I was sent to the hospital at least twice a week for months. No protein was ever found in my urine so pre-eclampsia was not diagnosed again until the week before my due date. I was admitted to hospital where I had blood tests which showed my liver enzyme levels were increasing, so although my kidneys were not affected by pre-eclampsia, my liver was. The doctors made the decision to do an emergency c-section which meant I couldn't have my community midwife with me as there was no time, but she texted me to make sure I was ok. When I saw her after the birth she was fantastic, she came to my home, checked my wound, ensured I was on the right medication and even stayed for a while to play with my son.*
>
> *Although both births didn't go to plan, I'm so thankful for my community midwife and if I ever decide to have another baby I know I would be well looked after and that the concept of 'with woman' is well and truly in place.*

Raised BMI in Pregnancy

Midwives hold a valuable position when it comes to contributing to and advancing the public health agenda for women, babies and families (DH 2010). A key priority for Public Health England is to find ways to reduce obesity within the general population (PHE 2017), due to concerns for individuals but also cost to the NHS. A midwife's role in the management of this agenda presents itself in the form of caring for women classified as obese and/or with a high body mass index (BMI) throughout pregnancy and labour (CDC 2017).

Women with a high BMI have significant health implications and are at greater risk of obstetric complications, such as gestational diabetes and pre-eclampsia. Guidelines recommend that a woman with a BMI over $35 \, \text{kg/m}^2$ should book in an obstetric unit (WHO 2017, RCOG 2018). However, Rowe et al. (2018) found that woman who have a BMI of 35–40 kg/m^2, are otherwise healthy and have previously given birth are just as safe in an alongside midwifery unit (AMU) as those with a low BMI.

Midwives are taught to find a balance between meeting the needs of the woman and providing individualised care, whilst also taking into account the environment and the challenges she may face (Garrod and Byrom 2007). Whilst birthing in AMU can reduce medical intervention, which may allow a woman to feel like she has greater control of the process, the AMU may not be suitable for some woman with a high BMI. In this instance, the midwife must adapt her care in order to provide personalised support for woman in the labour ward. In this environment the midwife needs to ensure that the correct equipment and appropriate bed is available, making sure to plan everything in advance.

This ability to understand the individual needs, whilst also having the skills to protect what is most precious to the women, means a midwife holds a position of trust and is afforded a level of communication that surpasses most other health-care professionals (HCP) (Holton et al. 2019). However, some midwives have reported that lifestyle issues are a low priority in maternity care, whilst others find it a sensitive topic (Smith et al. 2012). There are studies showing insensitivity on the part of midwives when trying to form rapport or help relax women with high BMI, using phrases such as *'there's a baby in there somewhere'* (Vireday 2002). It is imperative, therefore, that midwives continue to learn and develop their skills when communicating with women with high BMIs.

The public health issue of obesity is one of the more sensitive topics a midwife will need to address. It's a complex and nuanced issue that permeates society. For instance, in 2015 *London Overweight Haters Ltd* created and distributed flyers on the London Underground network designed to *'fat shame'*. The fliers included messages like *'we disapprove of your wasting NHS resources'* and *'we object to the enormous amount of food resources you consume'*. Whilst this is an extreme and horrendous example, it highlights the problems faced by overweight individuals and points to a potential for unconscious bias towards people with a high BMI.

Women are highly receptive to information about their weight and lifestyle during pregnancy and therefore how this information is communicated is vital (Christenson et al. 2019). In their Randomised Controlled Trial (RCT) related to weight management in pregnancy, Simpson et al. (2015), found that women in the intervention group benefitted from the social support of the midwives and, in particular, gaining knowledge in relation to weight in pregnancy. This was a truly significant trial from which the collaboration between the Royal College of Midwives (RCM) and Slimming World has been formed. This collaboration is designed to help women manage their weight in pregnancy and help midwives meet the public health agenda.

Supporting women with a high BMI can certainly be a challenge for a midwife as it adds another layer to an already complex situation. Education around communication in this scenario is almost as important as the medical care training due to the psychological connotations (Foster and Hirst 2014). We must educate midwives to better understand how a woman's individual circumstances may have led to a high BMI, whilst also being aware of societal pressures and opinions. In addition, midwives must become more astute, using terms like 'Body Mass Index', 'BMI' or 'weight category', which are less emotive than the medical terms widely used by fellow HCPs, like 'obese' or 'obesity'.

The role of the midwife is to advocate for the woman; in order to be successful in this they need to be receptive to the needs of the woman, being respectful, sensitive and honest, and creating an environment of trust and security (Pembroke and Pembroke 2008; Fuber and McGowan 2011).

Midwives' Stories

Rhiannon's Story

I took over the care of Deepa,* a primiparous woman with a booking BMI of 46, which is classified as extremely obese. She was on the cardiotocography (CTG), which records the baby's heartrate continuously. I ensured she understood the reasoning behind this.

Deepa was moving a lot during contractions and it was becoming increasingly more difficult to monitor the baby's heartrate continuously, so I asked if she would be happy for a fetal scalp electrode to be applied. Following a detailed explanation, Deepa was happy for this to be applied.

She was quite conscious about her body image, so I ensured that as few people as possible were in the room when this was applied. As labour progressed, the baby become quite distressed and a decision was made for a category 2 caesarean section. Deepa was very anxious about this, in particular about the spinal epidural and the fact that so many people would be in theatre when she was self-conscious. I reassured her that I would be with her at all times.

During siting of the spinal, I talked through exactly what was happening and stayed by her side the whole time so that she felt more secure. I ensured the team kept her as covered up as possible to try and help with her insecurities and made sure that Deepa felt comfortable at all times. Deepa reported that she felt a lot more relaxed knowing that I was there acting as an advocate for her.

After the baby girl was born, I was able to stay with Deepa when she went into the observation bay. This helped Deepa to feel more confident, particularly when breastfeeding. She said she would not have felt as happy asking for help with breastfeeding if it was a midwife she did not know due to her insecurities. I was able to show Deepa different positions such as the underarm hold and her confidence grew. By being able to build up a close and trusting relationship with Deepa, she was able to feel more at ease when going for a caesarean section. Her insecurities due to her high BMI were lessened through me listening to her wishes and ensuring that she felt comfortable at all times.

Olivia's Story

Women who have complications in pregnancy often are very appreciative of having a midwife by their side during their labour and delivery. Continuity of care often enhances their experiences and allows midwives to provide women-centred care. An example that stands out for me is Grace*'s story.

(Continued)

Grace had a raised BMI. She was admitted antenatally with a shortness of breath: a suspected pulmonary embolism in her 28th week of pregnancy. I first met her in triage where she was incredibly uncomfortable and finding it very hard to breathe, she leaned on me to mobilise while we awaited tests and doctor reviews.

The following day, I started my shift and she was in the observation bay; I took handover while she was having a nebuliser and joked about how she was stuck with me again for the day. A couple of days later, I was on the antenatal ward where she had remained as an inpatient. When I met her that morning, we joked about whether she would get out of hospital soon. That afternoon I was able to discharge her, and she said that she hoped she would see me when she came in to have her little boy. I said she needed to behave and keep him in for a bit longer. Just as she was about to go home, she squeezed my hand and I wished her all the best, hoping I would get to see her at some point again.

A few months later, I walked into a labour ward shift and looked at the board, which had Grace's name on it. She was now in her 37th week of pregnancy having had spontaneous rupture of membranes and was now having her labour augmented.

When I walked into the room to take over, she was breathing heavily on the gas; when the contraction settled, she looked up, saw me and smiled – she said she was very glad to see me. Knowing one another already ensured that I did not have to build up a relationship with her. Grace was incredibly tired but already having built a rapport, she felt she could keep her eyes closed tight during contractions and would give me a nod when I needed to take observations. She knew I would understand.

Grace had had an epidural sited when I took over her care and throughout the day it became less and less effective. She was not coping well with the labour and wanted a caesarean section. When the doctors came in to see her, she felt unable to express her wishes to have a caesarean section to them, so I was able to advocate this for her. As I already knew her, she trusted me to explain her wishes to the consultant. The doctor suggested having the epidural re-sited as she had high BMI and would need adequate analgesia even if she was having a caesarean.

Once the doctor left the room, Grace dissolved into tears. She asked me what I thought she should do and I was able to reassure her that we could hopefully get her comfortable. Following re-siting of the epidural, it became effective and she was pain free. Grace still felt that having an operative delivery would be the right decision for her. We asked the consultant to revisit Grace and further discussions ensued.

While preparing Grace for theatre, there was a time when everyone left the room and it was just the two of us. She told me she was scared and didn't want me to leave her. I reassured her that I would be staying with her and not going anywhere. When she went to theatre for an emergency caesarean section, I was able to be by her side for the whole time.

Following delivery, Grace was incredibly thankful and reassured that she had a familiar and known midwife to looking after her and didn't have to start again with someone new. This is a good example of how continuity can massively enhance women's experiences of their care. When women feel that they cannot express their needs and wishes for themselves, they sometimes need someone they know to advocate for them. Providing such care also goes back to the foundations of why I became a midwife and how this improves the satisfaction of being 'with woman'.

Postpartum Haemorrhage

Primary postpartum haemorrhage (PPH) is traditionally defined as blood loss of 500 ml or more within 24 hours of birth (WHO 2012), although a more useful definition is one based on the clinical impact on a woman of any blood loss (RCOG 2016b). Secondary PPH is defined as excessive or abnormal bleeding from the genital tract from 24 hours to 12 weeks post-delivery. Globally, PPH is the leading cause of maternal death in lower income countries, and accounts for a quarter of maternal mortality (Say et al. 2014). Within the UK, haemorrhage remains a leading cause of maternal death, with rates fluctuating between triennial national reports (Knight et al. 2019).

Whilst death is the most severe outcome following a postpartum haemorrhage, experiencing this obstetric emergency can impact the mother in many other ways; there will be an increased need for medical intervention and observation, including the possibility of a life-saving hysterectomy (Elmir et al. 2012, Mavrides et al. 2016), and rarely it may lead to organ damage due to reduced perfusion, such as Sheehan syndrome (Schrager and Sabo 2001). It can impact on the initial contact between mother and baby, which in severe cases may go on for several days if admittance to intensive care is required (Elmir et al. 2012; Knight et al. 2016). Whilst the factors associated with an increased risk of postpartum haemorrhage are known, and therefore women most at risk can be identified and appropriate management can be recommended (Mavrides et al. 2016), in developing countries there has been a trend in increasing postpartum haemorrhage rates (Knight et al. 2009). As such, it is likely that midwives will encounter this obstetric emergency at some point in their practice.

A severe postpartum haemorrhage is frightening for both midwives and the women in their care (Dahlen and Caplice 2014; Knight et al. 2016); woman may experience uncertainty as to whether or not they will survive the event (Elmir et al. 2012). The sheer volume of blood that can be lost in a PPH is shocking, and this can lead woman to worry not only for their own lives, but that of their baby and wider family (Elmir et al. 2012). Whilst there is an understandable focus on interprofessional training for the skills to manage this emergency situation, with courses such as PROMPT (Practical Obstetric Multi-Professional Training), it must not be forgotten that for some (possibly the majority) of woman who experience this it will come as an unexpected, out of the blue, event from which they may find it difficult to adjust. In this situation communication, as always, is key. Woman find a calm and professional approach reassuring (Knight et al. 2016); any explanations need to be clear, using non-medical language, ensuring the woman's partner is not forgotten (Knight et al. 2016). Individualised personal support from empathetic staff can help women adjust from high-dependency care to 'normal' postnatal care (Knight et al. 2016), but midwives need to be aware that woman who have had severe PPH may well experience flashbacks and nightmares because of this (for them) unprecedented event (Elmir et al. 2012).

Midwife's Story

Victoria's Story

On a day shift, I took over care of a woman who had a high-risk pregnancy. Susan* had a medical history of significant abdominal surgery including midline bowel surgery which would make a caesarean section extremely dangerous. In addition to this, she was pre-term at 36 weeks and 5 days and had prolonged pre-term rupture of membranes. She had an epidural and was fully dilated on her previous examination.

As we approached the time to start active pushing, Susan became increasingly anxious. It was important at this time to talk her through the whole process and I took care to emphasise that I would be with her throughout. After an hour of pushing with minimal descent of the fetal head, the registrar did a vaginal examination and found that the baby was in a direct occiput-posterior position meaning it may be difficult for baby to be born without assistance. As a result, a decision for a forceps delivery was made. As Susan's midwife, I focused on palpating contractions and being with her and her partner offering guidance and reassurance.

The doctors in the room were friendly and encouraging, informing Susan what was happening. Her baby was born in a good condition. Following delivery, unfortunately Susan had a post-partum haemorrhage of 1000 ml due to uterine atony. The emergency was well managed, and I made sure to explain to the couple what was happening and who people were, to ensure that Susan and her partner stayed calm with their baby. The bleeding settled, she was sutured, and I tidied the room up.

Despite the antenatal risk factors, the difficult delivery and the emergency, Susan and her husband stated that they had a good birth experience as they felt reassured throughout. Being present and 'with woman' is particularly important during complex and high-risk deliveries.

Multiple Pregnancies

Globally, the birth rate of twins varies considerably, with research identifying Africa as having the most and South East Asia the lowest, 18 and 10 pairs per 1000 births respectively (Smits and Monden 2011). Within the United Kingdom (UK) and United States (US), the birth rate of twins continues to fall, theorised as being due to changes in legislation reducing the number of embryos transferred to the woman during assisted conception. In the UK, the Office of National Statistics identified the multiple maternity birth rate as falling for the third consecutive year, 15.4 per 1000 women (ONS 2018) with those older than 45 years most likely to have a multiple pregnancy in 2018. The birth rate for twins in the US has fallen from 33.9 in 2014 to 32.6 per 1000 live births in 2018 (Statista 2018).

A woman's childbearing experience depends largely on whether her twins are monozygotic or dizygotic. Monozygotic twins (uniovular) have no genetic predisposition, are genetically identical, the same sex, with complications largely associated with the timing of splitting into two following fertilisation. The later the division, the more likely complications will occur due to reduced chorionicity and amnionicity.

Chorionicity and amnionicity relate to 'the number of placental masses, the appearance of the membrane attachment to the placenta and the membrane thickness' (RCOG 2016a).

- Monochorionic, diamniotic (MCDA) pregnancies, have one chorion and two amnions. In approximately two thirds of cases, splitting of the embryo will have occurred between four and eight days after fertilisation.
- Monochorionic, monoamniotic (MCMA) pregnancies, with one amnion and one chorion, are rare due to the embryo splitting later (9–12 days) (Denton and O'Brien 2017).

Dizygotic twins (binovular or fraternal) result from the fertilisation of two separate ova and sperm, have their own placenta (either separate or fused), amnion and chorion and are associated with fewer complications.

'Being with Woman' Having Twins

Whether complicated or healthy, all women with a twin pregnancy need to feel supported. The role of the midwife is crucial in creating a supportive relationship focused on care, compassion and education. Being 'with woman' is key to translate the complex and to help prepare women for being the mother of twins. It has long been known that care by one or a small number of midwives is more satisfying for women than being cared for by many (Rowley et al. 1995; Taylor et al. 2018). Coordinating family-centred support with the woman at the centre, defines being 'with woman' during her twin pregnancy.

Psychological support, understanding and expertise focused on continuity of care and advice has been shown to provide better outcomes for women and their families. Research identifies the importance of a dedicated service for multiple pregnancies focused on expert obstetric and midwifery care (NICE 2019; Ferriman et al. 2018; RCOG 2016a) with support from health professionals and charities such as the Multiple Birth Foundation and TAMBA. The continuity of midwifery support, to guide a woman with twins and her family through the childbearing continuum, is crucial.

Women with a twin pregnancy should be offered an ultrasound scan in the first trimester to assess gestation, amnionicity and chorionicity. Monochorionic twin pregnancies with a single placenta, one chorion and one or two amnions will require close monitoring, increased antenatal appointments, ultrasound scans and potential referral to tertiary services, since they are at risk of complications increasing the chances of morbidity and mortality. Early midwifery contact, or being 'with woman', is crucial for all pregnant women, particularly those with a twin pregnancy, due to the contact and support needed over the next weeks and months.

Stress, anxiety and uncertainty related to a twin pregnancy is often unexpected and/or exacerbated by complications (Beauquier-Maccotta et al. 2016); the effect of which is felt more acutely if pregnancy has been long awaited, following a period of fertility investigations and treatment or due to the death of one or both twins (Munk-Olsen et al. 2014). Complications often associated with reduced amnionicity and chorionicity include twin–twin transfusion syndrome (placental vascular anastomoses, occurring in approximately 1–3 per 10 000 births) (Blickstein 2006; Falletta et al. 2018), cardiac anomalies, congenital malformation (Fonseca et al. 2012) and growth anomalies. Referral to tertiary services, invasive procedures and prematurity add to the enormity of stresses experienced.

Depending on maternal and fetal wellbeing, enhanced monitoring and patient contact may result in a woman with a twin pregnancy being supported by multiple healthcare professionals, and a healthy lifestyle is particularly important. In a prospective study of 20 pregnant women with DCDA twins, Gandhi et al. (2018) reported an increase in calories during the last two trimesters to support energy needs; a referral to a dietitian with expertise in supporting women pregnant with twins may be important. Using a cross-sectional, online survey of 276 mothers of twins delivered in the last three years, Whitaker et al. (2019) explored advice from healthcare providers regarding physical activity and nutrition. Using statistical and content analysis, findings revealed that advice was minimal with many advising limited activity, not based on evidence. A need for further research was identified, focused on lifestyle behaviour in twin pregnancies.

Depending on chorionicity, monitoring the wellbeing of twins may increase the frequency of ultrasound scans and doppler studies. Particularly in monochorionic twin pregnancies, the support from a trusted midwife may make all the difference in relation to support and the interpretation of results or delivery of worrying or bad news. Using quantitative methodology, Masini et al. (2019) undertook a study examining a mixed cohort of twin pregnancies between 22 and 24^{+6} weeks (MC and DC) which were recruited to participate as the study focused on ascertaining whether dopplers of the transabdominal uterine artery differed in monochorionic, diamniotic and dichorionic twins. Analysis revealed reduced activity in monochorionic twin pregnancies compared to singleton pregnancies, which is important when detecting complications.

Bereavement obviously demands a heightened awareness as to how a mother of twins is likely to be feeling. Using a cross-sectional correlational approach, Druget et al. (2018) explored the psychological effect of losing one or both twins in a MC pregnancy. Twenty-eight Spanish women participated, with data collected via individual interviews and completion of a modified perinatal grief scale. Although findings may not be generalisable to women outside of Spain, they revealed the enormity of loss, whether one or two babies, resulting in long-term morbidity and the need for excellent support during pregnancy, birth and postpartum.

Being 'with woman' during birth and postpartum provides reassurance, expertise, continuity of advice and support for the whole family (Whitford et al. 2017). Feeding two babies often simultaneously demands time and patience, being 'with woman' as reflected in the vignette below provides considerable benefits for both the mother and midwife.

Midwives' Stories

Julia's Story

As lead midwife for multiple pregnancies, I have a responsibility to these women to make sure that they are well informed and understand their plan of care. This involves not only clinical duties, but also being the conduit for information, support and linking families together as a support network.

The role is enormously rewarding as I am 'their' midwife, and I am their first port of call. I offer a session of antenatal classes, which links the couples together but also gives them the information they require to make informed choices. This often makes clinic appointments a little more fluid as they already have a certain amount of knowledge prior to their consultation.

Some current statistics in one local hospital show that 65% of multiple pregnancies are delivered by lower segment caesarean section (LSCS). Around 50% of multiple births will be delivered before the arranged date of 37/40 weeks of pregnancy for non-identical twins and 36/40 gestational weeks for identical twins. About 30% of multiple births will be admitted to NICU for prematurity, which accounts for 2% of total births. These pregnancies and deliveries use the most of available resources, such as scanning every two to four weeks and of course admissions to NICU.

As lead midwife for multiples, I have had the pleasure of caring for some complicated pregnancies but also some wonderfully straightforward ones too.

Amy's Twin Story

It was just approaching midnight of my third night shift that week, when I answered a call from the antenatal ward. The midwife on the phone was very worried about one of the twin mothers who had been admitted earlier that day. Dichorionic diamniotic (DCDA) twins who were now in their 29th week had been scanned earlier that day and discovered they had intrauterine growth retardation (IUGR). The expectant mother Tina* was now receiving a course of steroids to mature their lungs in anticipation of an early delivery.

When Tina arrived on the labour ward some 10 minutes later, she was leaking clear liquor and having regular, strong uterine contractions. Chaos ensued as all available members of the multi-disciplinary team entered the room with a task to be completed. The on-call registrar exposed her abdomen and began scanning the twins to determine their positions. The anaesthetist questioned Tina about her medical history. A midwife prepared to gain venous access with a large bore cannula to administer a magnesium infusion ahead of delivery. A maternity assistant stood at the head of the bed with pen and paper poised to document each moment of care given. The neonatal team checked their equipment ready to provide neonatal life support to each twin if required.

When I entered the room Tina looked terrified as she consented to each aspect of care, endured the intense pain of the rapid contractions and desperately tried to stop herself crying whilst she waited for her husband to arrive. I had met Tina before and sometimes just a familiar face is enough to put you at ease. I squeezed past the other members of staff in the room and took her hand. She squeezed me so tight but gradually her breathing slowed, her panic settled, and she began to calm. Over the course of the next moments I never left her side, explaining the task each person was doing, offering reassurance and becoming the communication channel between the multi-disciplinary team (MDT) and Tina. This resulted in a much quieter atmosphere in the room, rather than multiple people speaking at the same time.

Upon examination the cervix was found to be 9cm dilated and Tina was transferred to obstetric theatre. I stayed by her side until her partner arrived and was able to be her companion and support. Tina delivered the first twin soon after we arrived in theatre and then delivered the second twin in a breech presentation and with a cord prolapse within just three minutes. The babies stayed in NICU for a number of weeks, but both made it home before their due date and are thriving despite their prematurity.

Olivia's Twin Story

Sometimes, when women are very high risk, having consultant-led care can be very daunting and midwives can play a role in making women feel more relaxed. Commencing a busy shift on labour ward two years after being qualified and looking after Rosie*, with a twin pregnancy at 29 weeks gestation who was fully dilated, seemed extremely daunting.

Rosie was fully dilated, and we were to wait for the on-call consultant to come into the hospital for delivery. This was a strange and frightening time for Rosie as she felt overwhelmed by the number of staff members in the room. This included me, the midwife from the night shift, the registrar, the shift leader and the full NICU team and there was a sense of anticipation for the delivery. During this sort of situation, it is the midwife's role to minimise the impact of such a full team and seek to support the woman through effective communication. I talked to Rosie and reassured her that it didn't matter who was in the room but that everyone there had their own job to support her and improve her experience.

Following the arrival of the consultant it was time to commence pushing. I helped Rosie deliver her first twin. However, Rosie had been counselled that for the second

(Continued)

twin it was a little bit more difficult as it needed to be guided down into the pelvis and an artificial rupture of membranes performed. Rosie knew that there was a possibility of cord prolapse and being transferred to theatre was a strong possibility. During this time, Rosie squeezed my hand tightly and looked into my eyes for reassurance. I gave a reassuring nod and smiled at her and she repeated it back at me. She knew that I would be there to support her.

The registrar ruptured membranes with the obstetric consultant watching closely, myself holding the Rosie's hand, with her partner standing close by with tears of worry in his eyes. The ultrasound equipment was placed on her abdomen and we watched the second twin, in a cephalic position descending into the pelvis. We all let out a sigh of relief and the consultant promptly left the room. The second twin slid out with no difficulties and was handed to the paediatricians although the baby was active and pink.

Once the placentas were delivered by me, the paediatricians left the room. It was just me and Rosie. Her partner had followed the babies to the neonatal unit. I helped Rosie to hand express some precious colostrum for her babies while she rested her head back and we talked about potential names for the twins. Everything now was calm following the storm.

Woman's Story

Angela*'s Story

I remember my mother had twins and the midwife saying to her after about a week, oh don't bother trying breastfeeding, it will be really difficult; but right from the beginning when I knew I was pregnant with twins I just wanted to give it a go. I'd fed my first baby myself and had felt very positive about breastfeeding and wanted to do the same for the twins. I wanted that closeness and bonding. Antenatally, my midwife had taught me that breastfeeding twins was perfectly possible to do, she made me feel that if other women had done it, it was not going to be a problem for me. In a few words, I found breastfeeding the twins a marvellous experience; in the end I would say that I could relax and enjoy it. My advice to other women is get as much help and advice as you can whilst you're in hospital and listen to the midwives. I got a lot of help, I mean every feed it was a case of a midwife coming along to support me, until I got the hang of it. I think by the time I left hospital I felt confident and was able to put them both on and feed them both. Seeing the same midwife really helps, I could create a relationship, a better understanding of what we'd done before and what we'd tried. One midwife I will never forget, she was there for me but didn't take over, she gave me the confidence to see that I could breastfeed my babies which made me feel complete, a loving, caring mother – I will never forget her.

Lessons Learnt

The above literature and illustrating stories are only a snapshot of the many complications of high-risk pregnancies and birth. Midwife's stories indicate the need for more vigilant care and a partnership with women and families in making decisions that will ensure a safer and more positive outcome for both the mother and her baby/babies. Women's vulnerability during their complex and sometimes difficult pregnancies and births is well portrayed in the vignettes above and the women's stories highlight the importance of support and nurturing that is perceived to be so valuable in these situations. The essence of the 'with woman' concept is clearly demonstrated.

'With Woman' in Special Care or Intensive Care Neonatal Units

The Role of the Family Support Nurse in NICU

Improved survival of preterm and term neonates with health problems has increased the number of neonates admitted to a neonatal intensive care unit (NICU). This impacts the level of care and information due to the lack of support for families that is provided by healthcare professionals in these busy units (Gooding et al. 2011). Women who give birth to preterm babies or babies requiring a NICU admission need individualised family-centred support as they are more stressed and anxious during this time (Shimizu and Mori 2017). Depression and anxiety are prevalent in these parents and emotional distress is not easily recognised by healthcare professionals. However, screening for depression (Rogers et al. 2012) and a family-focused approach by nurses in NICU, offering listening visits as a counselling approach, was found to be helpful (Segre et al. 2013, 2015; Chuffo and Segre 2018). Despite difficulties with finding time to implement nurse-led screening strategies developed by nurses in NICU, they were able to effectively screen long-stay women for depressive symptoms to identify and support those women most in need of counselling and care (Segre et al. 2014).

One of the issues that could ameliorate the conditions of having a baby in NICU is that parents are present during clinical rounds. They can express concerns, ask questions and remain fully informed about the complex needs and outcomes of their babies in long-term care (Boswell et al. 2015). This concurs with findings from outside the UK, which suggest that unique stress management amongst NICU parents to overcome emotional distress was created through effective communication with the medical team, seeking information, hope and reassurance by resorting to spirituality to maintain calm and fulfil a need to connect to their baby and enhance attachment (Heidari et al. 2017).

The long-term effects on mothers after having a baby in NICU have been found to have an impact of psychological distress up to one year after the event and results in mothers having a less positive perception of their child's wellbeing (Holditch-Davis et al. 2015). In one study, mothers of very low birthweight babies (VLBW) displayed anxiety during the hospitalisation of their infant in a NICU, which later affected their ability to recognise infant cues that adversely affected developmental outcomes (Zelkowitz et al. 2011). Another study indicates that paternal anxiety levels scored highly on a Clinical Interview for Parents of High-Risk Infant scale (CLIP) despite their silence, and hidden depressive symptoms need to be considered by healthcare professionals in NICU (Candelori et al. 2015).

Women's Views of Support in NICU

Parents' and healthcare professionals' views are dissonant on the type and consistency of care provided by nurses and doctors in NICU, in line with the parents' perceptions and needs. Parents expressed the need for support with establishing and developing the parent–infant relationship through a therapeutic relationship with nurses. This relationship was perceived by parents to facilitate information and education with infant care and develop their parent role whilst their baby was hospitalised in NICU (Franck and Axelin 2013). Midwives and neonatal nurses are best placed to actively promote resilience in parents to improve their mental health, by gaining confidence and competence and becoming advocates for their babies. This may be achieved through guidance for parents by NICU-based healthcare professionals, enabling them to learn how to live with events beyond their control, developing coping strategies and decreasing NICU-related stress. Evidence suggests that such strategies enable better maternal coping behaviours in their relationship with their baby, long after discharge from NICU (Rossman et al. 2017).

Mothers' experience of early skin to skin care (SSC) immediately following the birth of a premature infant indicates that they responded positively to this practice and it enabled normalisation of the birth experience. However, staff experience and support to encourage and maintain SSC had an impact on the mother–infant relationship outcomes (Gulla et al. 2017). Efforts to decrease maternal anxiety, enhance confidence in infant caring skills and improve breastfeeding rates could also be achieved through kangaroo care (Sweeney et al. 2017).

Once parents transition to home after discharge from NICU, they still face difficulties and challenges which require enhanced professional support

(Boykova 2016). It is important to note that mothers having a baby admitted to NICU perceived themselves to be less ready for home discharge if they had a history of mental health problems (McGowan et al. 2017). An interesting study examining the relationship of the mental health of mothers and extremely low birthweight infants suggests that exposure to anxiety and low maternal mood can adversely affect birthweight and impact their mental health as adults (Rangan et al. 2019) (Table 5.2).

Table 5.2 Concept analysis of 'with woman' with the compromised neonate.

Antecedents	Evidence	Attributes (A) and Consequences (C)
The role of the family support nurse	Shimizu and Mori (2017) individualised family-centred support	Depression, anxiety and emotional distress (A)
	Rogers et al. (2012) Segre et al. (2013, 2015) Chuffo and Segre (2018) screening for depression	Listening visits helpful (C) Counselling and care (C)
Care support	Boswell et al. (2015) stress management	Presence of parents during clinical rounds and effective communication (A) Reduced stress and were fully informed about care management of their baby (C)
	Heidari et al. (2017) support through spirituality	Parents seeking information, hope and reassurance (A) Spirituality to maintain calm and enhance attachment to their baby (C)
Long-term effects on parents	Holditch-Davis et al. 2015 psychological outcomes	Psychological distress up to one year after the event (A) Mothers having a less positive perception of their child's wellbeing (C)
	Zelkowitz et al. (2011).	Displayed anxiety during the hospitalisation of their infant in a NICU (A) Affected their ability to recognise infant cues that adversely affected developmental outcomes (C)
	Candelori et al. (2015).	Paternal anxiety levels score high (A) Despite their silence and hidden depression (C)

(Continued)

Table 5.2 (Continued)

Antecedents	Evidence	Attributes (A) and Consequences (C)
Women's views	Franck and Axelin (2013) support	Need for support to establish and develop parent–infant relation (A)
		Therapeutic relationship with nurses to promote resilience, improve their mental health, by gaining confidence and competence and becoming advocates for their babies (C)
	Rossman et al. (2017) coping strategies	Developing coping strategies and decreasing NICU-related stress (A)
		Long-term better maternal coping behaviours in their relationship with their baby (C)
	Gulla et al. (2017), Sweeney et al. (2017) physical contact	Early skin to skin care (SSC) (A)
		Enables normalisation of the birth experience and impact on the mother–infant relationship outcomes (C)
		Kangaroo care (A)
	Rangan et al. (2019) long-term outcomes	Decreases maternal anxiety, enhance confidence in infant caring skills and improve breastfeeding (C)
		Anxiety and low maternal mood (A)
		Can adversely affect birthweight and impacted infant's mental health as adults (C)

A Family Support Nurse's Story

It is acknowledged that NICU is a stressful and technological environment. In the middle of this overwhelming space is a very vulnerable baby surrounded by nurses, doctor's wires and alarms! The whole scene is totally unexpected, devastating, intimidating and crushing (parent's descriptions) to all parents. Families of babies that are born extremely early have not had the time to prepare for their arrival either emotionally or financially. To try and help parents and families adjust to the stressful situation that they have been thrust into, the unit employed me as a family support nurse.

My role is to be there for the parents/families and support them in whatever way I can. Just being there to listen in a non-judgemental way helps to ease the stress of the situation for the family. It is important for the parents to understand that we are

*there to care for their baby – the baby is not ours – and that they play a very impor-
tant part in their baby's growth and development. All their worries, opinions and
presence on the unit are extremely important to us and their baby. We see the parents as an integral part of our team. One of my roles is to ensure that all staff know
how to empower the parents to become confident in caring for their baby. Staff need
to know how sometimes too much encouragement can have a negative outcome,
such as the parents being overwhelmed. They need to find a balance. They need to
know that the parents can be frightened handling a fragile human being and that
sometimes the simplest tasks might need to be divided up into small stages.*

*Listening to parents cannot be underestimated. The focus for parents is the health
and wellbeing of their child but life goes on outside of NICU. They still need to pay
bills; they still need to care for any other children. They still need to do the shopping, laundry and cook dinner. Parents just have an overwhelming sense of guilt
and talking can sometimes help with these feelings. Having a person who understands the situation they find themselves in with the experience of talking to other
parents can alleviate some of the guilt they often feel.*

Jo's Story

*Women who are pregnant with twins, triplets or quads are more likely to have a
baby on the NICU. Clara* was aware that we would be admitting her babies on the
NICU unit. The parents had a tour of the unit and they had been counselled about
what to expect. Clara was carrying quads; the three girls were growing well but
the fourth, a boy, was very small. During the pregnancy, the parents had been
offered fetal selective reduction on two occasions which they refused. They
accepted that the boy could die in utero at any point.*

*A date for an elective section was made. Four teams were at the delivery for the
babies. The parents were blessed prior to the delivery and they wanted the priest
to be present in case the boy died. They wanted him blessed as soon as possible.*

*The delivery went well, and the girls progressed through NICU. The boy who was
IUGR had a slow journey. Clara knew what to expect in NICU. They stayed in
accommodation for a few weeks, then they travelled in each day. Although they
lived 20 miles away, dad worked locally to the hospital, so he would drop Clara at
the hospital in the morning. Then in the evening he would visit after work and
they would both go home in the evening.*

*Although Clara was aware and felt well counselled in the NICU unit, she was not
aware that the children could be discharged at different times. The girls had progressed well and were ready to go home. But the boy who was significantly smaller*

(Continued)

had a long time left to go on the unit. It was unfair for the girls to remain in hospital when they were clinically well. However, Clara would be the primary carer for the girls, so how was she going to be able to visit and stay the full day and care for three babies? Also, she would be doing the night feeds for three babies, so exhaustion was very probable.

The boy who remained in hospital was visited prior to his dad going to work and after his dad worked. Clara visited at the weekend. Clara and her husband felt guilty about not being with their son.

Lessons Learnt

The care that midwives and neonatal nurses provide for women and families whilst their infant is in a neonatal unit is vital in recognising anxiety, fear and depression during this time. Keeping parents involved and informed of their infant's progress is essential to alleviate some of these feelings through listening and counselling on how best to cope with the uncertainty of their baby's wellbeing. A therapeutic relationship between parents and professionals ensures more positive outcomes in the short- and long-term development of the infant in the special care environment.

References

American College of Obstetricians & Gynaecologists (ACOG) (2014). Hypertension in pregnancy. http://www.acog.org/Resources-And-Publications/Task-Force-and-Work-Group-Reports/Hypertension-in-pregnancy (accessed 26 June 2020).

Badakhsh, M., Hastings-Tolsma, M., Firouskohi, M. et al. (2020). The lived experience of women with a high-risk pregnancy: a phenomenology investigation. *Midwifery* 82. http://doi.org/10.1016/j.midw.2019.102625.

Beauquier-Maccotta, B., Chalouhi, G.E., Picquet, A.L. et al. (2016). Impact of monochorionicity and twin to twin transfusion syndrome on prenatal attachment, post-traumatic stress disorder, anxiety and depressive symptoms. *PLoS One* 11 (1): e0145649.

Behruzi, R., Hatem, M., Goulet, L. et al. (2010). Humanized birth in high risk pregnancy: barriers and facilitating factors. *Medicine, Health Care & Philosophy* 13: 49–58.

Bibeau, A. (2014). Interventions during labour and birth in the United States: a qualitative analysis of women's experiences. *Sexual & Reproductive Health Care* 5 (4): 167–173.

Blickstein, I. (2006). Monochorionicity in perspective. *Ultrasound in Obstetrics & Gynecology* 27: 235–238.

Boswell, D., Broom, M., Smith, J. et al. (2015). Parental presence on neonatal intensive care unit clinical bedside rounds: randomised trial and focus group discussion. *Archives of Disease in Childhood. Fetal and Neonatal Edition.* https:// fn.bmj.com/content/fetalneonatal/100/3/F203.full.pdf.

Bothamley, J. and Boyle, M. (2009). *Medical Conditions Affecting Pregnancy and Childbirth.* Abingdon: Radcliffe Publishing.

Boykova, M. (2016). Life after discharge: what parents of preterm infants say about their transition to home. *Newborn and Infant Nursing Reviews* 16 (2): 58–65. http:// doi.org/10.1053/j.nainr.2016.03.002.

Candelori, C., Trumello, C., and Babore, A. (2015). The experience of premature birth for fathers: the application of the clinical interview for parents of high-risk infants (CLIP) to an Italian sample. *Frontiers in Psychology* http://doi.org/10.3389/fpsyg.2015.01444.

Centre for Disease Control and Prevention (CDC) (2017). Defining adult overweight and obesity. https://www.cdc.gov/obesity/adult/defining.html (accessed 10 October 2017).

Chen, H., Guo, J., Wang, C. et al. (2020a). Clinical characteristics and intrauterine vertical transmission potential of COVID-19 infection in nine pregnant women: a retrospective review of medical records. *Lancet* https://doi.org/10.1016/S0140-6736 20): 30360 30363.

Chen, Y., Peng, H., Wang, L. et al. (2020b). Infants born to mothers with a new coronavirus (COVID-19). *Frontiers in Pediatrics* 8 (104) https://doi.org/10.3389/fped.2020.00104.

Christenson, A., Johansson, E., Reynisdottir, S. et al. (2019). "Or else I close my ears" How women with obesity want to be approached and treated regarding gestational weight management : A qualitative interview study. *PLOS One.* https://journals. plos.org/plosone/article?id=10.1371/journal.pone.0222543 (accessed 14 July 2020).

Chuffo, D.R. and Segre, L.S. (2018). A Nurse-Based model of psychosocial support for emotionally distressed mothers of infants in the NICU. *JOGNN* 47: 14–121.

Dahlen, H.G. and Caplice, S. (2014). What do midwives fear? *Women and Birth* 27 (2014): 266–270.

Denton, J. and O'Brien, W. (2017). *Multiple Pregnancy in Mayes' Midwifery* (eds. S. Macdonald and G. Johnson). Edinburgh: Churchill Livingstone.

Department of Health (2010). *Midwifery 2020: Delivering expectations.* https://www. gov.uk/government/publications/midwifery-2020-delivering-expectations (accessed July 2020).

Druget, M., Nuño, L., Rodó, C. et al. (2018). Emotional effect of the loss of one or both Fetuses in a Monochorionic twin pregnancy. *Journal of Obstetric, Gynecologic & Neonatal Nursing* 47 (2): 137–145.

Dudley, L., Metin Gulmezoglu, A., Henderson-Smart, D.J. et al. (2010). Magnesium sulphate and other anticonvulsants for women with pre-eclampsia. *Cochrane Database System Review.* https://doi.org/10.1002/14651858.cd000025.pub2.

Elmir, R., Schmied, V., Jackson, D., and Wilkes, L. (2012). Between life and death: Women's experiences of coming close to death, and surviving a severe postpartum haemorrhage and emergency hysterectomy. *Midwifery* 28 (2): 228–235.

Falletta, L., Fischbein, R., Bhamidipalli, S.S., and Nicholas, L. (2018). Depression, anxiety and mental health experiences of women with a twin-twin transfusion syndrome pregnancy. *Archives of Women's Mental Health* 21: 75–83.

Ferriman, E., Stratton, S., and Stern, V. (2018). *Twin Pregnancy*, obstetrics, gynaecology and reproductive medicine. 28 (8): 221–228.

Fonseca, A., Nazaré, B., and Canavarro, M.C. (2012). Parental psychological distress and quality of life after a prenatal or postnatal diagnosis of congenital anomaly: a controlled comparison study with parents of healthy infants. *Disability Health J* 5 (2): 67–74.

Foster, E. and Hirst, J. (2014). Midwives' attitudes towards giving weight-related advice to obese pregnant women. *British Journal of Midwifery* 22 (4) http://www.magonlinelibrary.com/doi/full/10.12968/bjom.2014.22.4.254 (accessed 23 October 2017).

Franck, L. and Axelin, A. (2013). Differences in parents' nurses' and physicians' views of NICU parent support. *Acta Paediatrica* 102: 590–596. http://doi.org/10.1111/apa.12227.

Furber, M. and McGowan, L. (2011). A qualitative study of the experiences of women who are obese and pregnant in the UK. *Midwifery* 27 (4): 437–444.

Gandhi, M., Gandhi, R., Mack, L.M. et al. (2018). Estimated energy requirements increase across pregnancy in healthy women with dichorionic twins. *The American Journal of Clinical Nutrition* 108 (4): 775–783.

Garrod, D. and Byrom, S. (2007, 2007). *The midwifery public health agenda: setting the scene*. In: *Essential Midwifery Practice: Public Health* (eds. G. Edwards and S. Byrom). Oxford: Blackwell.

Gooding, J.S., Cooper, L.G., Blaine, A.I. et al. (2011). Family support and family-centred care in neonatal intensive care units: Origins, advances and impact. *Seminars in Perinatology* 35 (1): 20–28.

Gulla, K., Dalho, R., and Bradley Eilertsen, M.-E. (2017). From the delivery room to the neonatal intensive care unit. *Mothers' experiences with follow-up of skin-to-skin contact after premature birth Journal of Neonatal Nursing* 23 (6): 253–257. https://doi.org/10.1016/j.jnn.2017.06.002.

Heidari, H., Hasanpour, M., and Fooladi, M. (2017). Stress management among parents of neonates hospitalized in NICU: a qualitative study. *Journal of Caring Sciences* 6 (1): 29–38. http://doi.org/10.15171/jcs.2017.004.

Holditch-Davis, D., Santos, H., Levy, J. et al. (2015). Patterns of psychological distress in mothers of preterm infants. *Infant Behaviour & Development* 41: 154–163. https://doi.org/10.1016/j.infbeh.2015.10.004.

Holton, S., East, C., and Fisher, J. (2019). Weight management during pregnancy: a qualitative study of women's and care providers' experiences and perspectives. *BMC Pregnancy and Childbirth* 17, 9 351. https://bmcpregnancychildbirth. biomedcentral.com/articles/10.1186/s12884-017-1538-7 (accessed on 14 July 2020).

Jordan, R.G. and Gabzdyl, E. (2019). *Prenatal & Postnatal Care: A woman-centered approach: Hypertensive Disorders of Pregnancy Ch 31*, 2e, 511–539. USA: Wiley Blackwell.

Knight, M., Callaghan, W.M., Berg, C. et al. (2009). Trends in postpartum hemorrhage in high resource countries: a review and recommendations from the international postpartum Hemorrhage collaborative group. *BMC Pregnancy and Childbirth* 9: 55. https://doi.org/10.1186/1471-2393-9-55.

Knight, M., Acosta, C., Brocklehurst, P. et al. (2016). Beyond maternal death: improving the quality of maternal care through national studies of 'near-miss' maternal morbidity. *Programme Grants for Applied Research* 4 (9): 1–151.

Knight, M., Bunch, K., Tuffnell, D. et al. (eds.) (2019). *Saving Lives, Improving mother's Care- Lessons to Inform Future Maternity Care from the UK & Ireland Confidential Enquiries in Maternal Deaths & Morbidity 2015–2017*. Oxford: National Perinatal Epidemiology Unit.

Lee, S. (2014). Risk perception in women with high risk pregnancy. *British Journal of Midwifery* 22 (1): 8–13.

Lee, S., Ayers, S., and Holden, D. (2012). Risk perception of women during high risk pregnancy: a systematic review. *Health Risk and Society* 14 (6): 511–531.

Lee, S., Ayers, S., and Holden, D.A. (2013). A metasynthesis of risk perception in women with high risk pregnancies. *Midwifery* https://doi.org/10.1016/j. midw.2013.04.010.

Li, N., Han, L., Peng, M. et al. (2020). Maternal and neonatal outcomes of pregnant women with COVID-19 pneumonia: a case-control study. *Clinical Infectious Diseases*. https://doi.org/10.1093/cid/ciaa352.

Lowe, N. (2019). Preventing women's deaths from pregnancy-related causes. *JOGNN* 48: 249–251.

Masini, G., Tordini, C., Pietrosante, A. et al. (2019). Prediction of pregnancy complications by second-trimester uterine artery Doppler assessment in monochorionic twins. *Journal of Clinical Ultrasound* 47 (7) available at https://doi. org/10.1002/jcu.22734 accessed on 7 July 2020.

Mavrides, E., Allard, S., Chandraharan, E. et al., Thomson AJ on behalf of the Royal College of Obstetricians and Gynaecologists. (2016). Prevention of postpartum haemorrhage. *BJOG* 124: e106–e149.

McGowan, E.C., Du, N., Hawes, K. et al. (2017). Maternal mental health and neonatal intensive care unit discharge readiness in mothers of preterm infants. *The Journal of Pediatrics* 184: 68–74. https://doi.org/10.1016/j.jpeds.2017.01.052.

Mor, G. and Cardenas, I. (2010). The immune system in pregnancy: A unique complexity. *American Journal of Reproductive Immunology* 63 (6): 425–433.

Munk-Olsen, T., Bech, B.H., Vestergaard, M. et al. (2014). Psychiatric diseases following fetal death: a population-based cohort study. *BMJ Open* 4 (6): e005187.

Narayan, H. (2015). *A Compendium for Antenatal Care of High-Risk Pregnancy.* Oxford: Oxford University Press.

National Institute of Health and Care Excellence (NICE) (2019). *Twin and triplet pregnancy, Guideline 137.* London: NICE.

Nippita, T.A., Porter, M., Seeho, S.K. et al. (2017). Variations in clinical decision-making for induction of labour: a qualitative study. *BMC Pregnancy & Childbirth* 17 Article number: 317.

Office of National Statistics (ONS) (2018). Birth characteristics in England and Wales: 2018. www.ons.gov.uk/peoplepopulationandcommunity/ birthsdeathsandmarriages/livebirths/bulletins/birthcharacteristicsinenglandandw ales/2018 (accessed 14 July 2020).

Pembroke, N.F. and Pembroke, J.J. (2008). The spirituality of presence in midwifery care. *Midwifery* 24: 321–327.

Public Health England (PHE) (2017). Health matters: obesity and the food environment. https://www.gov.uk/government/publications/health-matters-obesity-and-the-food-environment/health-matters-obesity-and-the-food-environment—2 (accessed 20 October 2017).

Public Health England (PHE) (2020). COVID-19: investigation and initial clinical management of possible cases 2020. https://www.gov.uk/government/ publications/wuhan-novel-coronavirus-initial-investigation-of-possible-cases/ investigation-and-initial-clinical-management-of-possible-cases-of-wuhan-novel-coronavirus-wn-cov-infection (accessed 5 March 2020).

Rangan, M., Banting, M., and Favotto, L. (2019). Maternal mental health and internalizing and externalizing psychopathology in extremely low birth weight adults. *Journal of Developmental Origins of Health and Disease*: 1–8. https://doi. org/10.1017/S2040174419000771.

RCOG (2020a). Coronavirus (COVID-19). Pregnancy and women's health. https:// www.rcog.org.uk/globalassets/documents/guidelines/2020-07-24-coronavirus-covid-19-infection-in-pregnancy.pdf (accessed 20 July 2020).

RCOG (2020b). Occupational health advice for employers and pregnant women. https://www.rcog.org.uk/globalassets/documents/guidelines/2020-09-10-occupational-health-statement-rcog-rcm-fom.pdf (accessed 20 July 2020).

Reed, R., Sharman, R., and Inglis, C. (2017). Women's descriptions of childbirth trauma relating to care provider actions and interactions. *BMC Pregnancy & Childbirth* 17: 21. https://doi.org/10.1186/s12884-016-1197-0.

Reinders, A., Cuckson, J.C., Lee, J.T. et al. (2005). An accurate automated blood pressure device for use in pregnancy and pre-eclampsia. *BGOJ* 112: 1–6.

Robinson, M., Pennell, C.E., McLean, N.J. et al. (2011). The over-estimation of risk in pregnancy. *Journal of Psychosomatic Obstetrics and Gynaecology* 32 (2): 53–58.

Robson, S. and Waugh, J. (2013). *Medical Disorders in Pregnancy: A Manual for midwives.* London: Wiley-Blackwell.

Roderiquez-Almagro, J., Hernandez-Martinez, A., Roderiques-Almagro, D. et al. (2019). Women's perceptions of living a traumatic childbirth experience and factors related to a birth experience. *International Journal of Environmental Research & Public Health* 16: 1654. https://doi.org/10.3390/ijerph16091654.

Rogers, C.E., Kidokoro, H., Wallendorf, M. et al. (2012). Identifying mothers of very preterm infants at risk for postpartum depression and anxiety before discharge. *Journal of Perinatology* 33: 171–176.

Rossman, B., Greene, M.M., Kratovil, A.L. et al. (2017). Resilience in mothers of very-low-birth-weight infants hospitalized in the NICU. *Journal of Obstetric Gynecologic & Neonatal Nursing* 46 (3): 434–445.

Rowe, R. Knight M, Kurinczuk, J. (2018). Outcomes for women with BMI>35kg/m^2 admitted for labour care to alongside midwifery units in the UK: A national prospective cohort study using the UK PLOS One Published on behalf of UK Midwifery Study System (UKMidSS) https://doi.org/10.1371/journal.pone.0208041 (accessed 29 June 2020).

Rowley, J.M., Hensley, M.J., Brinsmead, M.W., and Wlodarczyk, J.H. (1995). Continuity of care by a midwife team versus routine care during pregnancy and birth: a randomised trial. *Medical Journal of Australia* 163 (6). Available at: https://doi.org/10.5694/j.1326-5377.1995.tb124592.x Accessed on 17 July 2020.

Royal College of Obstetricians and Gynaecologists (RCOG) (2016a). Management of monochorionic twin pregnancy. Green-top Guideline No 51. London: RCOG.

Royal College of Obstetricians and Gynaecologists (RCOG) (2016b). Postpartum Haemorrhage, Prevention and Management. Green-top Guideline No 52. London: RCOG.

Royal College of Obstetricians and Gynaecologists (RCOG) (2018). Care of Women with Obesity in Pregnancy Green-top Guideline No. 2. https://obgyn.onlinelibrary.wiley.com/doi/pdf/10.1111/1471-0528.15386 (accessed 29 June 2020).

Say, L., Chou, D., Gemmill, A. et al. (2014). Global causes of maternal death: a WHO systematic analysis. *The Lancet Global Health* 2 (6): e323–e333.

Schrager, S. and Sabo, L. (2001). Sheehan syndrome: a rare complication of postpartum hemorrhage. *Journal of American Board of Family Practice* 14 (5): 389–391.

Segre, L.S., Chuffo-Siewert, R., Brock, R.L. et al. (2013). Emotional distress in mothers of preterm hospitalised infants: a feasibility trail of nurse-delivered treatment. *Journal of Perinatology* 33: 924–928. https://doi.org/10.1038/jp.2013.93.

Segre, L.S., Pollack, L.O., Brock, R.L. et al. (2014). Depression screening on a maternity unit: a mixed-method evaluation of nurse' views and implementation strategies. *Issues in Mental Health Nursing* 35 (6): 444–454. https://doi.org/10.310 9/01612840.2013.879358.

Segre, L.S., Orengo-Aguayo, R.E., and Chuffo-Siewert, R. (2015). Depression management by NICU nurses: Mothers' views. *Clinical Nursing Research* 25 (3): 273–290. https://doi.org/10.1177/1054773815592596.

Shimizu, A. and Mori, A. (2017). Maternal perceptions of family-centred support and their associations with mother-nurse relationship in the neonatal intensive care unit. *Journal of Clinical Nursing*. https://doi.org/10.1111/jocn.14243.

Simpson, S., Cassidy, D., and Elinor, J. (2015). Healthy eating and lifestyle in pregnancy. The HELP trial. *Pregnancy Hypertension: An International Journal of Women's Cardiovascular Health* 4 (3): 233. https://www.sciencedirect.com/science/article/pii/S0195666314007302 (accessed 29 June 2020).

Sinni, S.V., Wallace, E.M., and Cross, W.M. (2014). Perinatal staff perceptions of safety and quality in their service. *BMC Health Service Research* 14: Article number 591.

Smith, D.M., Cooke, A., and Lavender, T. (2012). Maternal obesity is the new challenge; a qualitative study of health professionals' views towards suitable care for pregnant women with a body mass index (BMI) $\geq$30 kg/m^2. *BMC Pregnancy and Childbirth* 12: 157. https://bmcpregnancychildbirth.biomedcentral.com/artic les/10.1186/1471-2393-12-157 (accessed 29 June 2020).

Smits, J. and Monden, C. (2011). Twinning across the developing world. *PLoS One* 6 (9): e25239. https://doi.org/10.1371/journal.pone.0025239 (accessed 14 July 2020).

Statista (2018). Birth rate for twins in the United States from 1980 to 2018 (per 1,000 live births). https://www.statista.com/statistics/276017/us-twin-birth-rate (accessed 14 July 2020).

Sweeney, S., Rothstein, R., Visintainer, P. et al. (2017). Impact of kangaroo care on parental anxiety level and parenting skills for preterm infants in the neonatal intensive care unit. *Journal of Neonatal Nursing* 23 (3): 151–158. https://doi.org/10.1016/j.jnn.2016.09.003.

Taylor, B., Cross-Sudworth, F., MacArthur, C. (2018). Better Births and continuity: midwife survey results. Birmingham: University of Birmingham.

The Magpie Trial Collaborative Group (2002). Do women with pre-eclampsia, and their babies benefit from magnesium sulphate? The Magpie Trial: A randomised placebo-controlled trial. *Lancet* 359 (9321): 1877–1890. https://doi.org/10.1016/s0140-6736(02)08778-0.

Theilen, L.H., Meeks, H., Fraser, A. et al. (2018). Long-term mortality risk and life expectancy following recurrent hypertensive disease of pregnancy. *American Journal of Obstetrics & Gynaecology* 107: e1–e6.

Tucker, K.L., Crawford, C., Greenfields, S.M. et al. (2017). Blood pressure self-monitoring in pregnancy. *BMC Pregnancy & Childbirth* 17 (1): S109–S110.

UK Obstetric Surveillance System (UKOSS) (2020). COVID-19 in pregnancy. Nuffield Department of Population Health, University of Oxford https://www.npeu.ox.ac.uk/ukoss/current-surveillance/covid-19-in-pregnancy (accessed 24 June 2020).

Vireday, P. (2002). Are you a size friendly midwife? Midwifery Today (pp. 28–32). Spring.

Whitaker, K.M., Baruth, M., Schlaff, R.A. et al. (2019). Provider advice on physical activity and nutrition in twin pregnancies: a cross sectional electronic study. *BMC Pregnancy and Childbirth*, available at: https://doi.org/10.1186/s12884-019-2574-2 (accessed on 7 July 2020).

Whitford H.M., Wallis, S.K., Dowswell, T., et al. (2017). Breastfeeding education and support for women with twins or higher order multiples. https://doi.org/10.1002/14651858.CD012003.pub2 (accessed 17 July 2020).

WHO (2012). WHO recommendations on prevention and treatment of postpartum haemorrhage. https://www.who.int/reproductivehealth/publications/maternal_perinatal_health/9789241548502/en (accessed 25 May 2020).

WHO (2017). Obesity. http://www.who.int/mediacentre/factsheets/fs311/en (accessed 29 June 2020).

WHO (2020). Coronavirus disease (COVID-2019) Situation report 113 – 12th May 2020. https://www.who.int/emergencies/diseases/novel-coronavirus-2019/situation-reports (accessed 25 May 2020).

Zelkowitz, P., Na, S., Wang, T. et al. (2011). Early maternal anxiety predicts cognitive and behavioural outcomes of VLBW children at 24 months corrected age. *Acta Paediatrica* 100: 700–704.

6

'With Woman' with Gestational Diabetes Mellitus

*Anna M. Brown, Julia Derrick; Amy Duncan (midwives);
and Joanne (woman)*

Introduction

This chapter examines the literature pertaining to gestational diabetes mellitus (GDM) and the compromised neonate because of either the at-risk pregnancy or a complicated labour and delivery. It debates the issues around support for woman and their neonates and how healthcare professionals strive to fulfil the concept of 'with woman' who has GDM. It explores midwives' and women's perspectives of unfolding events and the supporting measures that can be put in place to ensure more positive outcomes. The literature explores journeys of women with gestational diabetes and the implications for their neonates.

Gestational Diabetes Literature

GDM, which usually occurs in the second trimester of pregnancy, results from a glucose intolerance and increased insulin resistance. The condition results in increased risks, for both mother and her neonate, as an outcome of pregnancy (HAPO 2008; McCance 2011). A woman diagnosed with GDM will expect to be monitored more frequently, which may lead to interventions in pregnancy and labour. In addition, overexposure to the hyperglycaemic condition in utero results in a compromised fetus due to the mother's diabetes. After delivery, the neonate may display clinical complications of hypoglycaemia, hyperbilirubinemia, polycythaemia and respiratory distress syndrome (RDS), amongst others (NICE 2015).

Current published literature on the management of GDM and other pre-existing diabetic conditions in pregnancy suggest treatments that may ameliorate outcomes for both mother and neonates. Cheung (2009), Nolan (2011), carrying out a review of evidence for blood glucose monitoring, examined pharmacological management for GDM (such as glyburide, metformin and insulin) and dietary and exercise therapy. Good glycaemic control and healthy lifestyle measures should be taken to minimise development of obesity and Type 2 diabetes (T2D) in later life although appropriate medication may reduce these risks because of GDM (Sathyapalan et al. 2010).

Diagnosis of GDM

Approximately 5% of all pregnant women in England and Wales present with GDM or pre-existing or Type 1 diabetes, of which 87.5% are GDM with tendencies to develop long-term diabetes after pregnancy (NICE 2015). The evidence is unclear as to the most effective diagnostic procedure and glycaemic thresholds, in addition to the benefits of screening for GDM (HAPO 2008; Benhalima et al. 2015; Farrar et al. 2017). However, NICE (2008) supported by the World Health Organisation (WHO 2013), recommend thresholds based on the Hyperglycaemia and Adverse Pregnancy Outcome Study (HAPO 2008). In the previous 2008 NICE guidelines, universal rather than selective screening (Scott et al. 2002; Cosson et al. 2006; Tieu et al. 2010) for GDM were recommended, with the aim to improve diagnosis, treatment and subsequent outcomes for both the mother and the neonate (Brown et al. 2016). However, recent evidence from Tieu et al. (2017) showed that there is insufficient evidence to demonstrate that through universal screening and increased numbers of GDM women diagnosed there are improved fetal and maternal outcomes (Meek et al. 2015; Kennedy 2017). Updated NICE 2015 guidelines for diabetes care make recommendations for a risk assessment and testing for GDM if the following is identified: Body Mass Index (BMI) above $30\,kg\,m^{-2}$, previous macrosomic baby weighing 4.5 kg or above, previous gestational diabetes, family history of diabetes (first-degree relative with diabetes) and minority ethnic family origin with a high prevalence of diabetes (Erjavec et al. 2016).

Although there is no consensus as to what degree of glucose intolerance would diagnose a woman with GDM (Lindsay et al. 2017), the evidence suggests that early diagnosis will reduce the risks to mother and baby and improve perinatal outcomes (Yogev et al. 2009). NICE (2015) recommend that blood glucose control is assessed through HbA1c levels to ensure the impact of hyperglycaemia on the neonate is reduced by maintaining a level at $48\,mmol\,mol^{-1}$ (6.5%). NICE (2015) maintain that a level of risk for GDM cannot be determined through routine monitoring of HbA1c in women with GDM and is only predictive in the first trimester for women with pre-existing diabetes. In addition, NICE 2015 do not recommend fasting plasma glucose for diagnosis of GDM and suggest further selective testing, at 24–28 week's gestation, through self-monitoring of blood glucose using a glucometer. If glycosuria is found to be at 2+ as a single risk factor, this is followed by a two-hour 75 g oral glucose tolerance test (OGTT) and GDM is diagnosed if the OGTT results indicates that plasma glucose is $7.8\,\text{mmol}\,\text{l}^{-1}$ or above.

Managing GDM to Improve Outcomes

Women suffering from GDM are at increased risk of recurrence of this condition in subsequent pregnancies (Singh and Rastogi 2008; NICE 2008). Increased risk of developing GDM is associated with maternal and neonatal outcomes in some ethnic groups and older women (Carolan et al. 2012). Other adverse outcomes, such as increased hypertension and instrumental intervention during labour, may be associated outcomes of GDM and are increased risks if the woman also has a raised BMI of above $30\,\text{kg}\,\text{m}^{-2}$ (Simmons 2011).

The effect of treatment on GDM comparing therapeutic intervention, such as diet or insulin, to routine antenatal care have been examined through a systematic review and meta-analysis (Poolsup et al. 2014). Results suggest that treating GDM significantly reduced the risk of macrosomia, shoulder dystocia and gestational hypertension. Other studies have investigated the effects of a low glycaemic index diet on pregnancy outcomes in GDM and concluded that there were no significant differences in GDM between women on this diet and those on a conventional high-fibre diet, in terms of birthweight, prevalence of macrosomia, insulin treatment or adverse pregnancy outcomes (Louie et al. 2011). Walsh et al. (2012) found similar results but suggest that a low glycaemic index diet did have a positive effect on gestational weight gain and maternal glucose tolerance. These findings are supported by another meta-analysis of randomised evidence to explore how obstetric outcomes can be improved through diet and lifestyle interventions such as exercise and physical activity (Thangaratinam et al. 2012).

Midwives have a unique opportunity to provide information and education about management or prevention of GDM and fulfil the concept of 'with woman' suffering from this condition (Carolan et al. 2012). Health professionals should be able to correctly identify risk factors and successfully selectively screen for GDM (Kennedy 2017). However, Murphy (2010) suggested that this is not always the case and midwives may not correctly identify women at risk of GDM. Midwives have a valuable role to play in offering information, health promotion and support to empower women to make the right decisions for their care and help to normalise a medicalised experience of pregnancy, if the condition is recognised and carefully managed (Rogers and Hughes 2010). Brown et al. (2018) suggest that midwives can play a key role in educating women about healthy lifestyles, especially diet and nutrition, in a bid to reduce obesity in pregnancy that leads to risk factors associated with a raised BMI.

The experiences of midwives providing care and counselling to women with GDM were explored by Persson et al. (2011) who concluded that health professionals experienced increased demands to enhance monitoring of these women. Midwives were motivated to use different strategies, such as intensifying diabetes screening and management of mother and fetus, as a precaution in identifying all GDM women. The authors suggest that training in coaching/counselling sessions for the midwives would improve the number of women who were diagnosed with GDM. The authors recommend that midwives need to be vigilant and develop a strategy to work more closely with dieticians and nutritionists to reduce the risk of obesity in women with GDM. In addition, some evidence (Brown et al. 2018) suggests that those women who were 29 years old and younger were found to be at greater risk of developing the condition of GDM.

Women's Experiences of GDM Management

Education and support from midwives about diabetes in pregnancy, its management and associated comorbidities, such as adverse risks to both mother and neonate, is key to empowering women to understand and make decisions about their care. Parsons et al. (2014) and Nolan et al. (2011) provide evidence about perceptions and experiences amongst women with GDM and their expectations of care provision by midwives (Jagiello and Chertok 2015). Evidence suggests that women with GDM, requiring insulin treatment, experienced negative emotional impact lasting beyond pregnancy (Figueroa Gray et al. 2017). The authors imply that alternative treatment options for GDM and informed choices needed to be explored further. However, it appears that insulin treatment rather than dietary control resulted in higher levels of anxiety and stress in GDM women on insulin (Hui et al. 2014).

Midwives may be able to support women to self-manage GDM and meet their birth expectations through positive psychological interventions to manage and reduce adverse maternal and neonatal risks (Lawrence 2011). These findings concur with those from Carolan et al. (2012) and Carolan (2013) who suggest that women diagnosed with GDM experience a process of adjustment which is facilitated more effectively through midwifery support at each stage to self-manage the condition. Recognising the needs of women with GDM may influence their behaviour towards the diagnosis as they are interested in achieving optimal health for their baby, through interventions to improve glycaemic control and prevent development of T2D in the future. Midwives may fully embrace the 'with woman' concept in supporting women with GDM through their journey towards an optimal birth.

Implications for the Neonate of a GDM Woman

Colostrum expression prior to delivery has been accepted by women traditionally to stimulate lactation and avoid engorgement and is taught by midwives as hand expression in preparation for breastfeeding and promoting production of lactogenesis 2 (Chapman et al. 2013). Little evidence is available as to the benefits of colostrum harvesting in women who develop gestational diabetes, although anecdotally they are advised to express breastmilk in late pregnancy and store colostrum with the view of treating hypoglycaemia in the neonates and ameliorate the condition after delivery. Conflicting evidence is available as to the benefits or concerns in terms of antenatal breastmilk expression and associations with release of oxytocin leading to preterm birth (Cox 2006, 2010; Soltani and Scott 2012; Chapman et al. 2013; Fallon and Dunne 2015). In addition, little is known about the impact of colostrum supplementation after delivery and its effect on normalising hypoglycaemia in neonates born to women with GDM (Chertok et al. 2009; East et al. 2014; Fair et al. 2019). This latter part of this chapter seeks to explore these issues and review how antenatal colostrum harvesting in pregnant women impacts on outcomes for mothers and their babies and what role the midwives play in ensure they fulfil the 'with woman' concept in these situations (Alberdi et al. 2018).

The Role of Lactation in GDM Women

The role of lactation in GDM women has been explored by some researchers and it is suggested that breastfeeding has an impact on normalising blood glucose and increases sensitivity to insulin in early postpartum, although the long-term effects are not clear (Gunderson et al. 2012; Much et al. 2014). Studies have examined issues of duration and cessation for breastfeeding and identified that these are mainly related to supply of breastmilk and feeding ability, and support for women to build confidence with breastfeeding (Singh et al. 2009, Oakley et al. 2014, Brisbane and Giglia 2015, Morrison et al. 2015, Oza-Frank et al. 2016, Zelalem et al. 2016, Wallenborn et al. 2017, Bronwell et al. 2019). Women with gestational diabetes have been found to be at greater risk of developing type 1 diabetes after the pregnancy and late onset Type 2 diabetes and other co-morbidities, including obesity.

The physiology of lactation associated with women diagnosed with GDM indicates that there is a risk of delayed lactogenesis 2 (De Bortoli and Amir 2015) and therefore this group of women are less likely to successfully breastfeed (Rusmussen and Kjolhede 2004; Forster et al. 2011; Matias et al. 2014; Brownell et al. 2019). Other conditions in pregnancy which may delay lactogenesis 2 are late onset pre-eclampsia and other hypertensive disorders of pregnancy (Demirci et al. 2019). However, in a mother with GDM, impaired glycaemic control and increased insulin resistance results in hyperglycaemia. The high glucose levels cross the placenta into the fetal circulation, which stimulates increased secretion of insulin. The fetal response to hyperglycaemia and hyperinsulinemia is to lay down fat and protein storage, resulting in a macrosomic baby. This presents problems in terms of increased neonatal morbidity of shoulder dystocia and birth trauma and maternal morbidity of complicated/assisted delivery such as forceps delivery or caesarean section, perineal trauma and postpartum haemorrhage. In addition, the infant is five times more likely to experience hypoglycaemia after the delivery and twice as likely to develop neonatal jaundice in the first week of life (Kamana et al. 2015). RDS is also an increased risk, resulting in admissions to a neonatal intensive care unit (NICU) (Mitanchez et al. 2015).

The long-term effects of GDM have been documented in the literature which concludes that there is evidence to suggest that fetal exposure to hyperglycaemia increases risks and results in 'metabolic programming' of the neonate to develop diabetes and obesity in adulthood (Aune et al. 2014; Mitanchez et al. 2015). Controlled management of GDM and early breastfeeding of the neonate could reduce some of these risks in later life (Yessoufou and Moutairou 2011, Wszolek 2015, Lamba et al. 2016).

As with previous chapters, the literature is next examined through Rodgers' Concept Analysis to identify attribute and consequences of the 'with the GDM woman' concept (Table 6.1).

Table 6.1 Concept analysis of 'with the GDM woman' and compromised neonate.

Antecedents	Evidence	Attributes (A) and Consequences (C)
GDM outcomes for mother	Singh and Rastogi (2008) NICE (2008) increased risks for older woman and some ethnic groups	Hypertension (C) Increased intervention in labour and delivery (C) Intensified midwifery monitoring (C)
GDM treatment	Simmons (2011) limiting gestational weight gain Poolsup et al. (2014) insulin versus diet therapy	Midwifery advice and support with nutrition and diet (A) Improves obstetric outcomes (C) No significant differences in pregnancy outcomes (C)
Midwives' views	Carolan et al. (2012) midwives' role to provide information and education Persson et al. (2011) experiences of midwives providing care and counselling	Identifying risk factors correctly (A) Empowering women to make right decisions (C) Normalising a medicalised experience (C) Increased demands to enhance monitoring (A) Improved training and integrated care with dietitians and nutritionists (C)

(Continued)

Table 6.1 (Continued)

Antecedents	Evidence	Attributes (A) and Consequences (C)
Women's experiences	Nolan et al. (2011) and Parsons et al. (2014) expectations in meeting emotional needs	Education and support by MWs (A) Understanding and empowering women to make right choices (C)
	Figueroa Gray et al. (2017) GDM women requiring insulin treatment	Lasting negative impact on women (C)
	Hui et al. (2014) insulin vs diet control	Higher levels of anxiety and stress (A) Midwifery support with dietary control reassuring (C) Process of adjustment (A) Midwifery support at each stage to self-manage GDM (A) Interest in achieving optimal health (C) Positive psychological response, reduced adverse outcomes (C)
	Carolan (2013) psychological impact	
Lactation in GDM women	Gunderson (2012) and Much et al. (2014) effect of breastfeeding	Normalising blood glucose (A) sensitivity to insulin in early PP (C)
	Morrison et al. (2015) supply of breastmilk and feeding ability	Support for duration and cessation of breastfeeding (A) Improved confidence with breastfeeding (C)
	De Bortoli and Amir (2015) physiology of lactation	GDM impact on lactation (A)
	Demirici et al. (2018)	Late onset pre-eclampsia (A) Delay in lactogenesis 2 (C)
	Matias et al. (2014)	Less likely to successfully breastfeed (C)
	Kamana et al. (2015) impact of GDM	Macrosomic baby (A) Hypoglycaemia and neonatal jaundice (C) Respiratory distress syndrome (C)
	Mitanchez et al. (2015)	Long-term effects of GDM (A)
	Yessoufou and Moutairou (2011)	Support and early diagnosis reduces risks (C)

Conclusion

The above literature has examined the impact and consequences of GDM on women and their neonates. Studies have presented findings which suggest that overall, women experience higher levels of anxiety due to the condition as monitoring by health professionals is intensified during pregnancy and labour leading to more interventions. Midwives as lead professions should be able to identify risk factors correctly and support women with advice on treatment, diet and nutrition through improved training and collaboration with other expert professionals.

Women should therefore feel empowered to make the right decisions for their individualised care, resulting in a positive psychological response and reduced adverse outcomes. In addition, when midwives educate women to express breastmilk antenatally, the rates of successful feeding by the neonate in the immediate postnatal period are greatly increased.

A Specialist Midwife's Story

Julia's Stories

The public view of a midwife is the person who delivered their baby. The reality is that midwives are responsible for all aspects of care during pregnancy, birth and afterwards. As a midwife caring mainly for high-risk pregnancies, it can be easy to lose sight of this.

As a diabetes specialist midwife, working within a small team and seeing women and their families, and often subsequent pregnancies, the women become familiar with you and they are relaxed around you.

The remit of this role is to keep in touch with women and review their blood glucose levels, making diagnoses and offering counselling afterwards. Giving advice and liaising with other members of the multi-disciplinary team. The women attend clinics frequently, often weekly, so they perceive us as their main caregiver.

Women with pre-existing diabetes have more appointments during their pregnancy than most women with complex care. We quite often see these women weekly and develop a relaxed and friendly relationship with these women. Here are some of their stories.

Sarah* with high BMI: Sarah was a lovely lady who attended fortnightly. She had a raised BMI of 65. She was quite immobile and very difficult to weigh and take basic observations from. It would take three people to listen to the fetal heart rate and we would reassure her by making light of the situation. She was expecting her first child and was very excited.

She realised that her size was an obstacle and was quite embarrassed about it. Although her weight was an issue and had been addressed, she was still restricted to some extent to try to reduce her weight. She tried really hard to keep her blood glucose levels under control and did reasonably well.

Sarah delivered by caesarean section at 38/40 a beautiful baby with a birthweight within the normal range. She was so delighted with this child and we were so happy that she had made such an effort to keep good blood glucose control. We

(Continued)

visited her on the postnatal ward and wished her well. She returned a few weeks later to thank us.

Amy's GDM and Colostrum Harvesting Story

Earlier this year, I took over the care of Alice* who was admitted to hospital at 38 weeks for an induction of labour as she had gestational diabetes. Her last baby was delivered by emergency caesarean at 6 cm dilated, but this time she was aiming for a vaginal delivery. Being cautious about her previous experience, Alice had requested an epidural anaesthetic as soon as possible; in case another caesarean was needed, she wanted to have the epidural in situ. The artificial rupture of membranes had successfully induced her labour. So, advocating for the mother, I ensured we had the epidural sited as a matter of urgency.

Over the course of the day Alice stayed mobile in the bed and her contractions continued until she reached 8 cm dilated. However, the subsequent examination found no change in dilatation and her contractions had reduced to just one every 15 minutes. When the obstetric consultant attended the room, they discussed with Alice and her husband two options. Firstly, they offered to start an oxytocin infusion to increase the contractions, but with the risk of uterine rupture, or the option of another caesarean. Alice* reluctantly consented to the hormone infusion saying, 'I really don't want another caesarean, but this drip worries me.' After checking maternal and fetal wellbeing, I reassured Alice and suggested we could try another more holistic approach before starting the oxytocin infusion. We discussed the possibility of expressing some colostrum to try and increase the uterine contractions. Alice was keen to breastfeed her baby but was concerned that she may be forced to give artificial milk to help the baby maintain its blood sugars as a result of her GDM. Again, I explained the benefits of intrapartum hand expression and that this could result in the storage of some colostrum ready to give her baby if required. She was overjoyed that we had another option to try before the hormone infusion and was eager to try it. I communicated her desires with the obstetric team, advocating again for this mother, and taught her how to hand express. Over the next 20 minutes she harvested 2 ml of colostrum. Within 40 minutes her contractions had returned to 4 every 10 minutes and she was starting to experience a severe pressure sensation. She had a vaginal examination two hours later where the cervix was found to be fully dilated and the presenting part visible at the height of contractions. Alice went on to have a spontaneous vaginal delivery, the birth she was so keen to achieve, and when her baby struggled to latch initially, we were able to feed it the colostrum she had harvested. This baby maintained normal blood sugars and remained exclusively breastfeeding at the time of discharge.

A Woman's Story

Joanne's Story

Before becoming pregnant with my daughter, I had a discussion with my diabetic nurse and therefore I knew that as a Type 1 diabetic I would need to be under consultant care during pregnancy. As soon as I had a positive test, the community midwives told me that I would need to be referred to the diabetes consultant by my GP. I had just moved to a new house and surgery and unfortunately it took a few calls to the GP, but eventually they did agree to refer me, and I had a viability scan at around six weeks, followed by an appointment with a consultant and diabetes specialist midwife.

I found the diabetes midwife to be extremely helpful and approachable and met with her, along with a consultant, every four weeks throughout my pregnancy to review scan results and monitor my blood glucose levels. I had an app on which I uploaded my blood glucose levels daily, so it could be monitored. I could request a call back through this which I used a few times when I had concerns and the midwife always called back within a day and discussed my treatment with me, discussing it with the consultant if necessary. I was made aware that I would be induced between 37 and 39 weeks, even if everything was going well.

Managing my diabetes with pregnancy was very difficult. I found at the beginning my blood glucose levels weren't affected too much, then I had lots of high spikes usually followed by low readings where I was self-correcting with insulin. My insulin needs did increase, and I felt supported by doctors and midwives regarding my treatment.

Alongside consultant care, I was seen by a community midwife from about 10 weeks then throughout pregnancy. I would say that this was a little inconsistent as I saw three or four different midwives; however, it was reassuring to hear the baby's heartbeat and know that my own health separately from my diabetes was good.

From 28 weeks I had growth scans every 4 weeks, which were all fine, and I was also given some leaflets on induction. I did feel very daunted by this, as one leaflet was specific to diabetes (gestational, Type 1 and Type 2) and one was a general leaflet about induction. The leaflets seemed to contradict each other slightly and I was left with lots of questions and concerns. Towards the end of my pregnancy, I had a meeting with the diabetes midwife to discuss the induction process and I think it would have been helpful to me to have this face to face meeting much earlier, as I ended up giving birth less than a week later. My insulin needs dropped quite dramatically, and I was told that this could indicate the placenta failing; this led to induction at 36 + 4 weeks.

(Continued)

My induction was brought forward by a few days and I was given the pessary at about 10 p.m. I had my own room and a midwife, who was at a workstation just outside the room, was looking after me and one other lady. This was very reassuring, although I had been told I would have a 1:1 midwife. At the time of induction, I was 1 cm dilated, my husband went home as we were told it was likely the process would take at least two days. My contractions started quite quickly and were very intense. When the midwife monitored me, she said I was having 'tightenings', and was very calm, I think this helped me to keep relaxed. At 2 a.m., I was in a lot of pain and asked whether I should call my husband to come in; around this time my waters broke. I was still 1 cm dilated and the midwife said it was still likely to be at least 24 hours until I would be in active labour and advised that he didn't need to come in yet. Therefore, I decided to ask for pain relief and was given paracetamol and codeine. The pain seemed to intensify quickly, and I was given morphine. The midwife happily gave me an anti-sickness injection as I explained that I was very anxious about pain relief making me sick. I managed to relax for a while and at 5 a.m. I was 10 cm dilated and ready to go into the delivery room. I was told that I would be on a sliding scale for insulin; however, this didn't happen. I do feel that I could have been monitored a little more overnight, in particular between 2 a.m. and 5 a.m.

I was given gas and air and was pushing for around 1 hour 30 minutes, but I was exhausted. I remember insisting the midwife call a doctor and asking for forceps as I was sure nothing was happening and had no urge to push. At first the midwife said this wasn't needed, but soon the baby's heartrate was dropping so a doctor was called. The baby was in a difficult position and I was given the choice of ventouse, or spinal epidural and forceps. As I was so exhausted, I went for the pain-free option. At this time the midwife's shift was over; I actually think this was helpful as I had become rather frustrated when I felt the baby wasn't moving and I think seeing a fresh face helped! From there everything went very quickly, and my baby was safely delivered; the forceps were used for a lift out. Even though I had just had a baby, by this time I could not keep awake after a sleepless night and lots of medication! The midwife and a student helped the baby latch on and supported her whilst I slept.

Overall, I felt very supported by midwives during my pregnancy, in particular by the diabetes midwife. I would have liked to discuss birth options sooner and I do feel that perhaps the first midwife I had during delivery was slightly too relaxed.

Lessons Leant

There are some interesting stories above illustrating the concept analysis of the literature which explores midwives' and women's experiences of diabetes in pregnancy and outcomes for the baby and the mother. This is suggested in the literature as increased intervention in labour and delivery and intensified midwifery monitoring are identified in the cited studies. However, Joanne's story, as a diabetic woman, suggests that due to expected outcomes of prolonged labour after induction, she laboured silently in the early hours of the morning, without her partner present; dilating very quickly from 1 to 10 cm in three hours, which is very fast for a primigravid woman. Joanne's perception is that the midwife was '*slightly too relaxed*' and that '*I do feel that I could have been monitored a little more overnight, in particular between 2 a.m. and 5 a.m.*' This woman also commented that she would have liked to have discussed birth options sooner, gaining an understanding of what had happened and being empowered to make the right choices. Overall, however, she did feel well informed and supported by the specialist health professionals, who identified her risks correctly and planned a safe birth.

References

Alberdi, G., O'Sullivan, E.J., Scully, H. et al. (2018). A feasibility study of multidimensional breastfeeding support intervention in Ireland. *Midwifery* 58: 86–92.

Aune, D., Norat, T., Romundstad, P. et al. (2014). Breastfeeding and the maternal risk of type 2 diabetes: a systematic review and dose response: meta-analysis of cohort studies. *Nutrition, Metabolism & Cardiovascular Diseases* 24: 107–115.

Benhalima, K., Matthieu, C., Damm, P. et al. (2015). A proposal for use of uniform diagnostic criteria for gestational diabetes in Europe: an opinion paper by the European Board & College of Obstetrics and Gynaecology (EBCOG). *Diabetologia* 58 (7): 1422–1429.

Brisbane, J.M. and Giglia, R.C. (2015). Experiences of expressing and storing colostrum antenatally: a qualitative study of mothers in regional Western Australia. *Journal of Child Health Care* 19 (2): 2016–2215.

Brown, A.M., Rajeswari, D., and Bowles, A. (2016). Choice of planned place of birth for women with diet-controlled gestational diabetes mellitus. *British Journal of Midwifery* 24 (10): 702–710.

Brown, A.M., Rajeswari, D., Williams, P., and Lowndes, A. (2018). Managing gestation diabetes mellitus: audit data of outcomes for women and neonates. *British Journal of Midwifery* 26 (12): 775–786.

Brownell, E., Howard, C., Lawrence, R. et al. (2019). Delayed lactogenesis II predicts the cessation of any or exclusive breastfeeding. *Journal of Pediatrics* 161 (4): 608–614.

Carolan, M. (2013). Women's experiences of gestational diabetes self-management: a qualitative study. *Midwifery* 29: 637–645.

Carolan, M., Gill, K.G., and Steele, C. (2012). Women's experience of factors that facilitate or inhibit gestational diabetes self-management. *BMC Pregnancy and Childbirth* 12 (1): 99.

Chapman, T., Pincombe, J., and Harris, M. (2013). Antenatal breast expression: a critical review of the literature. *Midwifery* 29: 203–213.

Chertok, I.R., Raz, I., Shoham, I. et al. (2009). Effects of early breastfeeding on neonatal glucose levels of term infants born to women with gestational diabetes. *Journal of Human Nutrition and Dietetics* 22 (2): 166–169.

Cheung, N.W. (2009). The management of gestational diabetes. *Vascular Health and Risk Management* 9: 153–167.

Cosson, E., Benchimol, M., Carbillon, L. et al. (2006). Universal rather than selective screening for gestational diabetes mellitus may improve fetal outcomes. *Diabetes & Metabolism* 32: 140–146.

Cox, S. (2006). Expressing and storing colostrum antenatally for use in the new born period. *Breastfeeding Review* 14 (3): 11–16.

Cox, S. (2010). An ethical dilemma: should recommending antenatal expressing and storing of colostrum continue? *Breastfeeding Review* 18: 5–7.

De Bortoli, J. and Amir, L.H. (2015). Is onset of lactation delayed in women with diabetes in pregnancy? A systematic review. *Diabetic Medicine* 33: 17–24.

Demirci, J., Schmella, M., Glasser, M. et al. (2018). Delayed lactogenesis II and potential utility of antenatal milk expression in women developing late-onset preeclampsia: a case series. *BMC Pregnancy and Childbirth* 18: 68.

Demirci, J., Glasser, M., Fichner, J. et al. (2019). "It gave me confidence": first-time U.S. mothers' experience with antenatal milk expression. *Maternal & Child Nutrition*. http://doi.org/10.1111/mcn.12824.

East, C.E., Domlan, W.J., and Forster, D.A. (2014). Antenatal milk expression by women with diabetes for improving infant outcomes. *Cochrane Database of Systematic Reviews* (7): CD010408.

Erjavec, K., Poljicanin, T., and Matijevic, R. (2016). Impact of implementation of new WHO diagnostic criteria for gestational diabetes mellitus on prevalence and perinatal outcomes: a population-based study. *Journal of Pregnancy* 2016. https://dx.doi.org/10.1155%2F2016%2F2670912.

Fair, F.J., Waton, H., Gardner, R. et al. (2019). Women's perspectives on antenatal breast expression: a cross-sectional survey. *Reproductive Health* 15: 58. https://doi.org/10.1186/s12978-018-0497-4.

Fallon, A. and Dunne, F. (2015). Breastfeeding practices that support women with diabetes to breastfeed. *Diabetes Research and Clinical Practice* 110: 10–17.

Farrar, D., Simmonds, M., Bryant, M. et al. (2017). Risk factor screening to identify women requiring oral glucose tolerance testing to diagnose gestational diabetes: a systematic review and meta-analysis of two pregnancy cohorts. *PLoS One* 12 (4): e0175288.

Figueroa Gray, M., Clarissa, H., Kiel, L. et al. (2017). "It's a very big burden on me": women's experiences using insulin for gestational diabetes. *Maternal & Child Health Journal* 21 (8): 1678–1685.

Forster, D.A., Moorhead, A., Jacobs, S. et al. (2011). Advising women about diabetes in pregnancy to express human milk in late pregnancy (Diabetes and Antenatal Milk Expression DAME): a multi-central unblended randomised controlled trial. *The Lancet* 389: 2204–2213.

Gunderson, E.P., Crites, Y., Chaing, V. et al. (2012). Influence of breastfeeding during the postpartum oral glucose tolerance test on plasma glucose insulin. *The Obstetrician and Gynaecologist* 120 (1): 136–143.

HAPO. The HAPO Study Cooperative Research Group (2008). Hyperglycaemia and adverse pregnancy outcomes. *The New England Journal of Medicine* 358: 1999–2002.

Hui, A.L., Sevenhuysen, G., Dexter, H. et al. (2014). Food choice decision-making by women with gestational diabetes. *Canadian Journal of Diabetes* 38 (1): 26–31.

Jagiello, K.P. and Chertok, I.R. (2015). Women's experiences with early breastfeeding after gestational diabetes. *Journal of Obstetric, Gynecologic & Neonatal Nursing* 44 (4): 500–509.

Kamana, K., Shakya, S., and Zhang, H. (2015). Gestational diabetes mellitus and macrosomia: a literature review. *Annals of Nutrition & Metabolism* 66 (Suppl. 2): 14–20.

Kennedy, J. (2017). Diagnosis and screening of gestational diabetes: conflicts of policy. *MIDIRS Midwifery Digest* 27: 4.

Lamba, S., Simmy, C., and Manta, N. (2016). Effects of antenatal breastmilk expression at term pregnancy to improve postnatal lactational performance. *The Journal of Obstetrics and Gynecology of India* 66 (1): 30–34.

Lawrence, J.M. (2011). Women with diabetes in pregnancy: different perceptions and expectations. *Best Practice & Research Clinical Obstetrics & Gynaecology* 25: 15–24.

Lindsay, R.S., Mackin, S.T., and Scott, M.N. (2017). Gestational diabetes mellitus-right person, right treatment, right time? *BMC Medicine* 15: 163.

Louie, J.C., Markovic, T.P., Perera, N. et al. (2011). A randomised controlled trial investigating the effects of a low-glycaemic index diet on pregnancy outcomes in gestational diabetes mellitus. *Diabetes Care* 34 (11): 2341–2346.

Matias, S.L., Dewey, K., Quesberry, C.P. et al. (2014). Maternal prepregnancy obesity and insulin treatment during pregnancy are independently associated with delayed lactogenesis in women with recent gestational diabetes mellitus. *The American Journal of Clinical Nutrition* 99 (1): 115–121.

McCance, D.R. (2011). Pregnancy and diabetes. *Best Practice & Research Clinical Endocrinology & Metabolism* 25: 945–958.

Meek, C., Lewis, H., Patient, C. et al. (2015). Diagnosis of gestational diabetes: falling through the net. *Diabetologia* 58 (9): 2003–2012.

Mitanchez, D., Yzydorczyk, C., Siddeek, B. et al. (2015). The offspring of the diabetic mother- short and long-term implications. *Best Practice & Research. Clinical Obstetrics & Gynaecology* 29: 256–269.

Morrison, M., Collins, C., Lowe, J. et al. (2015). Factors associatede with early cessation of breastfeeding in women with gestational diabetes mellitus. *Women and Birth* 28 (2): 143–147.

Much, D., Beyerlein, A., Robbauer, M. et al. (2014). Beneficial effects of breastfeeding in women with gestational diabetes mellitus. *Molecular Metabolism* 3: 284–292.

Murphy, H.R. (2010). Gestational diabetes: what's new? *Medicine* 38 (12): 676–678.

National Institute of Health and Care Excellence (2015). Diabetes in pregnancy: management of diabetes and its complications from preconception to the postnatal period (Guidance NG3). www.nice.org.uk/NG3 (accessed 28 January 2018).

National Institute of Health and Care Excellence (2008). Diabetes in pregnancy: management of diabetes and its complications from preconception to the postnatal period (Guidance NG63). www.nice.org.uk/CG063 (accessed 28 January 2018).

Nolan, C. (2011). Controversies in gestational diabetes. *Best Practice & Research Clinical Obstetrics & Gynaecology* 25: 37–49.

Nolan, J.A., McCrone, S., and Chertok, I.R. (2011). The maternal experience of having diabetes in pregnancy. *Journal of the American Academy of Nurse Practitioners* 23: 611–618.

Oakley, L.L., Henderson, J., Redshaw, M. et al. (2014). The role of support and other factors in early breastfeeding cessation: an analysis of data from a maternity survey in England. *BMC Pregnancy & Childbirth* 14: 88. http://doi.org/10/1186/1471-2393-14.

Oza-Frank, R., Moorland, J., McMamara, K. et al. (2016). Early lactation and infant feeding practices difer by maternal gestational diabetes history. *Journal of Human Lactation* 32: 658–665.

Parsons, J., Ismail, K., Amiel, S. et al. (2014). Perceptions among women with gestational diabetes. *Qualitative Health Research* 24: 575.

Persson, M., Hornsten, A., Winkvist, A. et al. (2011). "Mission impossible"? Midwives' experiences counselling pregnant women with gestational diabetes mellitus. *Patient Education and Counseling* 84: 78–83.

Poolsup, N., Suksomboon, N., and Amin, M. (2014). Effect of treatment of gestational diabetes mellitus: a systematic review and meta-analysis. *PLoS One* 9 (3): e92485.

Rogers, K. and Hughes, C. (2010). Recognising the risks: the midwife's role in identifying women at risk of gestational diabetes. *MIDIRS Midwifery Digest* 20: 2.

Rusmussen, K.M. and Kjolhede, C.L. (2004). Prepregnant overweight and obesity diminish the prolactin response to suckling in the first week postpartum. *Pediatrics* 113 (5): e465–e471.

Sathyapalan, T., Mellor, D., and Atkin, S.L. (2010). Obesity and gestational diabetes. *Seminars in Fetal & Neonatal Medicine* 15: 89–93.

Scott, D.A., Loveman, R., McIntyre, L. et al. (2002). Screening for gestational diabetes: a systematic review and economic evaluation. *Health Technology Assessment* 6 (11): 1–161.

Simmons, D. (2011). Diabetes and obesity in pregnancy. *Best Practice & Research Clinical Obstetrics & Gynaecology* 25: 25–36.

Singh, S.K. and Rastogi, A. (2008). Gestational diabetes mellitus. *Diabetes & Metabolic Syndrome: Clinical Research & Reviews* 2 (3): 227–234.

Singh, G., Chouhan, R., and Sidhu, M.K. (2009). Effects of antenatal expression of breast milk at term in reducing breastfeeding failures. *Medical Journal Armed Forces India* 65 (2): 131–133.

Soltani, H. and Scott, A. (2012). Antenatal breast expression in women with diabetes: outcomes from a retrospective cohort study. *International Breastfeeding Journal* 7: 18. http://www.internationalbreastfeedingjournal.com/content/7/1/18.

Thangaratinam, S., Rogozinska, E., Jolly, K. et al. (2012). Effects of interventions in pregnancy on maternal weight and obstetric outcomes: meta- analysis of randomised evidence. *British Medical Journal* 344: e2088.

Tieu, J., Middleton, P., McPhee, A.J., and Crowther, C.A. (2010). Screening and subsequent management for gestational diabetes for improving maternal and infant health. *Cochrane Database of Systematic Reviews* 7: CD007222. https://doi. org/10.1002/14651858. CD007222.

Tieu, J., McPhee, A.J., Crowther, C.A. et al. (2017). Screening for geatational diabetes mellitus based on different risk profiles and settings for improving maternal and infant health. *Cochrane Database of Systematic Reviews*. https://doi.org/10.1002/14651858. CD007222.pub4.

Wallenborn, J.T., Perera, R.A., and Masho, S.W. (2017). Breastfeeding after gestational diabetes: does perceived benefits mediate the relationship? *Journal of Pregnancy*. https://doi.org/10.1155/2017/9581796.

Walsh, J., McGowan, C.A., Mahony, R. et al. (2012). Low glycaemic index diet in pregnancy to prevent macrosomia (ROLO study): randomised control trial. *British Medical Journal* 345: e5605.

World Health Organization (2013). Diagnostic criteria and classification of hyperglycaemia first detected in pregnancy. Report number: WHO/NMH/ MND/13.2. http://tinyurl.com/jjozagy (accessed 31 March 2018).

Wszolek, K. (2015). Hand expressing in pregnancy and colostrum harvesting- preparation for successful breastfeeding? *British Journal of Midwifery* 23 (4): 268–274.

Yessoufou, A. and Moutairou, K. (2011). Maternal diabetes in pregnancy: early and long-term outcomes on offspring and the concept of "Metabolic Memory". *Experimental Diabetes Research*. https://doi.org/10.1155/2011/218598.

Yogev, Y., Metzger, B.E., and Hod, M. (2009). Establishing diagnosis of gestational diabetes mellitus: impact of hypoglycaemia and adverse pregnancy outcomes study. *Seminars in Fetal & Neonatal Medicine* 14: 94–100.

Zelalem, T.H., Mohamed, E., Chavan, B. et al. (2016). Association between type of health professional at birth and exclusive breastfeeding. *Journal of Midwifery & Women's Health* 62: 562–571.

7

'With Woman' in Perineal Trauma

Angie Wilson (Specialist Midwife); and Ruth* and Emilia* (women)

Introduction and Background

Childbirth is for most women and their families an exciting and joyous event. It is a time to celebrate new life and to give thanks for the baby's safe arrival. Birth has the potential to be a transforming event in a woman's life and can be experienced and described as positive and growth enhancing or negative and traumatising for the woman. Birth is undoubtedly a life-changing event and the quality of care given to women has the potential to affect them both physically and emotionally. Recognising problems in the woman and acting on them promptly is imperative if she is to fulfil her role as mother, woman and wife/partner normally and effectively. Obstetric perineal trauma (OPT) and its subsequent morbidity is the most common complication of childbirth and occurs in approximately 53–85% of vaginal deliveries, most commonly occurring in the perineal body (Haelle et al. 2016; Begley et al. 2019; Preston et al. 2019). This figure has declined in recent years in line with the declining birthrate from 56% to 42% of all vaginal deliveries between 2017 and 2018 and 2013–2014 respectively (Hospital Episodes Maternity Statistics 2019). However, figures differ worldwide and are dependent on geographical locations, birth settings and cultural practices (O'Kelly and Moore 2017).

OPT is described as any damage to the genitalia during childbirth that occurs spontaneously or intentionally by surgical incision (episiotomy) (Kettle 2004: 1401). Trauma includes: bruising, grazing, tearing, stretching or indirectly by prolonged denervation during the second stage of labour. Anterior perineal trauma includes injury to the labia, anterior vaginal wall, urethra or clitoris and is usually associated with minimal morbidity. Posterior perineal trauma is any injury to the posterior vaginal wall, perineal muscles or anal sphincter complex in a third-degree tear and includes the epithelium in a fourth-degree tear (O'Kelly and Moore 2017;

Better Births: The Midwife 'with Woman', First Edition. Edited by Anna M. Brown.
© 2021 John Wiley & Sons Ltd. Published 2021 by John Wiley & Sons Ltd.

Farrar et al. 2014). Perineal trauma occurs during spontaneous or assisted vaginal delivery and may be more extensive following the first vaginal delivery (Sultan et al. 1994; RCOG 2019). Anal sphincter injuries (OASIs) during vaginal birth can occur naturally or as a result of obstetric intervention. Definitions of perineal trauma are described in full in Green Top Guidelines No. 29 (RCOG 2015).

In the UK, approximately 0–8% women experience a third- or fourth-degree tear following a vaginal delivery, now termed obstetric anal sphincter injury (OASI) (Webb 2018). The incidence for primiparous women is 6.1% compared with 1.7% in multiparous women (RCOG 2015). OASI is the major cause of anal incontinence (AI) in women with defaecatory disfunction (March et al. 2011; Farrar et al. 2014; Joris et al. 2019). Anal incontinence (AI), defined as involuntary loss of flatus, liquid or solid faeces, including faecal urgency (Norton et al. 2002), has been reported as a major cause of perineal morbidity by Sultan et al. (1993), Glazener et al. (1995) and Keighley et al. (2016). The incidence varies internationally and ranges between 0.5–17.3% of vaginal births dependent on the level of obstetric intervention (OECD Health at a Glance 2013). This type of trauma is associated with increased maternal morbidity (Dahlen et al. 2015; Reid et al. 2014; Farrar et al. 2014). The rate of OASIs in England has tripled from 1.8% to 5.9% from 2000 to 2012 (Gurol-Urganci et al. 2013) and would appear to have increased at a similar rate in other developed nations such as Australia (Dahlen et al. 2015). OASIs affect approximately 11–61% women worldwide (Reid et al. 2014; Antonakou et al. 2017).

The increase in OASIs cannot be explained by increased risk factors alone but may be attributed to better recognition, classification and reporting of OASI both in midwifery and obstetric practice. However, the change in clinical practice of a more liberal approach to perineal management, such as 'hands off/poised' as opposed to 'hands on' (manual perineal protection – MPP) and a reduction in obstetric practice of routine episiotomy with vacuum deliveries, may play a significant part in this increase in perineal trauma, specifically OASIs (Patterns of Maternity Care in English NHS Hospitals 2011/12 RCOG 2013, Evans et al. 2019).

Having a vaginal birth is a significant contributor in the aetiology of pelvic floor dysfunction (PFD) and may result in some or a combination of: urinary and/or faecal incontinence, and pelvic organ prolapse (Wilson 2014; Pierce-Williams et al. 2019). OASI is a cause of significant morbidity for up to 50% women, it can be both distressing and disabling and can have a devastating and longlasting effect on women's quality of life, physically, socially and psychosexually both in the short and long term (Williams et al. 2007; Keighley et al. 2016; Webb et al. 2016; Antonakou 2018; Evans et al. 2019).

Pain and infection continue to be the major cause of morbidity followed by varying degrees of anal incontinence with more severe trauma (Laine et al. 2012; Bick et al. 2012; Reid et al. 2014; Harvey et al. 2015; Keighley et al. 2016). Sexual dysfunction may result as a consequence of varying degrees of perineal trauma (Sayasanth and Pandeva 2010; Leeman and Rogers 2012). Dyspareunia and sexual difficulties are not uncommon, with up to 53% women reporting difficulties at eight weeks postpartum with 49% still having problems at 12–18 months (Buhling et al. 2006; Sayasanth and Pandeva 2010). These disabilities can affect the woman's attachment and relationship with her new baby, partner and family, and can influence how women perceive a subsequent pregnancy, labour and birth. Thus, the woman's subsequent fear of childbirth is often related to previous negative experiences of childbirth.

The impact of perineal trauma on the woman's psychological health in the early puerperium must also be considered by midwives. A distressing birth experience can create debilitating symptoms of psychological trauma which can necessitate debriefing and counselling. The woman may be poorly prepared for the impact perineal pain and discomfort has on successfully carrying out normal activities of daily living and integrating back into family life. Evidence also suggests that there is a relationship between a second-degree tear or more severe perineal trauma with perineal wound infection. This is associated with higher inflammatory markers, linked to depressive related mental health issues and postnatal depression, as demonstrated in higher Edinburgh Postnatal Depression Scale scores (Dunn et al. 2015). In addition, approximately 9% of women may experience postpartum post-traumatic stress disorder (PPTSD) following birth, due to a traumatic birth experience which includes third- or fourth-degree tears (Bailham and Joseph 2003; Evans et al. 2019).

The aim of this chapter is to identify how all midwives, doctors and the multidisciplinary team can make a significant difference to the woman's experience associated with perineal trauma and subsequent morbidity, enabling the woman self-advocacy and empowerment. Providing evidence-based information, enhancing women's knowledge and their ability to make informed choices and decisions about their perineal management, especially following OASIs, is imperative to their future morbidity and self-worth.

This chapter focuses on the therapeutic relationship and interpersonal skills between the woman and specialist perineal care midwife, and how the woman's attendance and consultation in a perineal care clinic (PCC) can empower and influence her experience of childbirth and perineal outcomes. Specifically, how the experience impacts on her future physical, psychosocial, sexual and mental wellbeing.

Midwives' Role in Supporting Women with Perineal Trauma

Better Births (NHS England, 2016) identified key components of care that midwives need to embrace collaboratively to enhance the woman's birth experience.

- Safer and more personalised care.
- Kinder, more professional and family friendly service.

- Providing access to information for every woman to enable them to make informed choices and decisions about their care.
- Care which needs to be centred around individual needs and circumstances.

These are the priorities of England's NHS Transformation programme, which are further supported by NICE impact maternity (NHS England 2018: 14) emphasising the priorities for the 'Personalisation and experience of care'. Better Births provides a vision for personalised care, centred on the woman, her baby and her family, around their needs and their decisions, where they have genuine choice, informed by unbiased information. The NMC Standards of Proficiency for Midwifery (NMC 2019a, b) advocate the delivery of skilled, knowledgeable, respectful, safe, competent and effective midwifery care. Woman want to be heard, have their experiences acknowledged, and to form an equal partnership with competent carers. Thus, midwifery, obstetric care and policy must be led by women's physical and social needs.

Within various models of midwifery care, discussed in Chapter 3, we ask ourselves: is midwifery truly sensitive to gender sensitive issues and care? Do midwives take these issues into account when caring for women with problems related to perineal trauma and later morbidity? Midwives' values have been shaped historically by male and medical dominance and the culture of midwifery within an NHS organisation. For women to feel empowered about the choices and decisions they make about their own perineal management and birth choices, midwives need to perceive that they themselves are empowered (Wilson 2009).

Midwives have been encouraged to facilitate informed choice and control for women through sharing and trusting relationships, which are largely shaped by the model of midwifery care, the midwife known to the woman and the building of a partnership in care whereby the trusting relationship is a conduit for being 'with woman' (Bradfield et al. 2019). Sensitive care means speaking out for and a de-silencing for women with sensitive problems. The process of reclaiming voices enables women and midwives to become aware of changes within themselves, bringing empowerment for both. Midwives often feel unable to speak out for women, especially if they perceive they have been under the influence of dominant models of care (Kirkham 1999). Midwives are women's advocates and need to give voice to those in their care, enabling them to break free from medical dominance.

Women's Experiences of Care after Perineal Trauma

Valuing women's experiences of perineal trauma extends back to the earlier work of Salmon (1999: 220) who stated that when women have been undergoing perineal repair, and other intimate procedures, women's views and experiences have been repeatedly neglected and undervalued by both doctors and midwives. 'Torture and punishment' are emotive words expressed by some women in their context of their experience of perineal suturing following delivery. This is further emphasised in Salmon's findings of women's experiences of interpersonal relationships while being sutured and whilst healing, perceiving that they were being patched up and not being cared for.

Moyzakitis (2004) reports that women have complained of a lack of information and explanation from professionals related to interventions and events, resulting in women's limited understanding, decision-making ability, choice and opportunity to be involved in their care. Three women in Sinivaara et al.'s (2004) study were concerned regarding the cosmetic appearance of their perineum, an area dismissed by some healthcare professionals. Coming to terms with their enduring perineal pain also highlights the emotions that their experiences portrayed, such as anger and deep emotional and physical hurt. The fact that these issues were not taken seriously and the failure to be heard influenced women's negative perception of their interchanges with their carers. Altered body image through perineal scarring has been associated with negative body presentation and there are sexual factors that many healthcare professionals feel uncomfortable discussing with women as a result of uncertainties of sexuality in their own lives (Carter and Green 2007).

The formation of the MASIC (Mothers and Anal Sphincter Injuries in Childbirth) foundation (MASIC 2017) provides evidence of the need to support woman and their families following OASIs and anal incontinence. Anal incontinence has been a taboo subject and described as the 'unvoiced' symptom, with less than 50% women reporting the symptom (Fowler et al. 2009). An OASIS syndrome was identified by Keighley et al. (2016) which was uniquely visualised in the form of a word picture. The size of the words, representing the strength of their emotions and feelings, depicted how women felt and experienced their trauma. Words such as *dignity loss, unclean, sexual horrors, mutilated,* shattered motherhood, *baby, hiding my condition*, being a failure and disfigurement were some of the thoughts and feelings identified by these women (words in italics represent strength of feeling). These experiences have been largely ignored by the healthcare profession. Similarly, a complex web of morbidity following OASI has been reported by Evans et al. (2019), who has drawn our attention again to the physical, psychological, healthcare and social impact on women's lives.

Rationale for a Perineal Care Clinic

Within the midwifery profession, midwives are working with an increasingly well-informed client group who readily question and seek an understanding as to why debilitating perineal trauma occurred in a previous birth. Consequently, there has been an increased demand from women who request an elective cae-sarean section (ECS) due to fear, avoidance of perineal pain/trauma, severe PFD, dyspareunia, long-term sexual difficulties and often negative consequences of previous OASI (Sekon 2010; Dahlen et al. 2015). With minimal time allocated in a busy antenatal clinic, it is often difficult to counsel women comprehen-sively. To address this area of maternal morbidity it was necessary to establish a clinic in a local trust where women's voices and concerns could be heard, a risk assessment and specialised perineal care pathway utilised and a perineal care plan provided. The Department of Health (1999), NHS Plan and social care pol-icy recommended direct public services to provide essential services which were to be accessible and appropriate to need. Thus, one of the first multi-disciplinary PCCs was established in 1999 in Lancashire to address this issue (Dugdale and Hill 2005). PCCs have slowly been introduced into NHS Trusts in varying for-mats since 1990 (Fitzpatrick et al. 2002; Pretlove et al. 2004; Thakar and Sultan 2007; Fowler et al. 2009; Bosanquet 2010; Webb and Parsons 2011; Keighley et al. 2016).

There are various models of PCCs. Some are multi-disciplinary or 'one stop' clinics where the woman is seen routinely six to eight weeks postnatal follow-ing OASI by a consultant urogynaecologist/obstetrician and if any symptoms of urinary or anal incontinence (AI) are reported, an endoanal ultrasound scan and anal manometry can be performed at that visit (Thakar and Sultan 2007: 75) or a further referral made. A midwife, physiotherapist, conti-nence nurse specialist, colorectal surgeon and psychosexual counsellor can also be available to the woman in some settings, providing a holistic approach to perineal care.

Conclusion

In conclusion to this review, it is clear that many women experience varying degrees of physical and psychological perineal trauma and pain, impacting on family relationships, sexual intercourse and future births. The midwives' role in 'being with women', supporting and empowering them throughout the whole birth process using current evidence-based perineal management in collaboration with the multi-disciplinary team, is paramount. The positive outcomes for women supported by good perineal management during childbirth cannot be underestimated.

As with previous chapters, Rodgers' concept framework of analysis has been applied to the above literature and presented in Table 7.1.

Table 7.1 Concept analysis of 'with woman' with perineal trauma.

Antecedents	Evidence	Attributes (A) and Consequences (C)
Physical factors	Antonakou et al. (2017) risks for sustaining a repeat OASIs	Risks and outcomes for all perineal trauma (A) Identifying risk factors and recognising problems associated with anal incontinence and morbidity (A) Modifying risk factors (C)
	Dahlan et al. (2014) rates of severe perineal trauma	
	Donners et al. (2017), Webb (2018) mode of delivery in subsequent birth after OASIS	Hiding condition and overcoming barrier of 'silence' (A) Supporting women and families – (MASIC) (C)
	Evans et al. (2019), Joris et al. (2019) impact of OASIS and delivery outcome	Distress and disability (A) Understanding and improving quality of life (C)
	Dunn et al. (2015) links with perineal injury and PND, PPTSD and PTSD	Identifying mental health issues (A) positive outcomes for mother, baby and family (C)
	Keighley et al. (2016) impact of perineal trauma on anal incontinence, sexual function and wellbeing	
Midwives' role in the prevention of perineal trauma	Begley et al. (2019) techniques to preserve the perineum intact	Calm controlled birth (A) slowing down birth, protecting the perineum, 'slow, blow and breath baby out' (C)
	Bick et al. (2012) midwifery practice in managing perineal trauma and outcomes	Careful instruction and communication with women at birth (A) Reduction in OASIS (C)
	Laine et al. (2012) protecting the perineum	Standardised perineal protection package including manual perineal protection and perineal inspection (A) Women's satisfaction and improved perineal morbidity (C)
	Pierce-Williams et al. (2019) hands on vs hands off technique	
	RCOG (2019) OASI Care Bundle	Skilled and competent assessment and repair of perineal trauma (A) Good healing and reduced perineal infection, pain and scar tissue (C)
	Wilson (2012) educational programme in perineal repair	

(Continued)

Table 7.1 (Continued)

Antecedents	Evidence	Attributes (A) and Consequences (C)
Clinical support and perineal care clinics	Bradfield et al. (2019) being 'with woman' in known midwifery model	Multi-disciplinary approach in OASIS management and other perineal trauma (A)
		Holistic approach to care (C)
	Fitzpatrick et al. (2002) valuable resource for investigating postpartum perineal injury	One-to-one women-centred evidence-based information (A)
		Empowerment, choice, control and enhanced decision-making ability for women focusing on normality (C)
	Fowler et al. (2009) setting up perineal trauma clinics	
		Fear and anxiety for next birth (A)
	Goetz et al. (2010) compassion and caring	Spontaneous vaginal birth, intact perineum at home (C)
		Building a therapeutic, empathetic relationship through good communication, compassion, caring and respectfulness (A)
	Percy and Richardson (2018) therapeutic relationship, building partnership and reciprocity	
		Debriefing, being 'listened to' valued, and concerns taken seriously, high level of satisfaction (C)
	Wilson et al. (2014) women's satisfaction and perineal outcomes - Clinical Audit	Perineal assessment and care plan, acting as advocate (A) vaginal birth and reduced caesarean section rate
Women's experiences	Carter and Green (2007) body image and sexuality	Negative experiences 'patched up', torture and punishment, feeling neglected and undervalued (A)
	Keighley et al. (2016) OASIs syndrome – word picture	Social support and interpersonal relationships, listening to and valuing women's experiences (C)
	Moyzakitis (2004) role of care providers, impact on self-image and relationships	Feeling unclean (anal incontinence), loss of dignity, psychosexual morbidity (A)
		Uncovering a hidden condition, by uncovering the barrier of silence (C)
	Salmon (1999) valuing women's experience and sensitive care	Loss of self, sexuality and negative body image (A) Midwives better understanding of sexuality and a de-silencing of perineal trauma (C)

Angie: A Specialist Perineal Care Midwife

My role as specialist perineal care midwife has developed through expanded and advanced practice skills, knowledge and expertise in perineal care, management and postpartum recovery over 40 years (Wilson 2009, 2012, 2017). Support from senior colleagues and consultants has been instrumental in establishing the midwifery-led PCC at a local trust.

The clinic was established in 2012 and is based on the Calgary–Cambridge Model, a professional consultation (modified medical interview) (Kurtz and Silverman 1996). This model acknowledges the importance of women's concerns and encourages them to become involved in the decision-making process. It aids a better partnership between midwife and woman and incorporates a holistic assessment when discussing the physical, emotional and social problems identified. The focus on the model is building a trusting relationship with the woman (Munson 2007). Following the consultation, I would refer to the multi-disciplinary team as appropriate to need, whereby an element of shared and integrated care is formulated.

The aims of the PCC are to: improve perineal outcomes and reduce the risk of severe perineal morbidity for all women before and following vaginal birth, provide a woman-centred, cost-effective service with a holistic approach to care where women can feel empowered to influence their own choices, decisions, birth and perineal outcomes.

The consultation offers women the opportunity to discuss and share their concerns and anxieties, where they can reflect and understand the problems associated with previous perineal trauma or fear of such occurrence in a confidential and relaxed environment in a local Children's Centre, facilitated once a week. Fifty minutes are allocated to each woman who are enabled to debrief, review their previous labour and birth with their hospital notes and discuss risk factors and circumstances associated with their previous birth/s. The consultation and risk assessment provides women with an individualised perineal birth plan which can be incorporated into their notes and shared with midwives and obstetricians during labour, birth and the puerperium. The discussion supports normal birth and enables women to focus on normality and feel empowered to make decisions about how they birth and whether they have a vaginal birth or choose an elective caesarean section (ECS) dependent on obstetric and clinical findings.

Prior to seeing the woman, her previous hospital notes are reviewed and important information/events related to previous labour/s and birth/s are noted on a perineal care proforma. Factors considered are: gestation at birth, length of second stage, complications such as shoulder dystocia, precipitate labour or long second stage, occipito-posterior position, instrumental delivery, baby's birthweight.

Episiotomy/degree of tear, compound presentation and risk factors for perineal trauma, i.e. OASI (Wilson 2017: 672). It is important to identify if an endoanal/ manometry ultrasound has been undertaken previously. This will show levels of anal sphincter healing and or weakness and is an important investigation to consider alongside the woman's physical symptoms and clinical history, aiding decision making as to vaginal delivery or elective caesarean section (Sultan et al. 2007: 102; Antonakou et al. 2017; Donners et al. 2017; Webb 2018). Urinary symptoms are also explored and level of continence, together with pelvic floor muscle strength and integrity.

A comprehensive assessment is important as it will enable the woman to make a fully informed decision as regards her mode of birth. Having established the woman's concerns and taken a full history, a perineal inspection is undertaken with consent to exclude excessive scar tissue. A vaginal examination is also undertaken to assess pelvic floor muscle tone. With all the information provided, the woman can make a fully informed decision based on the choices offered to her. A perineal care plan is incorporated into and shared in the woman's notes for staff information and evidence-based recommendations for labour and birth. A copy is available for the woman to access. All women have access to the patient information leaflets (PILS) 'How to minimise perineal trauma at the birth of your baby and postnatal perineal care' (Wilson 2018).

Women's Experience of the Perineal Care Clinic

The experience of women attending the PCC and their subsequent birth experience and perineal outcome is dependent on the therapeutic and interpersonal relationship, skill and expertise of the practitioner facilitating the clinic. Central to my philosophy of being 'with woman' in the clinic is developing a compassionate, respectful and therapeutic relationship using effective communication (Dewar and Christley 2013). For many of the women I see, only one visit is required. It is essential, therefore, that this relationship is established quickly; the first 90 seconds is essential in building a good rapport (Cooper et al. 2006). This may also include the partner or significant family member or friend. The encounter involves understanding the woman's concerns, experiences and consequences of often very difficult, complex and traumatic experiences. These may be due to OASIs, complex perineal tearing, wound dehiscence, sexual difficulties and long-term morbidity. It is important to understand the woman's concept of her childbirth in a personal and experiential way, sharing her values and perceptions (Siddiqui 1999).

Kirkham (1993) discusses the importance of authenticity of being, closely associated with effective, sincere communication, which is the foundation of building a therapeutic relationship. When the woman exposes her innermost concerns as regards her previous trauma and her fear of what may occur at her next birth, the interaction which takes place needs to embrace evidence-based information with effective and attentive listening, which needs to be deep and meaningful. This requires receptive and perceptive communication. While the woman debriefs, it is important to 'switch from a more intense interaction of communication at a deeper level, to a masterly inactivity of careful listening', showing empathy and understanding. This requires a skilled level of thinking and doing on the midwives' part because it relies on being one's self and in tune with the woman. In addition, 'presence' in the relationship requires full commitment from the midwife with the woman central to care and able to trust the midwife with her innermost concerns. The relationship, therefore, is not just beneficial to the woman, but it also serves to benefit the midwife and woman together during the encounter as the process of the relationship becomes enriching for both. When an effective relationship is developed, the midwife commits to acting as the woman's advocate, based on a utilitarian principle (Siddiqui 1999). The model of a therapeutic relationship therefore encompasses the interrelationship between concepts, building a partnership, intimacy and reciprocity (Percy and Richardson 2018).

When a woman is deeply affected by a traumatic experience of OASI, for example, the midwife needs to express empathy and caring emotions, understanding and acknowledging the woman's experience and current concerns; this is the cornerstone to compassionate care. Compassionate midwifery has been defined as the interrelationship of authentic presence, noticing another's suffering, displaying empathy, sympathy and pity, connectiveness/relationship, emotion work, a motivation to help/support, empower women and alleviate suffering through negotiation by utilising knowledge and skills and connecting with the woman. The midwife must be genuine, authentic and act with kindness – compassion being the core of care (Menage et al. 2016; Permanente 2013; Compassion in Practice: Department of Health 2012).

Dignity, respect and compassion for the woman are consistent themes which are the underpinning values of the NHS Constitution (Department of Health 2013), the philosophy of the International Confederation of Midwives (2014) and Standards of Proficiency for Midwives (NMC 2019a, b). Dignity for the women visiting the clinic is about valuing how she feels, thinks and behaves, treating them as worthy and in a respectful manner. This includes providing choice, control and woman-centred care in a non-judgemental way, acting as the woman's advocate (Hall and Mitchell 2016). Bradfield et al. (2019) emphasises the development of a respectful partnership or professional relationship between midwife and woman and this is often based on the type of sensitive information shared through the woman's journey from an antenatal encounter to follow up appointments postnatally.

Cultural safety is also about respecting woman from different ethnic backgrounds and cultural practices such as women with previous female genital mutilation (FGM). The quality of care in the PCC will affect the woman's emotional wellbeing; thus, the consequences of individualised care can be experienced as empowering, healing, reassuring and emotionally supportive (Moberg 2015; Hall and Mitchell 2016). Sharing evidence-based information and working in partnership with women provides a platform for empowerment and confidence building where they have the freedom and are enabled to choose and decide for themselves, thus supporting them in their mode of birth and perineal management. These concepts are embedded in the Midwives' Codes and Standards (NMC 2019a, b).

Effectiveness of One-to-One Consultation in a PCC

Eight hundred and fifty-eight women have attended the PCC between 2012 and 2020.

Three clinic audits have been undertaken during this period to identify the woman's level of satisfaction when attending the clinic, during subsequent delivery and the severity of perineal trauma using the RCOG (2015) classifications of perineal trauma. This section provides a brief overview of one clinic audit undertaken between 2013 and 2014. During this period, 58 women were seen in the clinic and 48 subsequently delivered. The women were purposively selected for the audit. Evidence was collected from Euroking, the maternity database, women's case notes and semi-structured questionnaires. Thirty-nine (81.25%) women who had visited the clinic presented with a history of a third-degree tear (classifications ranging from 3a to 3c). None of these women had experienced a fourth-degree tear. The remaining women presented with problems associated with: episiotomy scar tissue, fear of tearing, vaginismus, vulvodynia and vaginal reconstruction. Birth outcomes for the 48 women attending the clinic are as follows: 35 (72.9%) women had spontaneous vaginal delivery (SVD), 4 (9%) women had an instrumental delivery and 9 (18.75%) women had an elective caesarean.

Perineal outcomes for the women who had delivered identified: 12 (25%) women had an intact perineum including 9 having a caesarean; 2 (4.1%) women had labial grazes; 5 (10.4%) women had a first degree tear; 23 (47.9%) women had a second degree tear; and 6 (12.5%) women had an elective episiotomy. There were no third- or fourth-degree tears in this audit cohort of women, compared to 2.6% women within the Trust having a spontaneous vaginal delivery (total deliveries 2896). Second-degree tears were more prevalent (Wilson 2014).

Qualitative data taken from the questionnaires revealed the women's high level of satisfaction following their visit to the PCC. This showed that undertaking a comprehensive assessment had assisted women in making their choice of delivery which contributed in part to the reduction of OASIs with nine women electing to have a planned caesarean section. Ninety percent of women found a one-to-one consultation useful to a large extent in explaining the circumstances which contributed or predisposed to their previous perineal problems, particularly OASIs. Time provided, and feeling that they were given the opportunity for someone to listen to and take their concerns seriously, made a significant impact on the women's level of satisfaction.

Visual illustrations and models enabled women to move forward in a positive way. Having time to discuss and be heard about their concerns especially related to more personal problems, such as comfortable and enjoyable sexual intercourse. This was very important to some women. Having a perineal assessment and vaginal examination (VE) to assess pelvic floor muscle strength and feedback encouraged women to have a vaginal birth.

Reviewing previous labour notes and planning how to minimise trauma in their next delivery was reassuring and empowering. Having detailed and referenced information gave women real insight into their birth options and 90% of women were more able to make decisions as regards their next birth. The consultation also enabled women to be more proactive in their own care, giving them time to reflect and plan for their future birth.

Areas of good practice and improvement/recommendations:

□ Benefit to women, maternity services, education and research.
□ Holistic inter-professional approach to perineal care.
□ Specialist consultation.
□ Reduces potential for short-and long-term perineal morbidity and sexual problems.
□ Reduces potential for litigation – best practice adopted.
□ Women were highly satisfied with the service.
□ Provision of ongoing education, teaching and research activities for students, midwives and doctors.

Since the three audits, all women who book antenatally are risk assessed for perineal trauma, and all women are referred to the PIL booklet 'Minimising perineal trauma at your birth and caring for your perineum after the birth of your baby' (Wilson 2018). This document is accessible electronically on the 'Maternity Notes' application on their phones. Evidence regarding perineal protection (NICE 2018, Laine et al. 2012 and RCOG 2015, 2019) has been highlighted in the Trust Perineal Care Pathway (Table 7.1).

Angie's Stories

Harriot*'s Story

Harriot, 29 years old, Gravida 2 Para 1. Clinic referral from consultant and seen at 32 weeks' gestation. Harriot's notes read before the appointment and the following was identified:*

History of a previous 3c perineal tear in 2012. Spontaneous vaginal delivery (SVD) at 39 weeks' gestation with a compound presentation of male infant, Jack, weighing 3690g (8 lb 2 oz). Second stage of labour not extended. Tear in notes illustrated as a button-hole tear, with an intact perineum. No problems identified post-delivery. An endoanal ultrasound scan and manometry showed that the internal and external anal sphincter muscles were complete with good maximum resting pressure and squeeze.

At the appointment, Harriot was particularly anxious and worried about her history of a 3c tear and did not want this happening again. I reassured her that between us we would do our very best to minimise this type of trauma occurring again. On assessment, Harriot was well and had no problems to date. She was asymptomatic regards urinary and anal incontinence and had no problems with constipation. Harriot explained it was six to seven months before she could comfortably have sexual intercourse (SI) due to pain and resulting scar tissue. I acknowledged this and offered her advice and support in this area of concern.

I emphasised her reduced risks of a repeat third-degree tear as she was asymptomatic with good ultrasound findings. Harriot was requesting a caesarean section (C/S). We discussed the advantages and disadvantages of a vaginal delivery (VD) vs C/S. I undertook a perineal and vaginal assessment with consent. There was no visible evidence of any perineal scar tissue and her perineum felt stretchy. Her pelvic floor tone was fair with an Oxford score of 3/5 (0: none – 5: very strong). We discussed the benefits of pelvic floor exercises (PFEs) and strengthening her pelvic floor. We discussed a comprehensive perineal care plan and how she and her midwife in labour could reduce the risk of perineal tearing. The plan was inserted into Harriot's labour notes and instructions for a senior midwife at birth to acknowledge her previous history. A copy was entered into Harriot's hand-held notes.

Harriot found this information very useful and was grateful for the information. She was more inclined to want a vaginal birth at this point in the consultation.

Harriot's Birth Outcome

Harriot had an unplanned spontaneous vaginal birth, kneeling at home! (born before arrival (BBA)) at 38 week's gestation, delivered by her husband. A boy Arthur weighing 3860g (8 lbs 8 oz). An intact perineum!

Evaluation questionnaire comments:

> *I felt more in control in this labour with this new knowledge – did not tear! Wish I was told this for the first labour. It was also useful as I ended up having a home delivery and no midwife as the labour was so quick. At least having the consultation meant I could control something! Breathing, blowing out and position and to be confident to allow baby to come at his own speed. The care plan was useful. There was a lot of info and it can be easily forgotten. Now and again I would read through the plan as a way of preparing myself mentally for the labour.*

It is reassuring to women that they can have a vaginal birth with minimal or no perineal trauma following OASI. Support, encouragement, reassurance and the woman's self-esteem and self-belief are paramount in the outcome.

Sarah*'s Story

Sarah, aged 36 years. Referred by consultant and seen in the clinic at 31 weeks gestation. Having read Sarah's notes prior to her visit to the clinic she had a history of ventouse delivery for fetal distress in 2012 at 41 weeks gestation with shoulder difficulty (not shoulder dystocia). Manual removal of placenta. Labour 16 hours with a 3-hour second stage. Third-degree tear (3b). Male infant (Daniel) weighing 8 lbs 4 oz. Sarah stated that she had been extremely traumatised by the whole birth experience. She was not sure she could go through the experience again and really wanted an elective C/S this time. She had physiotherapy post-delivery for some stress urinary incontinence (SUI). She could not resume sexual intercourse for 6–12 months due to physical and psychological trauma. There was no dyspareunia.

On assessment, Sarah was well and the pregnancy was progressing normally. She was asymptomatic regards urinary and anal incontinence. There was no evidence of SUI.

I undertook a perineal and vaginal assessment with consent. Sarah had a tight fourchette, but no visible scar tissue. The Oxford score was 5/5, excellent, her physio had worked. She was relieved and pleased to learn this information. I advised perineal massage to soften and stretch the tight fourchette. We discussed VD vs C/S and her chances of reoccurrence of another third-degree tear: 3–7% chance based on her history, but no guarantee she would not sustain perineal tearing again. We discussed strategies for a birth plan and how to minimise perineal trauma at her next birth if she had a vaginal delivery.

(Continued)

Sarah's Birth Outcome

Sarah had decided to have an elective C/S.

Questionnaire comments – value of clinic visit:

> *Understood better what happened last time, but too scared to risk the same happening again. Information was empowering in my own self-care with practical information I could do to help myself. I kept my options open till late on but unfortunately could not face what might happen. Too traumatised from the first time.*

It is evident that despite all the reassurance and assistance we can provide women in our care, a traumatic birth experience and OASI still leave some women fearful of a reoccurrence. Advice, reassurance, support and choice in mode of delivery is vitally important to the woman to have a satisfying and fulfilling birth experience.

Women's Stories

Ruth*'s Story

I am mum to three fantastic boys, Elijah 5, Jonah 2, and Isaac nine months. I am also a paediatric speech therapist, specialising in specific learning difficulties.

Growing up, I knew I wanted to be a mother, but there was always a certain level of anxiety when thinking of birth! My mum had a traumatic birth with my brother, and often tells me the story of how her surgeon nearly fell asleep when stitching her afterwards! This was my extent of awareness of perineal damage, and this shaped my preconceptions about childbirth; this and episodes of One Born Every Minute.

I met my husband, Peter, at university. He has always been the calming influence on my anxious nature. We started our family after eight years together. I spent the next two months reading as many books and Net Mum articles as I possibly could. Symptom spotting, and ensuring I ate all the recommended foods and took all the necessary steps to ensure we were fully prepared. Despite the vast and sometimes overwhelming information about the antenatal and labour process, I did not come across enough information that would prepare me for the possibilities of perineal trauma.

After a hospital tour, I came away feeling positive about welcoming my first little boy into the world. I was prepared as I could be, or so I thought. I had attended 'active birth preparation classes' for a few weeks, I had packed my overnight bag with impossibly small baby clothes and ensured I carried my yellow hospital notes at all times.

My first birth happened really quickly. Not what I was expecting. I spent most of my labour at home on the birthing ball, using my breathing techniques. When I arrived at the hospital, I was already 8 cm dilated, and I could feel a sense of urgency. It seemed to be happening much quicker than I had anticipated. Suddenly I did not feel calm or prepared! My waters went, and the midwife attached me to a monitor, there was meconium present in my waters, but Elijah's heartrate wasn't raised. I stopped listening to my instincts and panicked. I started to push Elijah and did not listen to my lovely midwife . . . I pushed when I knew it wasn't right and unfortunately sustained a third-degree tear. I feel very naive when I say that I did not know enough about perineal damage. I did not factor perineal damage into my birth story. I received some fantastic care form the physio department at the hospital. I feel extremely fortunate that there were no immediate complications from my damage.

Fast forward almost two years and I became pregnant with our second child, Jonah. As the birth drew closer, I became more and more anxious. My midwife referred me to the PCC. I did not fully understand what the benefit of this appointment would be. I can honestly say that the confidence I gained from that appointment was invaluable. It was, for me, the most important appointment of my pregnancy. It was the first time that I had been examined since being discharged from physio, and I was storing up a lot of anxiety about how my next labour would impact on my previous tear.

The specialist midwife discussed Elijah's birth at length; she was the first health professional to do so. Although I had discussed my birth experience with friends, I had not discussed my third-degree tear, nor the fear I had about it happening once more. It felt great to talk to someone with such in-depth knowledge. I was able to ask the questions required to put my mind at ease. Perhaps the most important aspect of my meeting with my specialist midwife was my examination; she was able to tell me how my scar tissue had developed, and thanks to the fantastic surgeon at the hospital all was well and there were no concerns about me proceeding with a vaginal delivery. I was also concerned about a 'full' feeling I was having and the possibility of a prolapse. I was too scared to check for myself. I was informed that I had a varicose vein, which explained some of the discomfort I was feeling. We discussed how this would

(Continued)

need to be taken into consideration should I need an episiotomy. This informa-tion was written very clearly on my hospital notes, so that the midwives involved would be aware.

Furthermore, the specialist midwife provided me with advice to avoid perineal damage. I thought that it was certain that I would tear badly again., I had read a lot of Mumsnet posts about women who had gone on to tear again in subsequent births, and then suffer the dreadful lasting complications that go with this. I was so relieved to learn that this did not have to be the case for my second birth; there are always ways to reduce these risks. My specialist midwife has this incredible, calm manner. She educated me so that I was able to approach Jonah's birth feeling empowered! I was so incredibly grateful that a service such as this existed, and a health professional as passionate and dedicated as this midwife was ensuring that women had access to it.

My birth preparation and plan were so clear in my mind. I believe that out of all the reading you try to cram in before having a baby, the advice given regarding minimising my risk of perineal trauma was by far the most vital! Jonah's birth was much longer, but much calmer. Towards the end of labour, I was feeling very tired but focused on avoiding damage. My midwives were fully aware that I was under specialist perineal care and were very on board with the advice she had passed on, particularly using a warm compress to lower the risk of tearing on delivery. I was so pleased with the outcome of Jonah's birth; I had avoided a repeated third-degree tear. I was so pleased, in fact, that we decided to do it again! When we found I was pregnant with our third child I sought an appointment with my specialist perineal midwife, as I knew how invaluable it had been before. Meeting with my specialist midwife again allowed me to feel a level of control. I also attended the fantastic hypnobirth-ing class. This couple's class was so insightful. My husband and I came away from the session in such a positive mood. I was so thankful for the class mid-wife for providing this useful class. I was sure my third birth would be my most straightforward.

My third pregnancy was going well, and I was the most relaxed I had been during any of my pregnancies. When I saw my specialist midwife, I was around 32 weeks. We discussed my birth history, and any fears I had about this birth. I was consider-ing using the birthing pool. I had considered this with my other births, but circum-stances did not permit me to continue. After discussing the pool at length with the specialist midwife, I could see the utmost importance of giving birth 'on dry land' as my midwives would need to be hands on during delivery, to try to avoid me tearing. This was such an important meeting for me. I was able to make my birth plan under my specialist midwives' guidance, talking through my fear of the baby coming too quickly, I was concerned that this baby (being my third) would also take me by surprise. I was reassured, and given some fantastic advice regarding slowing things down until I was ready to deliver him. This gave me confidence going forward.

At my 38 weeks check I was now measuring 41 weeks gestation, my baby's head measuring on the 98th centile. My GP mentioned the idea of revising my birth plan, possibly to include a c section. I went into a bit of a spin. I had my birth plan straight in my mind and now I was facing the possibility of a completely different birth to the one I had envisaged. I wasn't sure if I could go ahead with a vaginal delivery, with fresh anxieties about my baby's size. My main concerns were about him getting stuck and becoming distressed, needing an instrumental delivery and of course a repeated third-degree tear due to his head size.

I felt incredibly lucky that I could contact my specialist midwife. I sent her a flustered email and she explained to me she would ring me that afternoon. I spoke with her and she reassured me; reminding me of all the information she had previously shared with me, using birthing positions to aid a smooth delivery, and remaining calm enough to 'breath my baby out' re-instilling that confidence and giving me back my control. She reminded me of my options and recommended that I book to see the consultant at the hospital to discuss it further. My anxiety immediately reduced; I knew that I could tackle this again. The advice from my specialist midwife to 'stay calm and positive, trust and believe in your body and slowly birth your baby' was all I needed.

I was very grateful for being in hospital because my baby boy was coming quickly. My husband and I reached the fantastic midwife-led suite and met with our midwives. The midwives were looking over my notes when I informed them I knew he was coming. I ensured I told them I had been in the PCC and that included details of my previous tear and varicose veins. They noted the sticker on the front of my notes, drawing attention to my attendance at the clinic. With a combination of my hypnobirthing image (my boys on the beach in Devon), good old fashioned gas and air, and my specialist midwives' mantras in my head I was able to have my most relaxed and controlled birth so far. I repeatedly heard my specialist midwife telling me to breathe my baby out, and that my body knew what it was doing. I trusted my body.

Isaac arrived in this world just an hour after arriving in delivery. I was so ecstatic to have delivered my boy safely. He wasn't that big, only 8 lb 9 oz! He was, however, very beautiful. He is the most chilled out baby of the three, and I am convinced this

(Continued)

is due to how relaxed and ready I felt for his arrival. I had trusted my body and was so proud of what I had achieved!

I am and forever remain indebted to my specialist midwife for the wonderful care she gave me throughout my second and third pregnancies. I have no doubt that my stories would have been very different had I not had access to the PCC. I believe that every pregnant woman should have access to the vital advice offered regarding perineal care. This has been made possible through the booklet 'How to minimise perineal trauma at your birth and caring for your perineum after the birth of your baby'. The advice regarding care following birth is something that women might not otherwise have access to. I do feel very strongly that the care my specialist midwife provided and the midwifery team at the hospital is incredible. As I said to my midwife after Isaac's birth: 'everyone should have a specialist perineal care midwife'.

Emilia*'s Story

I was first referred to the specialist midwife perineal clinic after the birth of my first baby. I'd had a lengthy second stage labour and had required an episiotomy. The wound had not healed very well, and I had painful scar tissue which was affecting me. The specialist midwife helped me to deal with this, she advised me on how to manage the scarring and lessen the discomfort it was causing me.

In the later weeks of my second pregnancy, I started to feel quite nervous about the labour and was really keen to see the specialist midwife again to get further advice on how to minimise trauma the second time round. After seeing her I felt much better prepared. I felt reassured to know that there was a plan in place and that help would be available postnatally if required. I felt that my concerns were understood and taken seriously. Thanks to this I felt very calm and more confident during the birth, so much so that the labour progressed so smoothly and easily that my baby was born at home. Also, because I was relaxed there wasn't any bruising, so I was in a lot less pain postnatally. Thanks to the specialist midwife's plan, I was able to have confidence that the healing process would also be optimised. When I saw her after the birth she took every care to try to avoid me suffering with the problems I had had the first time and she referred me to the consultant and physiotherapist for further reassurance. I also felt more empowered to seek help and knowing that there was someone who cared was a real comfort. With the help of my specialist midwife and hypnobirthing, I have been able to have a really special birth experience this time.

Lessons Learnt

The role of the specialist perineal care midwife can make a significant difference to the lives and future birth experiences of women who have previously experienced debilitating physical and psychological problems because of perineal trauma, especially OASIs. Listening to, and acknowledging, women's concerns compassionately, careful assessment and providing evidence- based information and choice does have an empowering effect on women's decisions about their following birth. It has been demonstrated that the rate of OASI can be reduced significantly as evidenced in one small cohort of women attending the clinic in 2013–2014. The zero incidence of repeat OASI in this cohort has been very reassuring and it continues to remain extremely low. This has in part reduced the numbers of women having unnecessary caesarean sections which has cost implications for the NHS. This finding is consistent within other Trusts who have implemented PCCs, demonstrating that the careful assessment of women with previous OASI can safely opt for a vaginal birth.

References

Antonakou, A. (2018). The long-term physical, emotional and psychosexual outcomes related to anal incontinence after severe perineal trauma at birth. *European Journal of Midwifery* 2 (8): 8.

Antonakou, A., Papoutsis, D., and Tapp, A. (2017). The incidence and risk of factors for a repeat obstetric anal sphincter injury (OASIS) in the vaginal birth subsequent to a first episode of OASIS: a hospital-based cohort study. *Archives of Gynecology and Obstetrics* 295: 1201–1209.

Bailham, D. and Joseph, S. (2003). Post-traumatic stress following childbirth – a review of the emerging literature and directions for research and practice. *Psychology, Health & Medicine* 8: 159–168.

Begley, C., Guilliland, K., Dixon, L. et al. (2019). A qualitative exploration of techniques used by expert midwives to preserve the perineum intact. *Women and Birth*. https://doi.org/10.1016/j.wombi.2018.04.015.

Bick, D.E., Ismail, K.M., and Macdonald, S. (2012). How good are we at implementing evidence to support the management of birth related perineal trauma? A UK wide survey of midwifery practice. *BMC Pregnancy and Childbirth* 12: 57. http://biomedcentral.com/1471-2393/12/57.

Bosanquet, A. (2010). A day in the life of a specialist perineal midwife. *Midwives* 4: 58.

Bradfield, Z., Hauck, Y., Kelly, M., and Duggan, R. (2019). "It's what midwifery is all about": Western Australian midwives' experiences of 'being with woman' during labour and birth in the known midwife model. *BMC Pregnancy and Childbirth* 19: 29.

Buhling, K., Schmidt, S., and Robinson, J. (2006). Rate of dyspareunia after delivery in primiparae according to mode of birth. *European Journal of Obstetrics and Gynaecology* 124: 42–46.

Carter, S. and Green, A. (2007). Body image and sexuality. In: *Foundations of Nursing Practice – Leading the Way*. Ch 8 (eds. R. Hogston and B. Marjoram), 247–270. UK: Palgrave Macmillan.

Cooper, N., Forrest, K., and Cramp, P. (2006). *Essential Guide to Generic Skills*. Blackwell Publishing Ltd.

Dahlen, H., Priddis, H., and Thornton, C. (2015). Severe perineal trauma is rising, but let us not overact. *Midwifery* 31: 1–8.

Department of Health (1999). The NHS Plan: A new direction for English Public Health? *Critical Public Health* 11 (1): 75–81.

Department of Health (2012). *Compassion in Practice: Nursing, Midwifery and Care Staff. Our Vision and Strategy*. London: The Stationary Office.

Department of Health (2013). *The NHS Constitution*. London: The Stationary Office.

Dewar, B. and Christley, Y. (2013). A critical analysis of compassion in practice. *Nursing Standard* 28 (10): 46–50.

Donners, K.M., Kluivers, K.B., and de Leeuw, J.W. (2017). Choice of mode of delivery in a subsequent pregnancy after OASIS – a survey amongst Dutch gynaecologists. *International Urogynecology Journal* 10: 1537–1542.

Dugdale, A. and Hill, S. (2005). Midwifery-led care: establishing a postnatal perineal clinic. *British Journal of Midwifery* 13 (10): 648–653.

Dunn, A., Sudeshna, P., Ware, L., and Corwin, E. (2015). Perineal injury during childbirth increases risk of postpartum depressive symptoms and inflammatory markers. *Journal of Midwifery and Women's Health* 60 (4): 428–436.

Evans, E., Falivene, C., Briffa, K. et al. (2019). What is the total impact of an obstetric anal sphincter injury? An Australian retrospective study. *International Urogynecology Journal*. https://doi.org/10.1007/s00192-019-04108-3.

Farrar, D., Tuffnell, D.J., and Ramage, C. (2014). Interventions for women in subsequent pregnancies following obstetric anal sphincter injury to reduce the risk of recurrent injury and associated harms (review). *The Cochrane Database of Systematic Reviews* (11) (Art. No. CD010374).

Fitzpatrick, M., Cassidy, M., Ronan, P., and Ronan O'Connell, P. (2002). Experience with an obstetric perineal clinic. *European Journal of Obstetrics, Gynecology, and Reproductive Biology* 100: 199–203.

Fowler, G., Williams, A., Murphy, G. et al. (2009). Education – how to set up a perineal clinic. *The Obstetrician and Gynaecologist* 11: 129–132.

Glazener, C.M.A., Abdalla, M., Stroud, P., and Naji, S. (1995). Postnatal maternal morbidity: extent, causes, prevention and treatment. *British Journal of Obstetrics and Gynaecology* 102: 286–287.

Goetz, J., Keltner, D., and Simon-Thomas, E. (2010). Compassion: an evolutionary analysis and empirical review. *Psychological Bulletin* 136 (3): 351–374.

Gurol-Urganci, I., Cromwell, D.A., Edozien, L.C., and Mahamood, T. (2013). Third-and fourth degree perineal tears among primiparous women in England between 2000 and 2012: time trends and risk factors. *British Journal of Obstetrics and Gynaecology* 120: 1516–1525.

Haelle, T., Salvesen, K., and Volloyhaug, I. (2016). Obstetric anal sphincter injury and incontinence 15-23 years after vagina delivery. *Acta Obstet Gynaecol Scand* 95(8): 941–947.

Hall, J. and Mitchell, M. (2016). Dignity and respect in midwifery education in the UK: a survey of lead midwives of education. *Nurse Education in Practice* 21: 9–15.

Harvey, M.A., Pierce, M., Alter, J.E. et al. (2015). Obstetrical anal sphincter injuries (OASIS): prevention, recognition and repair. *Journal of Obstetrics & Gynaecological Can* 37 (12): 1131–1148.

Hospital Episodes Statistics 2018-2019 (2019). HES Publications.

International Confederation of Midwives (2014). www.internationalmidwives.org (accessed 23 March 2020).

Joris, F., Hoseli, I., Kind, A. et al. (2019). Obstetric and epidemiological factors influence the severity of anal incontinence after obstetric anal sphincter injury. *BMC Pregnancy and Childbirth*. http://dx.doi.org/10.1186/s12884-019-2238-2.

Keighley, M.R.B., Perston, Y., Bradshaw, E. et al. (2016). The social, psychological, emotional morbidity and adjustment techniques for women with anal incontinence following obstetric anal sphincter injury: use of a word picture to identify a hidden syndrome. *BMC Pregnancy and Childbirth* 16: 275.

Kettle, C. (2004). Perineal care. *Clinical Evidence*. http://www.clinicalevidence.com/ceweb/conditions/pac/10401: p. 1401 (accessed 23 March 2020).

Kirkham, M. (1993). Communication in midwifery. In: *Midwifery Practice: A Research-Based Approach* (eds. J. Alexander, V. Levey and S. Roch), 1–19. London: Macmillan.

Kirkham, M. (1999). The culture of midwifery in the National Health Service in England. *Journal of Advanced Nursing* 30 (3): 732–739.

Kurtz, S.M. and Silverman, J.D. (1996). The Calgary-Cambridge referenced observation guides: an aid to defining the curriculum and organising teaching in communication training programmes. *Medical Education* 30 (92): 83–89.

Laine, K., Skjeldestad, F.E., Sandvik, L., and Staff, A.C (2012). Incidence of obstetric anal sphincter injuries after training to protect the perineum: cohort study. *British Medical Journal* 2 (5): e001649. https://doi.org/10.1136/bmjopen-2012-001649.

Leeman, L. and Rogers, G. (2012). Sex after childbirth, postpartum sexual function. *Obstetrics & Gynecology* 119 (3): 647–655.

March, F., Rogerson, I., and Landon, C. (2011). Obstetric anal sphincter injury in the UK and its effects on bowel, bladder and sexual function. *European Journal of Obstetric Gynacological Reproductive Biology* 153: 223–227.

MASIC (Mothers with Anal Sphincter Injuries in Childbirth) (2017). Foundation. Charity Commission for England. http://www.opencharities.org/charters/1169632 (accessed 23 March 2020),

Menage, D., Bailey, E., Lees, S., and Coad, J. (2016). Concept analysis- a concept analysis of compassionate midwifery. *Journal of Advanced Nursing* 73 (3): 558–573.

Moberg, K.U. (2015). How kindness, warmth, empathy and support promote the progress of labour: a physiological perspective. In: *The Roar behind the Silence: Why Kindness, Compassion and Respect Matter in Maternity Care* (eds. S. Byrom and S. Downe). London: Pinter and Martin Ltd, chapter 13.

Moyzakitis, W. (2004). Exploring women's descriptions of distress and/or trauma in childbirth from a feminist perspective. *The Royal College of Midwives Evidence Based Midwifery* 2 (1): 8–14.

Munson, E. (2007). Applying the Calgary-Cambridge model. *Practice Nursing* 18 (9): 464–468.

National Institute for Health and Care Excellence (2018). NICE impact maternity. London.

NHS England (2016) Better Births. The National Maternity Review. England. www.england.nhs.uk/ourwork/futurenhs/mat-review (accessed 5 March 2020).

NHS England (2018). Maternity Transformation Programme. London.

NMC (2019a). Standards of Proficiency for Midwives. NMC: London.

NMC (2019b). The Code. NMC Codes and Standards. Professional standards of practice and behaviour for nurses, midwives and nursing associates. NMC: London.

Norton, C., Christiansen, J., Butler, U., and Harai, D. (eds.) (2002). *Incontinence: Second International Consultation on Incontinence*. Plymouth: Health Books.

OECD (2013). *Health at a Glance. OECD Indicators*. OECD Publishing Paris. https://doi.org/10.1787/health_glance-2013-en.

O'Kelly, S.M. and Moore, Z.E.H. (2017). Antenatal maternal education for improving postnatal perineal healing for women who have birthed in a hospital setting. *Cochrane Database of Systematic Reviews* (12) (Art No. CD012258).

Percy, P. and Richardson, C. (2018). Introducing nursing practice to student nurses: how can we promote care, compassion and empathy? *Nurse Education in Practice* 29: 200–205.

Permanente, K. (2013). Leadership & Vision. Tiny.cc/Leadership_vision (accessed 23 March 2020).

Pierce-Williams, R.A.M., Saccone, G., and Berghella, V. (2019). Hands-on versus hands-off techniques for the prevention of perinea; trauma during vaginal delivery: a systematic review and meta-analysis of randomised controlled trials. *The Journal of Maternal-Fetal & Neonatal Medicine*. https://doi.org/10.1080/14767058.2019.1619686.

Preston, H.L., Alfirevic, Z., Fowler, G., and Lane, S. (2019). Does water birth affect the risk of obstetric anal sphincter injury? Development of a prognostic model. *International Urogynecology Journal* 30: 909–915.

Pretlove, S.J., Thompson, P.J., and Toozs-Hobson, P.M. (2004). The first 18 months of a new perineal trauma clinic. *Journal of Obstetrics and Gynaecology* 24 (4): 399–402.

RCOG (2013). *Patterns of maternity care in English NHS hospitals 2011/12*. London: RCOG Press.

RCOG (2015). The management of third-and fourth-degree Perineal Tears. Green Top Guidelines. London.

RCOG (2019). OASIS Care Bundle. New information resource on Obstetric Anal Sphincter Injury launched. News 29 October. London.

Reid, A., Beggs, A., and Sultan, A.H. (2014). Outcome of repair of obstetric anal sphincter injuries after three years. *International Journal of Gynecology & Obstetrics* 127: 47–50.

Salmon, D. (1999). A feminist analysis of women's experiences of perineal trauma in the immediate post-delivery period. *Midwifery* 15 (4): 247–256.

Sayasanth, A. and Pandeva, I. (2010). Postpartum sexual dysfunction: a literature review of risk factors and mode of delivery. *British Journal of Medical Practitioners* 3 (2): 316–321.

Sekon, L. (2010). Changing patient's needs: issues and ethics of maternal requested caesarean section. *RCSI Medical Student* 3 (1): 61–64.

Siddiqui, J. (1999). The therapeutic relationship in midwifery. *British Journal of Midwifery* 7 (2): 111–114.

Sinivaara, M., Suominen, T., and Routasalo, P. (2004). How delivery ward staff exercise power over women in communication. *Journal of Advanced Nursing* 46(1): 33–41.

Sultan, A.H., Kamm, M., and Hudson, C.N. (1993). Anal sphincter disruption during vaginal delivery. *The New England Journal of Medicine* 329: 1905–1911.

Sultan, A.H., Kamm, M.A., Hudson, C.N., and Bartram, C. (1994). Third degree anal sphincter tears: risk factors and outcome of primary repair. *British Medical Journal* 308: 887–881.

Sultan, A.H., Thakar, R., and Fenner, D. (2007). *Perineal and Anal Sphincter Trauma* Investigations of anorectal function. Ch 9, 102. Springer-Verlag. London. Ltd.

Thakar, R. and Sultan, A.H. (2007). Postpartum problems and role of a perineal clinic. In: *Perineal and Anal Sphincter Trauma* (eds. A.H. Sultan, R. Thakar and D. Fenner) Ch. 6, 65. Springer-Verlag. London. Ltd.

Webb, S. (2018). Subsequent birth after obstetric anal sphincter injury. *Midwives* 21: 34.

Webb, S. and Parsons, M. (2011). The specialist perineal midwife: making a difference. *MIDIRS Midwifery Digest* 21: 351–352.

Webb, S., Yates, D., Manresa, M. et al. (2016). Impact of subsequent birth and delivery mode for women with previous OASIS: systematic review and meta-analysis. *International Urogynecology Journal.* https://doi.org/10.1007/s00192-016-3226-y.

Williams, A., Herron-Marx, S., and Hicks, C. (2007). The prevalence of enduring postnatal perineal morbidity and its relationship to perineal trauma. *Midwifery* 23: 392–403.

Wilson, A.E. (2009). A quasi-experimental study to evaluate an educational programme in perineal repair for midwives and students. PhD Thesis. University of Surrey, Guildford. Ch 5, p. 101.

Wilson, A.E. (2012). Effectiveness of an educational programme in perineal repair for midwives. *Midwifery* 28: 236–246.

Wilson, A.E. (2014). Maternity Unit Clinical Audit: Perineal Care Clinic. Royal Surrey County Hospital NHS Trust, Guildford, Surrey.

Wilson, A.E. (2017). The pelvic floor. In: *Mayes' Midwifery(Eds: Macdonald, S. & Johnson, G.).* Ch. 40, 672–674. London: Elsevier.

Wilson, A.E. (2018). How to minimise perineal trauma at your birth and caring for your perineum after the birth of your baby. Patient Information Leaflet. Royal Surrey County Hospital Foundation Trust, Guildford, Surrey.

Wilson, D., Milsom, I., and Freeman, R. (2014). UR-choice: can we promote mothers-to-be with information about the risk of pelvic floor dysfunction? *International Urogynecology Journal* 25 (11): 1449–1452.

8

'With Woman' from a Mental Health Perspective

Nadine Page (Mental Health Specialist), Erin Pascoe (Specialist Midwife);
Aisha-Sky Lindsay (midwife); and Helena* (woman)

Introduction

The early days of motherhood are generally considered to be a time of great joy and emotional wellbeing for a woman. However, it is not uncommon for women to experience what is referred to as the 'baby blues', which is a short period of feeling low, anxious and irritable. Women may experience mood swings, over-react to things and burst into tears more easily. It starts 3–4 days after delivery and usually stops by the time the baby is around 10 days old. These feelings are normal as hormones adjust to not being pregnant, and no treatment is needed. Sadly though, for many women, motherhood increases their vulnerability to mental illness such as postnatal depression (PND). PND may be mistaken for baby blues at first, but the signs and symptoms are more intense and last longer, eventually interfering with the mother's ability to care for her baby and cope with other daily activities of living. PND is a non-psychotic depressive illness that affects 10–15% of women in the first 12 months after birth and remains one of the leading causes of direct maternal death in the UK as a result of suicide (Knight et al. 2019). Occurring at a critical time when the mother is forming a relationship with her baby, if left untreated, PND can have detrimental consequences on infant cognitive and emotional development in both the short and long term (Jacques et al. 2019). Inadequate identification and treatment are associated with significant human and economic costs. Thus, early detection and intervention has been highlighted as key to reducing these adverse outcomes and their associated costs (NICE 2014 updated 2017).

Principles of Care in Pregnancy and the Postnatal Period

Continuity of carer is a principle that has been lauded as the gold standard of care for all women during the antenatal, intrapartum and postnatal period. MacArthur et al. (2014) surmised that midwife-led, flexible postnatal care, tailored to the needs of the woman, could help to improve women's mental health and reduce probable PND. The advent of Better Births (NHS England 2016) once again has highlighted the importance of this principle. However, with current staffing crises in the NHS, continuity has been extended to a pregnancy circle of care – the idea being that a woman would get to know a small group of midwives that she may encounter at various contacts during her pregnancy. When considering continuity of carer/s in the detection and support of depression for a pregnant or newly delivered mother, having an established relationship and baseline of a woman's character and nature would hope to more quickly identify if any change in mental state was occurring. One key priority when providing care for women with PND is that care is coordinated; a review of the literature by Huang et al. (2017) found that a collaborative approach was more effective and rendered more positive outcomes than traditional management and disjointed care by healthcare providers. Anecdotal evidence, shared with the author as a perinatal mental health midwife, echoes the research, but more important is that the women do not have to repeat their story to multiple professionals and a focus on moving forward is paramount.

Recognising Depression in Pregnancy and the Postnatal Period; Assessment and Referral

The NICE Guidelines (2014 updated 2017) have established the routine enquiry of mood during pregnancy and the postnatal period. The Whooley Questions and GAD-2 scale are part of the initial booking appointment, helping to establish a baseline and open a general discussion about a woman's mental health and wellbeing. Good practice would have midwives enquire about mood at every contact with the woman. Answering positively to any of the mood or anxiety questions should then prompt further discussion about what support the woman wishes to explore to address their issues. Other assessment tools can be considered, such as the Edinburgh Postnatal Depression Scale (EPDS) or the Patient Health Questionnaire (PHQ-9) to aid the professional in sourcing the right support for the woman.

Research conducted in Australia by Schmied et al. (2013) highlighted that it was previously not thought to be an integral part of the midwife's roles and responsibilities to screen and provide support for women with PND, but a culture shift has acknowledged that midwives are frequently the primary contact for women in the perinatal period. As such, women often develop safe and confiding relationships with their midwife, ideally placing them to assess and support and refer on where appropriate. Further studies by Small et al. (2014) Marnes and Hall (2013), Myors et al. (2012), Johnson and Galal (2014), Austin et al. (2013) and Homer et al. (2009) found that women are more likely to accept mental health support from a midwife. Onward referral for support can vary depending on services available to the woman's locality. Options include the GP, Perinatal Mental Health Midwives, Parent Infant Mental Health Service, Improving Access to Psychological Therapies, (IAPT) providers for counselling or cognitive behaviour therapy (CBT), and in extremis a Perinatal Mental Health Team.

Treatment Options, Monitoring and Support in the Postnatal Period

Varying options for the treatment of PND are available; the acceptance of these treatments by women vary depending on many factors. PND remains a stigmatised condition despite professionals and charities/social media campaigns aiming to bring the issue into everyday conversation to try and reduce this. However, the development of Perinatal Mental Health Care Pathways has at its heart the key messages in the Equality Act (McColgan 2010) that try to reduce inequalities between patients to ensure that access to and provision of services are provided in an integrated way to prevent health inequalities.

All professionals – regardless of level of expertise or training – are able to explore the principles of self-help and care with a woman. Discussing general wellbeing factors – such as good nutrition, sleep hygiene, exercise and family and friend networks alongside charitable support services – can help to establish a baseline of what a woman currently has in terms of support, and what they may wish to engage with to address their concerns and recover. Leahy-Warren et al. (2011) commented that midwives need to understand and acknowledge the significant contribution that social support, particularly from family and friends, has in positively influencing a first-time mother's mental health and wellbeing in the postpartum period.

Psychological interventions can be essential in a woman's recovery from PND. These interventions may be provided in primary, secondary or tertiary care. Timely referral should be made for any woman with suspected PND to an evidence-based NICE (2014 updated 2017) recommended psychological intervention. If a woman accesses psychological support through IAPT (Improving Access to Psychological Therapy) services, then a waiting time standard applies for perinatal referrals (NHS England, NHS Improvement, NCCMH 2018). Many variants of psychological intervention can be used in treating PND, a diagnostic tool is often used in the triage process to identify which type of therapy for example, CBT or one to one counselling, may be deemed appropriate. Research by Appleby et al. (1997) showed that therapy can be as beneficial as medication as a treatment option for PND. Some women may choose to seek private therapy sources if this option is available to them. They may have received therapy from a professional previously and wish to re-engage in the services of this person as they have a shared history, making the recovery process easier as they have an established relationship.

Antidepressants are generally well tolerated in pregnancy and breastfeeding by both women and their infants. Antenatal and PND is associated with adverse fetal, maternal and infant outcomes and should be treated (McAllister-Williams et al. 2017). Antidepressants continue to not be licensed in pregnancy and breast-feeding, and therefore the evidence that has been gathered is minimal in human case reporting and animal studies (Grigoriadis et al. 2013). Women should also be fully informed of the background population risk of potential side effects (NICE 2014 updated 2017). Research facilities such as UK Teratology Information Service (UKTIS 2017) provide the best evidence possible detailing the potential risks of medication during pregnancy and potential impact into the postnatal period. Similarly, there are minimal studies investigating the transmission rate of medication through breastmilk, but prescribing should consider the safest option possible in conjunction with the continuation of breastfeeding should the woman wish to. Clear guidance around prescribing should be available to all obstetric teams and GPs so that women do not feel an increase in stigma when making the difficult decision to choose medication to help their recovery.

It is widely acknowledged that there has been inequality in provision of special-ist perinatal mental health services throughout the UK. There has been a big push from NHS England under their implementation of the Five Year Forward View for Mental Health (NHS England 2016) programme to fund the start-up of services in localities. Their aim was that by 2020/21 all women would have access to special-ist services, but at the time of writing the report 85% of localities did not meet NICE (2017) guidelines.

Women's Perspective

There is limited research on the woman's perspective of support around PND in the UK. Viveiors and Darling (2018) completed some research in Canada around this topic and highlighted that barriers to accessing perinatal mental health ser-vices are: fear and stigma, broken referral pathways, distant location services, lack of number/capacity of specialised services, baby-centeredness and discharge from midwifery care at six weeks. Anecdotal evidence provided to the author as a peri-natal mental health midwife from patients is that having the extra support during a pregnancy or the postnatal period can make a huge difference to their recovery. Having a professional who does not judge, who can empathise, sympathise and troubleshoot their concerns – whilst appreciating the limitations of their mental health at the time – can have a positive impact, especially when contemplating a future pregnancy (Seimyr et al. 2013).

Hurt (2018) in her Master's thesis looked at the midwives' role in supporting pregnant and postnatal women experiencing depression. When gathering the responses from midwives, four common themes emerged: mother and baby PND services, continuity of midwifery care, community-based care and midwives being valued and supported. When compared to the research previously cited by Viverios and Darling (2018), it appears that both women and midwives have identified near identical themes and suggestions to service improvement. Whilst the Five Year Forward plan goes some way to addressing the imbalance, this is only looking at service provision in the UK, whereas the research has come from further afield, highlighting the fact that PND and perinatal mental health is an important topic across the globe.

Table 8.1 presents the analysis of key citations for the literature pertaining to mental health wellbeing in pregnant and postnatal women.

Conclusion

The literature has examined antecedents to mental health during pregnancy and in the postnatal period and indicates that evidence focuses on principles of mental healthcare, assessment of depression, professional's perspectives and those of woman experiencing perinatal depression.

It is recognised that changes in care patterns and collaborative care models, such as midwife-led, flexible and tailored care to meet the needs of women experiencing depression, could reduce and improve the mental health of women. In addition, clarity of care roles and cohesive guidance for practitioners, supported by education and training, could provide continuity of care and improved trusting relationships between healthcare professionals and the women accessing maternity services.

Of most importance, as indicated in the literature above, is correct assessment of depression pre- and post-delivery of the baby. This will ensure early detection, support from midwives and effective referral to allied healthcare professionals, leading to improved outcomes and mental wellbeing for childbearing women. Such social support will consequently enhance maternal/parental self-efficacy and reduce PND in the early days post-partum. Women's views suggest that creating a relationship with midwives which nurtures advocacy, is women centred and enables informed choice is a safe environment in which women feel encouraged to disclose their anxieties and feelings of depression. Ultimately, the evidence suggests that

Table 8.1 Concept analysis of mental health factors.

Antecedents	Evidence	Attributes (A) and Consequences (C)
Principles of care	MacArthur et al. (2014) redesigned care	Midwife-led, flexible and tailored to needs care (A) Improves women's mental health and reduces probable depression at four months postpartum (C)
	Huang et al. (2017) care models	Collaborative care models (A) Effective in depression management in primary care populations (C)
	Myors et al. (2013) collaboration and integrated services	Funding and resources and a shared vision, aims and goals (A) Role clarity (A) Pathways and guidelines (C) Continuity of care, building relationships and trust (C) Training, education and support for staff for MH services (C)
Assessment of depression	Schmied et al. (2013) role of midwife	Previous history of depression and poor partner relationship (A) Depression and anxiety postpartum and up to five years later (C) Identification support and referral (C)
	Marnes and Hall (2013) routine screening	Identification of women at risk of MH disorders (A) Earlier detection and improved outcomes (C) Midwives primary point of contact (C)
Professional perspectives	Austin et al. (2013) Australian guidelines	Holistic, woman- and family-centred approach (A) Effective management of MH and mood disorders in the perinatal period (C)
	Leahy-Warren et al. (2011) social support	Cognisance by MWs of the importance of social support for first-time mothers (A) Enhances maternal parental self-efficacy and reduces PND in early postpartum period (C)
Women's perspectives	Viveiros and Darling (2018) midwifery care	Seek continuity of care, women- centred care, informed choice and advocacy (A) MWs enhance the uptake of perinatal mental health by developing relationships with women that create safe conditions for disclosure (C) Improved information about MH symptoms, treatment and services (C) Identifying when women need additional social support (C)

women want to seek the support and continuity of care from their midwives but need the space and relationship in which this can be achieved.

Some of the accounts and stories below help to illustrate the literature discussed and analysed in this chapter.

Specialist Midwife's Story

Erin's Story

Gill came to the antenatal clinic as she had had a diagnosis of chronic emotionally unstable personality disorder (EUPD), depression and significant self-harm and suicidal ideation. This was her second pregnancy. In her first pregnancy she was emotionally stable, until the postnatal period where she experienced an exacerbation of her diagnosis and required significant time in various inpatient settings to stabilise her.

At six weeks of pregnancy she was admitted to A&E having been found by the side of the railway with the intent to kill herself. Social services were already working with the family and were subsequently alerted to this new pregnancy.

Gill was heavily medicated on various anti-psychotic, benzodiazepine and anti-depressant medications, but they appeared to be having little effect at this point. She was booked by maternity services but during her first trimester had a voluntary admission to an inpatient setting to try and stabilise her. Gill was prone to overdose on her prescribed medication throughout her pregnancy.

There were many professionals already involved in Gill and her family's care. This included community mental health psychiatrist and nurse, inpatient psychiatrists and nurses and social services. As the perinatal mental health midwife, I took over Gill's antenatal care alongside an obstetric consultant to help provide the extra support she would need, and the time required to liaise and meet with these other professionals to provide clear, joined up care.

As Gill had had extensive exposure to mental health services since her teenage years, she had a very different view of the support she was receiving from mental health services – or her perceived lack thereof. This was echoed by her family also. A common trait of women with an EUPD diagnosis is something called 'splitting'. This is where a woman will play various professionals off against each other to try and detract attention away from their issues. The key to combating this is effective communication within the multi-disciplinary team and not to assume certainty of information disclosed by the woman. This can potentially cause tension in the relationship with the woman if she becomes aware that all professionals are communicating with each other. Having an appreciation of the relationship that the woman and her support network has with various professionals is essential to keep Gill the centre focus of the care that is provided, and also to understand the role that the members of the team have to play in delivering maternity care to Gill.

(Continued)

During the pregnancy, Gill's medication was reviewed frequently and the dose altered accordingly depending on her presentation. Her frequent overdoses were also taken into consideration and the access to medication discussed and managed where possible, although this became much more challenging for the periods of time when she was at home. Gill was keen to undergo electro convulsive therapy (ECT) during her pregnancy, a treatment she had received previously with good effect. The multi-disciplinary team discussed this at length as it is not a common treatment to recommend during pregnancy. The ECT was also arranged to occur in Gill's local hospital on the labour ward rather than in an outpatient setting as is the usual practice. The ability to have anaesthetic support from the obstetric anaesthetic team was deemed prudent and should there be any adverse effect to the unborn baby during or after the treatment process then action could be taken immediately. This required effective communication and commitment from the various members of the multi-disciplinary team and ECT team to facilitate this unusual request. As the perinatal midwife I tried to be present for the majority of Gill's ECT treatments, to support the staff on the labour ward who had never witnessed this, for Gill to have a 'known' midwife present in the post general anaesthetic period, and to liaise with her partner with permission, to inform him that both mum and unborn baby were well post treatment.

Arrangements for delivery were discussed at length and a plan formulated with the support from the whole multi-disciplinary team that was felt to be best for Gill and her family. Delivery was safe and uncomplicated from an obstetric point of view. During her postnatal ward admission, Gill was supervised continuously due to her fluctuating mood during pregnancy. Discharge home with her baby was achieved, but within a few days Gill's mental health deteriorated again, and she began to self-harm and took another overdose. The baby was brought to A&E under advisement to be monitored as Gill had been breastfeeding, although temporarily stopped following the overdose. An admission to a mother and baby unit was arranged following this event, under a medical section, to monitor her mood and interaction with her baby.

Continuity of care remained very important during this inpatient admission, despite the facility being out of area. By attending review meetings up to the 28 days postnatal, I was able to help provide some history and context that was essential to help work with this family, and link back with the local team to update them. Gill and her family also felt reassured to have a familiar face in these situations as the meetings can be very intimidating with many professionals present to support them.

A case such as this does take an emotional toll on all professionals involved. The importance of communication, respect and understanding of each other's roles and boundaries in knowledge and understanding helped to keep us working together and keep the family at the centre of our work. It also helped to increase the feeling of shared responsibility for Gill's care and her family, which could otherwise feel very overwhelming.

Being Gill's midwife was an extremely challenging period in my career. Her complexity required flexibility and enormous compassion, something she didn't feel she received from all professionals. I felt the gravity and power of the midwife–mother relationship, and how to temper this to maintain effective working relationships with the multi-disciplinary team. We are privileged as midwives to quickly become a trusted person within a woman's life and trying to respect the position they hold you in, but also putting their best interests and that of the baby first, can sometimes push that trust to its limits.

Gill continued to require intense support from various inpatient mental health facilities during the first year post her child's birth. She continues to be supported by the community mental health team but has found new focus and is hopefully reaching a period of stability whilst she pursues this path.

A Midwife's story – Aisha's Story

There is no amount of knowledge/information/advice that will ever prepare you for parenthood. I'd been a qualified midwife for five years when my son was born, and I thought from my experience in the profession that I knew what to expect . . . oh how wrong I was! A few days into parenthood I started questioning all the advice I'd given parents in the postnatal period. All of the knowledge I thought I had, I now believed didn't apply to my situation; I was questioning everything I did, everything that my partner did, in fear of failing this little human that was relying on us so heavily. After the initial shock of parenthood, the first six months of my son's life was a rollercoaster of emotions, but I understood that this was just me getting used to my new role as a parent and the challenges of establishing breastfeeding. I was lucky that my son would wake every two hours over night and I very quickly got used to that mentally (although I had very wrongly assumed that my previous years of shift work had prepped me well physically: this was a new level of tiredness). When six months approached, he was awake a lot more throughout the night and for longer periods of time, he was more difficult to settle, and we found this quite hard

(Continued)

going. My son was breastfed and refused a bottle and dummy and I felt like the pressure was on me to get him back to sleep. The sleeplessness continued right up until he was almost two years old. This is when I think the postnatal depression (PND) started to become an issue.

Reality of parenthood, the sleep deficit, the pressure we feel to get everything perfect, the social pressure to just spring back and carry on with life as if nothing has changed, ensuring I did everything differently to my own mother . . . these were all contributing factors to my postnatal depression. I went to my GP nine months into my son's life and expressed that I wasn't feeling myself (I thought maybe I had hypothyroidism), and when she told me that I was suffering with severe anxiety and depression and I should strongly consider medication, without hesitation I declined. I didn't want to believe that taking a tablet would make anything better, all I thought I needed was a few good night's sleep and everything would be better. Unbelievably, I struggled on through the sleepless nights and hazy days for a further nine months following this consultation until I eventually admitted it and commenced medication.

Prior to this, I returned to work after 14 months of being away from midwifery, (I couldn't even fathom the idea of doing any 'Keeping In Touch' days) and that's when the PND really hit me hard. The night shifts on top of everything else took its toll on my body and my mind. I didn't feel safe at work, I was told by a midwife who I look up to that my 'spark' had disappeared, I felt like my passion for midwifery was missing. This job that I'd worked so hard for and knew I was made for was no longer enjoyable. I was looking for ways out, different jobs I could do that didn't involve long shifts, when all I needed to do was speak up about how I was feeling and ask for help but that, I felt, was shameful. I didn't want to seem as though I wasn't coping. I'm still not really sure what I was trying to prove and who I was trying to prove it to, but I just wish I had done everything sooner rather than suffering just because I was ashamed. It was around 15 months that I also stopped breastfeeding which I believe exacerbated how I was feeling. Perhaps the change in hormones when breastfeeding comes to an end is something we should be more knowledgeable about as midwives.

I eventually went back to the GP because I felt like not only my parenting skills were being affected, but also my ability to stay focused at work, and my social skills were taking a big hit and nothing was changing very quickly. I was finding it increasingly difficult to hold a conversation, even with the closest of family. I felt like my brain was failing me and at any moment there was a risk that something bad was going to happen either at home or at work. The role of the midwife to be 'with woman' just didn't seem possible; I was present in body but not in mind.

As a midwife, I should have known better and I will always feel guilty that I should have sought help sooner. When it comes to any form of depression, it is so important to talk, seek help and, most importantly, to not be ashamed. Since having my son, there have been dramatic cuts to the health visiting service with optional drop-in clinics as opposed to prearranged home visits. I worry that there will be more and more wasted opportunities for health visitors to pick up on those mothers that are afraid to shout for help. Perhaps I would have spoken up sooner if a healthcare professional had come to me and asked me how I was feeling?

Being a midwife, now I am a mother has not changed the way I care for a labouring woman at all; I appreciate that every woman's experience is different. What has changed is the way in which I deliver not only postnatal information but, equally as important, antenatal information on expectations following birth. In my opinion, we focus a lot on providing information on what to expect in labour and information on the mechanics of breastfeeding for postnatal information. I'm not assuming that everyone will feel the way I did, but perhaps we should be more honest with women on how difficult it's going to be over the next few years.

NB. The 'perfect parent' does not exist; we can only try our best, and if the best means asking for help, then we should do it more often.

A Woman's Story

Helena*'s Story

I wonder what he or she will look like. What shall we name our baby? I can't wait to meet him or her! What do you think of this wallpaper? Shall we hang up this night lamp? Oh! Look how cute these tiny socks are! So much to think of, but so exciting! These are a few of the many things my husband and I asked ourselves or spoke about in the weeks leading up to Benji's birth. Whilst at times it was stressful, for most of the pregnancy I found myself feeling excited and 'baby ready'. I very often felt that I was in overdrive, fuelled by all the preparation excitement. Even as my waters broke, it didn't feel scary – I was nervous but a good kind of nervous.

Fast forward to 10:50 p.m. on 30 October. 'He's beautiful, he's perfect' my husband said, but what I felt was indescribable. The pain I had just endured was out of this world; something I never imagined I would feel. Holding my baby in my arms was

(Continued)

just as indescribable but the feeling of pain crippled my body and I couldn't yet fathom what had just happened.

The next few days were a dream. People floated in and out, brought presents, balloons and oohed and aahed at this little human being. All I could think of was the pain I felt every time I moved an inch. Having had stitches, I felt uncomfortable and dirty. Everything felt like a hassle, even getting up to use the bathroom was a feat. Yet in between the struggles mummy duties set in. Feeding, changing, burping, soothing and the familiar feeling of dread and fear. What do I do? How do I do it? I felt so scared. The midwives and staff on the hospital ward were extremely caring and supportive and I felt I could turn to them at any given moment; however, when the lights were switched out at night, the fear crept in again.

After a week in hospital, we were set to go home. All packed and ready to go. Baby dressed and snuggly placed into the car seat. Balloons tied to the stroller. Bags stuffed with presents. But instead of feeling happy to go home, I felt terrified. Being back home was a blessing, surrounded with my personal belongings made me feel more at ease but it felt so odd to bring this little baby into our home. He's ours! It really does feel like a dream, but no one ever told me that this dream would soon turn into my biggest nightmare.

The next weeks that followed were one big blur. I lost track of what day it was and what time it was and could barely string a sentence together because I was just so petrified of being with my son especially being with him alone – even if it was just for a minute or so. How was I mother if I needed my own mother to comfort me and be with me the whole time? Everything was terrifying – what on earth have we done? These thoughts exacerbated by the hour and I just felt that I could not do this. Why did we have a baby? Can't my mother bring him up for the first few months? I don't want him. And these thoughts fuelled the vicious cycle of feeling guilty and like a horrible person – not at all like a mother. The whole experience of these weeks was so frightening because Benji just would not settle. He did not sleep. He simply cried, no, he screamed, for the majority of the day and night. Oh newborn babies sleep so much, people said. It's easy in the first weeks, feed, sleep and repeat. This was far from my experience – the screaming was deafening, and I just wanted out.

My whole world felt like it had been overturned, tossed around upside down and turned inside out. I did not want this. I did not feel happy. I did not feel like myself. Did I even love my baby? How could I not want him? I needed the support and thankfully I found it. The midwifery service was excellent, I could confide in the midwives who called me and spoke to me on the phone but also came home to visit. I leaned heavily on my own mother and my relatives – who were my saving grace. How people manage without any or little support is beyond me – they are to be admired because these first weeks were a nightmare. Until today I have immense respect for single mothers who raise newborn babies by themselves. Whilst I had the support of my husband, this too was a stress in itself. We were both extremely stressed out and feeling all over the place. We needed sleep. We needed help. We were a mess. Seeing each other in this situation just made things worse. It felt like we had made a big mistake.

A few months in and things slowly settled. We came to the conclusion that my son needed medication for acid reflux, and this immediately started to have an effect on him. He calmed down a little and was more settled. I really do believe that the less my anxiety was present, the less anxious my baby was. This little human being was inside me for nine months and so close to me, everything I channelled in was passed onto him. In my pregnancy I learnt a lot about the '4th trimester' and babies' first weeks outside the womb. How scary must it have been for Benji to be out in this big world, no longer in his mothers' tummy, cosy and safe? I started to think more on these lines and all I wanted to do was protect him. I will never forget the day I realised I loved him. I cried myself to sleep thinking: how did it take me so long to love him?

Today, 11 months later I look back with pride at how I overcame what to me was the biggest traumatic experience I have ever faced. I look back with a little bit of shame at how it took me so long to love this amazing little boy. I look back with gratitude at the undivided support I had, especially from my family and my mother. How I hope to be half the woman she is and have such love for her children. Today I cannot really remember the details of how I didn't sleep, how I could not leave Benji alone for a minute without him screaming the room down and how I hated the start of a new day. Today I look at him with so much love, this little, funny, charming, happy, gorgeous little boy who teaches me so much every day.

Lessons Learnt

The heartfelt stories above are truly moving. The raw emotions that women feel when faced with such overwhelming feelings of anxiety and depression are clearly described in these accounts. The stories from a midwife, a midwife who also became a mother and the mother having her first baby, illustrate the impact of perinatal depression from different perspectives. What each story has in common, is the need to recognise the reality of caring for women or the consequences of living with depression whilst caring for a newborn infant.

The care and support that these women received was of vital importance in alleviating to some extent, the fear and uncertainty caused by the impact of birth on their mental wellbeing. Professionals and family alike play a crucial role in supporting these women on their journey to recovery. Lessons can be learnt from the above accounts on how best both can be 'with woman' during this very real and debilitating experience.

References

Appleby, L., Warner, R., Whitton, A., and Farahger, B. (1997). A controlled study of fluoxetine and cognitive behavioural counselling in the treatment of postnatal depression. *British Medical Journal* 314: 932.

Austin, M.-P., Middleton, P., Reilly, N., and Highet, N. (2013). Detection and management of mood disorders in the maternity setting: the Australian clinical practice guidelines. *Women and Birth* 26 (1): 2–9.

Grigoriadis, S., Vonder Porten, E., Mamisashivli, L. et al. (2013). The impact of maternal depression during pregnancy on perinatal outcomes: a systematic review and meta-analysis. *The Journal of Clinical Psychiatry* 74 (4): 293–308.

Homer, C., Passant, L., Brodie, P. et al. (2009). The role of the midwife in Australia: views of women and midwives. *Midwifery* 25 (6): 673–681.

Huang, H., Tabb, K., Cerimele, J. et al. (2017). Collaborative Care for Women with depression: a systematic review. *Psychosomatics* 58 (1): 11–18.

Hurt, D. (2018). Midwives knowledge of perinatal depression and their role in supporting pregnant and postnatal women experiencing depression: An appreciative inquiry. Thesis for Masters of Midwifery Research, Faculty of Health, University of Technology, Sydney.

Jacques, N., de Mola, C.L., Joseph, G. et al. (2019). Prenatal and postnatal maternal depression and infant hospitalization and mortality in the first year of life: a systematic review and meta-analysis. *Journal of Affective Disorders* 243: 201–208. https://doi.org/10.1016/j.jad.2018.09.055.

Johnson, J. and Galal, S. (2014). Mental health-what's that got to do with midwives? *Australian Nursing and Midwifery Journal* 21 (8): 44–45.

Knight, M., Bunch, D., Tuffnell, D. et al. (2019). MBRRACE - saving lives, improving mothers' care. Lessons learned to inform maternity care from the UK and Ireland Confidential Enquiries into Maternal Deaths and Morbidity 2015–17.

Leahy-Warren, P., McCarthy, G., and Corcoran, P. (2011). First-time mothers: social support, maternal parental self-efficacy and postnatal depression. *Journal of Clinical Nursing.* https://doi.org/10.1111/j.1365-2702.2011.03701.x.

MacArthur, C., Winter, H., Bick, D. et al. (2014). Effects of redesigned community postnatal care on women's' health 4 months after birth: a cluster randomised controlled trial. *Lancet* 359: 378–385. https://doi.org/10.1016/S0140-6736(02)07596-7.

Marnes, J. and Hall, P. (2013). Midwifery care: a perinatal mental health case scenario. *Women and Birth* 26 (4): 112–116.

McAllister-Williams, R.H. et al. (2017). British Association for Psychopharmacology consensus guidance on the use of psychotropic medication preconception, in pregnancy and postpartum. *Journal of Psychopharmacology* 31 (5): 1–34.

McColgan, A. (2010). Equality Act. www.legislation.gov.uk (accessed 20 July 2020).

Myors, K., Schmied, V., Johnson, M., and Cleary, M. (2012). Collaboration and integrated services for perinatal mental health: an integrative review. *Child and Adolescent Mental Health Journal* 18 (1): 1–10.

Myors, K. et al. (2013). Collaborative and integrated services for perinatal mental health: an integrative review. *Child & Adolescent Mental Health* 18(1): 1–10.

NHS England (2016). Five year forward view for mental health. https://www.england.nhs.uk/wp-content/uploads/2016/02/Mental-Health-Taskforce-FYFV-final.pdf (accessed 4 July 2020).

NHS England (2017). Implementing Better Births: Continuity of carer; five year forward view. https://www.england.nhs.uk/wp-content/uploads/2016/07/fyfv-mh.pdf (accessed 4 July 2020).

NHS England, NHS Improvement, National Collaborating Centre for Mental Health (2018). The perinatal mental health care pathway. https://www.england.nhs.uk/publication/the-perinatal-mental-health-care-pathways/ (accessed 4 July 2020).

NICE (2014/2017). Antenatal and postnatal mental health: clinical management and service guidance - Clinical guideline [CG192]. Updated August 2017. www.nice.org.uk/guidance/cg192 (accessed 10 July 2020).

Schmied, V., Johnson, M., Naidoo, N. et al. (2013). Maternal mental health in Australia and New Zealand: a review of longitudinal studies. *Women and Birth* 26 (3): 167–178.

Seimyr, L., Welles-Nystrom, B., and Nissen, E. (2013). A history of mental health problems may predict maternal distress in women postpartum. *Midwifery* 29 (2): 122–131.

Small, R., Watson, L., Gunn, J. et al. (2014). Improving population level maternal health: a hard nut to crack? Long term findings and reflections on a 16-community randomised trial in Australia to improve maternal emotional and

physical health and birth. *PLoS One*. https://doi.org/10.1371/journal.
pone.0088457.

UK Teratology Information Service (UKTIS) (2017). 6. UK Teratology Information
Service [Internet]. UK:UKTIS [updated 2017.12.08; cited 2018.01.02]. http://www.
uktis.org. (accessed 12 July 2020).

Viverios, C.J. and Darling, E.K. (2018). Barries and facilitators of accessing perinatal
mental health services: the perspectives of women receiving continuity of care
midwifery. *Midwifery* 65: 8–15.

9

'With Woman' in Prison

Anna M. Brown; Clare Cochrane (Specialist Midwife); and Women

Introduction

This chapter explores the meaning of 'with woman' in prisons from midwives' and women's perspectives. It is an attempt to identify the adjustments that midwives make in a unique environment for incarcerated women, with complex needs, serving a prison sentence. It also examines the perspectives of these women in terms of maternity services available to them and how the 'with woman' concept is perceived.

According to the Prison Reform Trust (2018), 5% of the prisoner population imprisoned each year across the UK are women. Of these, 19% are involved in self-harm incidents as a result of the traumatic impact of incarceration and over half at 53% are reported to have suffered domestic abuse and experienced emotional, physical and sexual abuse as a child. An estimated 17 240 children are separated from their mothers by imprisonment each year. In 2018, 7745 women were incarcerated, with most of these – 82% – being sentenced for non-violent offences.

Little is known about maternity services for pregnant, labouring and postnatal women in prisons in the UK. A review by Birth Companions in 2016 resulted in a Birth Charter for women in prisons in England and Wales and some recommendations have been made (Delap et al. 2016). Currently, about 600 pregnant women are in prison and approximately 100 babies are born to these women each year in the UK and Wales. There are at present six mother and baby units (MBUs) in prisons in which babies can stay with their mothers until they are 18 months old (Delap 2016). Despite these units, however, about half of the women giving birth whilst serving a prison sentence have their babies removed at birth, resulting in anxiety/apprehension and grief of separation (Wismont 2000; Birmingham et al. 2006; Chambers 2009).

Many of these women are a vulnerable obstetric risk and frequently have complex care needs, inadequately met by the prison services, resulting in high-risk pregnancies (Foley and Papadupolous 2013). These risks are compounded by additional factors such as inadequate antenatal care, poor lifestyle choices – such as substance misuse, smoking and unhealthy nutrition – and health issues such as sexually transmitted diseases and poor mental health (Price 2005; Birmingham et al. 2006; WHO 2007). An external review towards the Birth Companions publication (2007) indicated that 'birth companions' for women from prisons during their labour provided emotional support (Marshall 2010) and enabled prison officers to focus on their role in maintaining security (Rowles and Burns 2007). Maternity services for these women need to be reviewed to identify training and educational needs of midwives and prison officers supporting these women and their current needs.

Interventions and Impact on Outcomes

Primarily, not many studies document the experiences and outcomes of child-bearing women in prisons. Shaw et al. (2015) carried out a systematic review which suggests that no robust studies exist to examine the effectiveness of interventions to improve outcomes amongst incarcerated women and their babies born during their prison sentence. In 2004, Bell et al. published results of outcomes for incarcerated women compared to controls in the USA. They found that women in prison during pregnancy had progressively higher odds of having a preterm infant and lower birthweight compared to a control group. However, public health intervention in correctional facilities during and after release may improve these odds (Morse et al. 2019). These results are reiterated in a systematic review by Knight and Plugge (2005a) of incarcerated women in the UK; although when compared with other disadvantaged groups, perinatal outcomes appear to improve for imprisoned women in terms of birthweight of their babies. Similarly, in the USA, Howard et al. (2009) found that timing of incarceration may have beneficial effects on birthweights of infants born to pregnant women in prison during the first trimester as compared to those in the second trimester. However, this effect was not associated with black or Hispanic women but white women only. More recently, a study from Australia (Dowell et al. 2019) suggests that there are no improved birthweight outcomes for mothers imprisoned during pregnancy but they are at an increased risk of having low birthweight babies. In addition, they have a higher prevalence of risk exposure to alcohol and substance misuse, mental health issues and physical injuries.

In addition to physical outcomes for antenatal women in prisons, there is evidence to suggest that high levels of stress and anxiety can have a negative impact on the mother and her unborn infant (Mukherjee et al. 2014). Galloway et al.

(2014) suggest that women in prisons are five times more likely to experience mental illness than their male counterparts. However, women who were given the opportunity to keep their babies up to 18 months in a MBU inside the prison had better mental health than those women who were not offered a place (Dolan et al. 2019). Unfortunately, those participants from the prison who were not offered the supportive environment of the MBU were more likely to have had mental health disorders and came from complex and chaotic backgrounds (Glover 2014).

Mental health incidences appear lower for women in MBUs due to the mother–infant interaction (Borelli et al. 2010), and forging relationships (Simkiss et al. 2013); a relationship which, if disrupted, can impact children long term (Epstein 2014). These findings are reiterated by study findings on Iranian women prisoners (Anaraki and Boostani 2014), which also support earlier data that children's presence in the prison had positive impact on the mothers to reduce loneliness, promote a sense of calm, provide a sense of comfort and security and encourage rehabilitation (Benoit 2004). Some other research, however, also examines a different perspective to that generally indicated in the studies above and suggests that women in the MBUs felt isolated and lonely if these units were underutilised (Western et al. 2014). The units were not supervised appropriately, lacked provisions and equipment to facilitate children, whilst the women felt more vulnerable due to the presence of their infants (Rose et al. 2016; Fritz and Whiteacre 2016). However, intervention programmes to improve the unit environment, staff supervision and timely intervention from the relevant professionals improved communication and outcomes for the mothers and their babies (Cassidy et al. 2010).

Women's Views and Experiences

Very little evidence exists of incarcerated women's perceptions and views of maternal care services for pregnant or postnatal women in prisons. Most of the literature is published from the USA, although a recent integrative review suggests that the experiences of incarcerated pregnant women is that they are victimised, marginalised and socially excluded (Baldwin et al. 2019).

Chambers in 2009 carried out a qualitative study exploring the effects on mother–infant bonding when women in prisons are aware of the possibilities of separation after birth from their infant. The findings suggest that emotional damage to the mother and her baby has a detrimental effect on this fragile bond and pregnant and postnatal women in prisons have to be treated with this in mind. Some evidence is available to document the resulting long-term outcomes for incarcerated pregnant and childbearing women and their babies (Knight and Plugge 2005b; Albertson et al. 2012; Bard et al. 2016; Paynter et al. 2019). Some literature documents that efforts have been made to support women to improve their parenting skills through educational programmes

(Sleed et al. 2013; Shlafer et al. 2014, Rossiter et al. 2015; Tenkku-Lepper et al. 2018) and initially to breastfeed their infants (Allen and Baker 2013; Abbott and Scott 2017). The Baby Friendly Hospital Initiative recommends that despite the prospects of mothers and neonates being separated after birth, all mothers are shown how to breastfeed (WHO 2009, UNICEF 2012) and Shlafer et al. (2018) suggests that initiation by incarcerated women was more likely when these women discussed breastfeeding with and were supported by their doula or 'birth companion'.

Some studies that have explored imprisoned women's views about breastfeeding indicate that breastfeeding could potentially improve these women's wellbeing and improves their self-worth (Huang et al. 2012). However, overall little is known about effective interventions that would reduce negative outcomes and improve the significance and value of compassion to impact the chances and quality of the lives of these women and their neonates once they leave prison (Baldwin 2018).

Maternity Services for Women in Prisons

The Birth Charter (Kennedy et al. 2016) recommends that pregnant women in prison should have access to the same standard of antenatal care as women in the community. They should be housed, fed and moved in a way to ensure the wellbeing of mother and baby (Ferszt and Clarke 2012; Shlafer et al. 2017). During childbirth, women should be accompanied by officers who have had appropriate training and clear guidance and they should receive appropriate and humane care during transfer between prison and hospital. In addition, women with babies in prison should be encouraged and supported in their chosen method of infant feeding and should be given the same opportunities and support to nurture and bond with their babies as women in the community.

There is limited research on midwives' knowledge of the care of imprisoned women during pregnancy and the postpartum period. Most of the available research is published in the USA (Goshin et al. 2019) suggesting that there is a need for education and training to fulfil this need. One study from Australia (Baldwin et al. 2019) indicates that few studies exist which focus on midwifery support for pregnant women in prisons and the services available to them.

One area in the south east of England reports that maternity services have been offered in a prison for some time now to include three-hour midwifery clinics held in the prison twice weekly, with one obstetric clinic held there every five weeks. In addition, a mobile ultrasonic service is held in a fortnightly session to screen women for anomalies and growth of the fetuses. A safeguarding midwife is also linked to these clinics and attends mother and baby board meetings at the prison to plan care for the unborn and delivered babies of these women in prison. A postnatal MBU which can accommodate 12 mothers and 13 babies has been successfully set up for a number of years (Cochrane 2019). The midwives supporting women in prison have clear aims of providing enhanced antenatal and postnatal care and ensuring that all care provision is evidence based and that difficult situations are managed with compassion and honesty – especially with those women who are separated from their baby.

The above literature was examined through Rodger's Concept Analysis framework to identify antecedents, attributes and consequences of the 'with woman' concept; the results are demonstrated in Table 9.1.

Table 9.1 Rodgers' Concept analysis of 'with woman' in prison.

Antecedents	Evidence	Attributes (A) and Consequences (C)
Physical health	Bell et al. (2004), Howard et al. (2009) low birthweight and preterm birth more prevalent for incarcerated women	Presence, advocacy (A)
	Morse et al. (2019) public heath intervention improves odds	Facilitation of clinics (C) Comfort (A)
	Ferszt and Clarke (2012), Howard et al. (2009, 2011), Shlafer et al. (2017) healthcare needs in prison/ nutritional needs	Limited use of restraints, healthy diet (C)
Psychological health	Wismont (2000) apprehension, grief and subjugation frequently observed amongst detained women	Relatedness (A)
	Birmingham et al. (2006) depressive disorders and emotional damage due to anxiety and trauma of separation from their baby is evident.	Decreasing anxiety (C) Increasing reassurance (C)
	Schroeder and Bell (2005), Chambers (2009), Allen and Baker (2013), Abbott and Scott (2017)	Enablement (A) Advocacy (A) Personal transformation (C)
	women who have been had support from a prison-based doula or birth companion are more likely to initiate breastfeed even when mothers and neonates are to be separated	Better birth experience (C) Supportive environment (A) Improved mental health (C)
	Marshall (2010), Shlafer et al. (2018) the effects of a doula intervention and/birth companions	
	Dolan et al. (2019), Fritz and Whiteacre (2016), Glover (2014) decreased effect on MH through MBUs	

(Continued)

Table 9.1 (Continued)

Antecedents	Evidence	Attributes (A) and Consequences (C)
Emotional well being	Price (2005) isolation and lack of personal autonomy due to health and gender inequalities in prisons Baldwin et al. (2019) victimised, marginalised and socially excluded Benoit (2004), Epstein (2014), Simkiss et al. (2013), Anaraki and Boostani (2014), Borelli et al. (2010) mother–infant relationship in MBU	Understanding (A) Compassion (A) Giving personal attention (C) Mother–infant relationship outcomes (A) Reduced loneliness, promote a sense of calm, comfort and security (C) Encourages rehabilitation (C)
Knowledge	Huang et al. (2012) women's views and understanding about breastfeeding Sleed et al. (2013), Rossiter et al. (2015), Tenkku-Lepper et al. (2018) educational programmes on parenting skills	Improved wellbeing and improved self-worth (C) Greater understanding (A) Practical skills/self and baby (A)
Midwifery/ prison services	Delap et al. (2016), Delap et al. (2016), Goshin et al. (2019) outcomes for incarcerated women and their neonates Knight and Plugge (2005b), Rowles and Burns (2007) pregnant imprisoned women as compared to other disadvantaged women when they are supported by a professional Cassidy et al. (2010) interventions	Lack of training, guidance and support for midwives (A) Better perinatal outcomes (C) Improved facilities and relevant and timely support (A) Improved communications and outcomes (C)

Conclusion

Many pregnant prisoners are single and unsupported and may have financial struggles. They tend to come from minority groups and are generally uneducated. The risk factors for many of these women are substance misuse, sexually transmitted infections, smoking and poor nutritional status, together with mental health issues because of domestic abuse and violence. Pregnancy and childbirth increase these risks due to previous inadequate antenatal care and poor obstetric history, resulting in continuing ill health and safeguarding concerns when their babies are born.

Examination of the cited literature indicates that midwifery support has a crucial role to play in improving conditions and outcomes of pregnant women in prisons. Facilitation of clinics to support and advocate for these prisoners provides reassurance and decreases anxiety through the compassion and continuity of carer approach. As a result of compassionate and understanding approaches by midwives, the women's wellbeing and self-worth improves, resulting in better perinatal outcomes and enhancing practical care skills for themselves and their babies.

The literature suggests that prison reforms are now an agenda for perinatal women in the criminal justice system and the Royal College of Midwives' (RCM 2014, 2019) position is to ensure that maternal and newborn health is not compromised by imprisonment. This also includes those women who have experienced miscarriage, stillbirth or who have been separated from their babies whilst in prison, who should have access to counselling and a referral to mental health support if appropriate. A collaborative approach between the criminal justice system and healthcare providers is recommended to ensure that women in prison have the same access to healthcare as anyone else accessing maternity services. In addition, every effort is made towards ensuring mothers and babies are kept together wherever possible, in MBUs, and in the best interests of the child so that long-term health and social consequences of separation are ameliorated.

Specialist Midwife's Stories – Clare's Stories

Jill*'s Story

I first met Jill when she was pregnant with her fifth child. She sat before me as an emaciated 25-year-old woman, she had a number of teeth either missing or broken, her facial skin marked by acne and limp blonde hair. She had a Body Mass Index of 17.

Jill was in prison for the first time, admitting to me that 'she had been in front of a judge, one too many times' for shoplifting. She had received a sentence of six months. She told me her most favoured items she stole were tins of baby formula powder and large blocks of chocolate. She sold these items to the local corner shop proprietor for £5 and £1 respectively. Most of the money was spent on cocaine. Jill described her typical day: on waking, she would take cocaine; lunch would be a cheese sandwich on white bread; dinner she and her partner would have a takeaway pizza or fried chicken followed by cocaine.

Jill was articulate and bright. She told me that she and her partner had met as teenagers and he was the father to all her children. She described him as a

(Continued)

'functioning' drug addict. He was able to hold down a job and this provided them with a flat to live in. Jill spoke about her first two children being removed as her cocaine habit grew and she was unable to care for them adequately. Instead of getting help after the children were removed, her drug use spiralled out of control.

Prison gave Jill an opportunity to eat three regular meals a day, to break her daily habit of cocaine. She gained weight, her skin healed and her hair looked lush. On one antenatal appointment, Jill stated 'she didn't realise she could feel this good'. Clear headed, healthier and on our final appointment before her release, Jill stated that she was looking forward to a future without drugs. She finally had the right 'head space'. Her goal was not only to stay off drugs, but to also support her partner to get off drugs, and they would be able to parent this child. We talked about the temptations in going back into the community, about the importance of continuing her maternity care with her local hospital and working with Children's Services. Jill felt that she was finally well equipped and ready to go back into the community.

I next saw Jill six weeks later back in prison. Pale, emaciated and unwell. She had broken her bail conditions and would now be in prison for the birth of this baby. We talked at length about her first week after release. Her partner had not been paying the rent whilst she had been in prison, so they had lost their flat. They had been housed in a bed and breakfast and the landlord knew of her drug and theft history. Jill felt unhappy with the change in circumstances and there was the temptation of drugs everywhere. She said to me 'life's hard and my partner was using in front of me'. Jill started using cocaine again, four days after her release from prison.

Jill gave birth to a beautiful daughter. She had not been successful in gaining a position on the Mother and Baby Unit at the prison. Children's Services were successful in getting an interim care order and baby was to be placed with a foster carer. Jill had one request: could her baby be placed with the same foster carer as her last baby. She described the foster carer as loving and kind. She had provided Jill with photos and updates on the heath and care of her children. This foster carer was available and very happy to care for Jill's baby. The foster carer came to the hospital and met with Jill and her partner and there I observed an openness and genuine kindness between them.

Removing a child from their mother will never be easy, and neither should it be. Jill was brave but also incredibly sad. Afterwards, we hugged and cried together. Jill has lost her five children and the amount of pain this has caused her is something I can only imagine. Jill said that she did not want to have any more children until she was free of drugs. Before she left hospital, Jill agreed to have a contraceptive implant. This was a huge deal for Jill, as she was needle phobic. I stayed with her during this procedure and held her hand tightly.

Postscript 2019

I have seen Jill twice more in prison. She comes, says hello, and always gives me a hug. When we last spoke, she told me that she had an approved place in a residential drug rehabilitation unit. She described it as her first real chance of change and she was not going to waste it. Her partner was also now in prison; he had continued to use drugs and had lost his job.

Hayley*'s Story

Hayley was 28 weeks pregnant when she came to prison for the first time. She had pregnancy notes with her as she had attended most of her appointments at her booking hospital. This is the exception rather than the rule with the women in prison. Often, they have not had any maternity care prior to coming to prison. I would describe Hayley as timid, withdrawn and she appeared very suspicious of me.

This was Hayley's first ongoing pregnancy and she was always very happy to talk about the pregnancy and the health of the unborn baby. When I would direct the conversation onto her own health and wellbeing, Hayley would always withdraw and refuse to answer. This also included the refusal to discuss the father or the fact that she tested positive to cannabis and cocaine when she arrived at prison.

Hayley usually attended her appointments with a novel in hand. She loved reading and we would discuss the latest novel. Hayley was also helping in the Education Centre, working alongside women, where English was not their first language. She had A level qualifications.

Hayley applied to the MBU at the prison requesting that she be allowed to care for her baby whilst she completed her sentence. It is at these boards that I often find out, for the first time, the exact nature of their crime and sentence. A social report is presented by the allocated social worker for the unborn outlining the family history, circumstances, concerns and positives. At times, what is stated in these reports is vastly different from what the woman has shared with us. I understand the reasons why they may do this but for the board to be effective and in order to safeguard a vulnerable baby, I need to know the facts and to hear from Hayley an honest and, at best, truthful account.

(Continued)

Hayley had suffered an appalling level of domestic abuse. She had found herself in a situation that she did not believe that she was worthy of getting out of. The drugs appeared to be a way of numbing the pain from the physical, sexual and emotional abuse.

Hayley spoke to the board, not about the past but about the future. Coming to prison had been the most positive thing that had happened to her in a long time. In prison she 'felt safe' and cared for. She stated that she was 'able to breathe normally'. Prison gave her time to think and plan. Hayley talked fondly of a sister that had always been supportive; about a mother who she had an 'up and down' relationship with but that they had been making real progress in rebuilding a stronger bond. She talked about her education and what training she wanted to do to increase her chances of employment once baby was older.

Hayley was successful in gaining a place on the MBU. I cared for them for the five weeks postnatal period, when Hayley and baby left prison. They were going to live with Hayley's mother.

Postscript

Hayley had been a victim of significant and prolonged domestic violence. She continued to withhold the information around the details of the baby's father. I must respect her decision. I referred and encouraged Hayley to access several support agencies within the prison. This was to provide Hayley with the known professionals around domestic abuse and mental health. I saw my role as enabling Hayley to have the opportunity to be in a safe environment to talk about the past, to talk about decision making processes and building better relationships.

Women's Stories

Due to security reasons for women in prisons, it was extremely difficult to be provided with any first-hand accounts from these women.

Lessons Learnt

The above stories highlight the importance of the midwife's role in support and advocating for pregnant women who are in prisons. Women in these situations are more prone to anxiety and depression and providing some continuity of care, from specialist midwives who facilitate visits and clinics, decreases anxiety and provided some reassurance.

Hayley's story gives some insight into women's vulnerable state and the appealing situations they find themselves in resulting in a prison sentence. With encouragement and support, however, Hayley appeared to '*feel safe and cared for*' and rebuild her life.

Jill's story illustrates how despite the support given she was unable to change her drug abusing habits at the cost of losing her baby. However, the midwife's continued physical and psychological support ('*we hugged and cried together*') was instrumental in enabling Jill to find her way on the road to recovery. Through the midwife's empathetic support and selfless giving of her time and efforts, both these accounts illustrate the true sense of being 'with woman'.

References

Abbott, L. and Scott, P. (2017). Women's experience of breastfeeding in prison. *MIDIRS. Midwifery Digest* 27 (2): 217–223.

Albertson, K., O'Keeffe, C., Lessing-Turner, G., et al. (2012). Tackling health inequalities though developing evidence-based policy and practice and childbearing women in prison: a consultation. Project report. Sheffield Hallham University. Sheffield.

Allen, D. and Barker, B. (2013). Supporting mothering through breastfeeding for incarcerated women. Journal of Obstetric. *Gynecologic, & Neonatal Nursing* 42 (Supp 1): S103.

Anaraki, N.R. and Boostani, D. (2014). Mother-child interaction: a qualitative investigation of imprisoned mothers. *Quality and Quantity: International Journal of Methodology* 48 (5): 2447–2461. https://doi.org/10.1007/s11135-013-9900-y.

Baldwin, L. (2018). Motherhood disrupted: reflections of post-prison mothers. *Emotion, Space and Society* 26: 49–56.

Baldwin, A., Sobolewskab, A., and Capper, T. (2019). Pregnant in prison: an integrative literature review. *Women and Birth* 32 (3): 195–203.

Bard, E., Knight, M., and Plugge, E. (2016). Perinatal health care services for imprisoned pregnant women and associated outcomes: a systematic review. *BMC Pregnancy and Childbirth* 16 (1): 285.

Bell, J.F., Zimmerman, F.J., Cawthon, M.L. et al. (2004). Jail incarceration and birth outcomes. *Journal of Urban Health* 81 (4): 630–644.

Benoit, D. (2004). Infant-parent attachment: definition, types, antecedents, measurement and outcome. *Paediatrics and Child Health* 9 (8): 541–545.

Birmingham, L., Coultson, D., Mullee, M. et al. (2006). The mental health of women in prison mother and baby units. *The Journal of Forensic Psychiatry & Psychology* 17 (3): 393–404.

Borelli, J.L., Goshin, L., Joestl, S. et al. (2010). Attachment organisation in a sample of incarcerated mothers and associations with substance abuse history, depressive symptoms, perceptions of parenting and social support. *Attachment & Human Development* 12 (4): 355–374. https://doi.org/10.1080/14515730903416971.

Cassidy, J., Ziv, Y., Stupica, B. et al. (2010). Enhancing attachment security in the infants of women in a jail-diversion program. *Attachment & Human Development* 12 (4): 333–353. https://doi.org/10.1080/14616730903416955.

Chambers, A.N. (2009). Impact of forced separation policy on incarcerated postpartum mothers. *Policy, Politics & Nursing Practice* 10 (3): 204–211.

Cochrane, C. (2019). Personal communication and information provided about women in prison.

Delap, M. (2016). Caring for perinatal women in prison: how the launch of the Birth Charter will help women and staff. *British Journal of Midwifery* 26 (6): 390–392.

Delap, M., Bourke, G., and Page, L. (2016). Maternity care for women in prisons in England & Wales. *British Journal of Midwifery* 24 (7): 462.

Dolan, R., Shaw, J., and Hann, M. (2019). Pregnancy in prison, mother and baby unit admission and impact on perinatal depression and 'quality of life'. *The Journal of Forensic Psychiatry and Psychology* 30 (4): 551–569.

Dowell, C.M., Mejia, G.C., Preen, D.B., and Segal, L. (2019). Low birth weight and maternal incarceration in pregnancy: a longitudinal linked data study of Western Australian infants. *SSM-Population Health* 7: 100324: 1–12. https://doi.org/10.1016/j.ssmph.2018.11.008.

Epstein, R. (2014). Mothers in prison: The sentencing of mothers and the rights of the child. *Howard League What is Justice? Working Papers.* https://howardleague.org/wp-content/uploads/2016/04/HLWP_3_2014.pdf (accessed 14 September 2019).

Ferszt, G. and Clarke, J. (2012). Health care for pregnant women in US state prisons. *Journal of Health Care for the Poor and Underserved* 23 (2): 557–569.

Foley, L. and Papadupolous, I. (2013). Perinatal mental health services for black and ethnic minority women in prison. *British Journal of Midwifery* 21 (8): 553–562.

Fritz, S. and Whiteacre, K. (2016). Prison nurseries: experiences of incarcerated women during pregnancy. *Journal of Offender Rehabilitation* 56 (1): 1–20.

Galloway, S., Haynes, A., and Cuthbert, C. (2014). An unfair sentence: All babies count: Spotlight on the Criminal Justice System. Barnardo's and NSPCC. https://library.nspcc.org.uk/HeritageScripts/Hapi.dll/filetransfer/2014AnUnfairSentenceAllBabiesCountSpotlightOnTheCriminalJusticeSystem.pdf (11 April 2019).

Glover, V. (2014). Maternal depression, anxiety and stress during pregnancy and child outcome; what needs to be done. *Best Practice & Research. Clinical Obstetrics & Gynaecology* 28 (1): 25–35.

Goshin, L.S., Sissoko, D.R.G., Neumann, G. et al. (2019). Perinatal Nurses' experiences with and knowledge of the care of incarcerated women during pregnancy and the postpartum period. *JOGNN* 48: 27–36. https://doi.org/10.1016/j.jogn.2018.11.002.

Howard, D.L., Strobino, D., Sherman, S.G., and Crum, R.M. (2009). Timing of incarceration during pregnancy and birth outcomes: exploring racial differences. *Maternal and Child Health Journal* 13: 457–466.

Howard, D.L., Strobino, D., Sherman, S.G., and Crum, R.M. (2011). Maternal incarceration during pregnancy and infant birthweight. *Maternal and Child Health Journal* 15: 478–486.

Huang, K., Altas, R., and Parvez, F. (2012). The significance of breastfeeding for incarcerated pregnant women: an exploratory study. *Birth* 39 (2): 145–155.

Kennedy, A., Marshall, D., Parkinson, D. et al. (2016). *Birth Companions: Birth Charter for Women in Prisons in England & Wales*. London: Birth Companions.

Knight, M. and Plugge, E. (2005a). Risk factors for adverse perinatal outcomes in imprisoned pregnant women: a systematic review. *Birth & Maternal Care* 5: 111. https://doi.org/10.1186/1471-2457-5-111.

Knight, M. and Plugge, E. (2005b). The outcomes of pregnancy among imprisoned women: a systematic review. *British Journal of Obstetrics and Gynaecology* 112 (11): 1467–1474.

Marshall, D. (2010). Birth companions: working with women in prison giving birth. *British Journal of Midwifery* 18 (4): 225–228.

Morse, D.S., Wilson, J.L., Driffill, N.J. et al. (2019). Outcomes among pregnant recently incarcerated women attending a re-entry transitions clinic. *Journal of Community Psychology* 47: 679–697.

Mukherjee, S., Dudith, P.V., Bahelah, R. et al. (2014). Mental health issues amongst women in correctional facilities: a systematic review. *Women & Health* 54 (8): 816–842.

Paynter, M.J., Drake, Cassidy, C., and Snelgrove-Clarke, E. (2019). Maternal health outcomes for incarcerated women: a scoping review. *Journal of Clinical Nursing* 28 (11–12): 2046–2060.

Price, S. (2005). Maternity services for women in prison: a descriptive study. *British Journal of Midwifery* 13 (6): 362–368.

Prison Reform Trust (2018). Women's policy framework. www.prisonreformtrust. org.uk/PressPolicy/Comment/InsideTime/ItemId/622/vw/1 (accessed 9 January 2020)

Rose, E., Gardiner, A., Daniel, B. et al. (2016). The Rose Project: Best for babies. The University of Sterling. http://hdl.handle.net/1893/24007 (accessed 12 October 2019).

Rossiter, C., Power, T., Fowler, C. et al. (2015). Mothering at a distance: what incarcerated mothers value about a parenting programme. *Contemporary Nurse* 50 (2–3): 238–255.

Rowles, S. and Burns, S. (2007). Birth Companions External Review Report. www. birthcompanions.org.uk/publications.html (accessed 5 April 2019).

Royal College of Midwives (2014). Women in custody: position statement. http://tinyurl.com/hcwnd7r (accessed 5 April 2019).

Royal College of Midwives (2019). Position statement: Perinatal women in the criminal justice system. www.rcm.org.uk (accessed 12 October 2019).

Schroeder, C. and Bell, J. (2005). Labour support for incarcerated pregnant women: the doula project. *Prison Journal* 85 (3): 311–328.

Shaw, J., Downe, S., and Kingdon, C. (2015). Systematic mixed-method review of interventions, outcomes and experiences for imprisoned pregnant women. *Journal of Advanced Nursing* 71 (7): 1451–1463.

Shlafer, R., Hellerstedt, W.L., Secor-Turner, M. et al. (2014). Doulas' perspective about providing support to incarcerated women: a feasibility study. *Public Health Nursing* 32 (4): 316–326.

Shlafer, R., Stang, J., Dallaire, D. et al. (2017). Best practices for nutrition care of pregnant women in prison. *Journal of Correctional Health Care* 23 (3): 297–304.

Shlafer, R., Davis, L., Hindt, L. et al. (2018). Intention and initiation of breastfeeding among women who are incarcerated. *Nursing for Women's Health* 22 (1): 64–78.

Simkiss, D.E., MacCallum, F., Fan, E.E.Y. et al. (2013). Validation of the mothers object relations scales in 2-4-year-old children and comparison with the child-parent relationship scale. *Health and Quality of Life Outcomes* 11 (49) https://doi.org/10.1186/1477-7525-11-49.

Sleed, M., Baradon, T., and Fonagy, P. (2013). New beginnings for mothers and babies in prison: a cluster randomised controlled trial. *Attachment & Human Development* 15 (4): 349–367.

Tenkku-Lepper, L.E., Trivedi, S., and Anakwe, A. (2018). Effectiveness of a prison-based healthy pregnancy curriculum delivered to pregnant inmates: a pilot study. *Journal of Correctional Health Care* 24 (3): 243–252.

UNICEF (2012). The baby friendly initiative. WHO, Geneva, Switzerland. http://unicef.org.uk/babyfriendly (accessed 11 April 2019).

Western, B., Braga, A. and Kohl, R. (2014). A longitudinal survey of newly-released prisoners: methods and design of the Boston reentry study. https://scholar.harvard.edu/files/brucewestern/files/brs_research_design.pdf (accessed 11 April 2019).

Wismont, J. (2000). The lived pregnancy experience of women in prison. *Journal of Midwifery and Women's Health* 45 (4): 292–300.

World Health organisation & United Nations Children's Fund (2009). *Baby Friendly Hospital Imitative: Revised, Updated and Expanded for Integrative Care*. Geneva: WHO.

World Health Organisation, United Nations Office on Drugs & Crime (2007). *Interventions to Address HIV in Prisons: Drug Dependence Treatment*. Geneva: WHO.

10

'With the Older Woman'

Clare Edney (Midwife), Anna M. Brown; and Kate* and Lucy* (women)

Introduction

Whilst total births in England and Wales are currently falling (from a recent high of 729 674 in 2012 to 679 106 in 2017), the standardised mean age of childbirth is now 30.5 years – the highest ever recorded (Office of National Statistics (ONS) 2019). Within the data, the shift towards older motherhood is clear: births to women over 35 years of age have been rising steadily since the 1970s, with those aged 40 years or more at their greatest proportion since 1944 (ONS 2019). Therefore, advanced maternal age (AMA) has been generally defined as 35 years and older in nulliparous women (Guedes and Canavarro 2014). This trend is reflected across Northern Europe and many higher socio-economic countries globally (OECD 2018). Researchers have suggested multiple trigger factors: the advent of easily accessible contraception, improved education and career opportunities for women, spiralling living costs (Sutcliffe et al. 2012), difficulties finding a suitable partner, (Waldenstrom 2016) and increased availability and uptake of in vitro fertilisation (IVF) and other reproductive technologies (HFEA 2018). Celebrity births to older women are also increasingly common and widely publicised on social media platforms (Decker 2019; Mills et al. 2015).

Despite the Internet and social media appearing to 'normalise' births to older mothers (Campbell 2011; Wood 2008), there is no question that it becomes more difficult to conceive and birth a healthy baby as a woman gets older. There is clear data that chromosomal abnormalities and rates of miscarriage significantly increase after the age of 35 (Loane et al. 2013). Evidence of pregnancy complications varies widely, but most studies show increased incidence of gestational diabetes, preterm birth, hypertension, pre-eclampsia, stillbirth and neonatal unit admission (Fuchs et al. 2018; Kenny et al. 2013; Laopaiboon et al. 2014). These risks are reflected in

Better Births: The Midwife 'with Woman', First Edition. Edited by Anna M. Brown.
© 2021 John Wiley & Sons Ltd. Published 2021 by John Wiley & Sons Ltd.

dramatically increasing rates of induction of labour (IOL) in England – currently 32.6% across all age groups, compared to 20.4% in 2007–2008 (NHS Digital 2018). For primiparae who deliver vaginally, there is a significant association between the risk of serious pelvic floor injury and AMA (Rahmanou et al. 2016). All studies demonstrate that women over 40, particularly primigravidae, are significantly more likely to require or request caesarean section (Bayrampour and Heaman 2010; Kahveci et al. 2018; Rydahl et al. 2019) with rates in England currently at 45% versus 28% for the general population (NHS Digital 2018).

Following the National Maternity Review (2016), the government implemented initiatives to ensure that more low-risk women see a midwife they know for the duration of their maternity care (NHS 2019). This is driven by data demonstrating lower rates of stillbirth with improved continuity of carer (NHS England 2017). However, 'high-risk' mothers do not fall into this category and are generally offered 'shared' care between midwives and obstetricians. There is, however, no consensus on the age at which women should be treated as high risk. In his 1960 article 'The elderly primigravida', O'Sullivan noted that most writers adopt the definition of the older primigravida as 35 years of age or over, but some prefer 40 years. Whilst contemporary authors seem to prefer the phrase 'advanced maternal age', most of the global literature continues to use the same age threshold. However, literature searches demonstrate that the range can be as wide as 32 years (Aasheim et al. 2013) to 48 years plus (Fitzpatrick et al. 2016).

In England, NICE antenatal care guidelines (2008) note that women at higher risk of complications, such as those aged 40 or older, should be offered 'additional care', but what form this should take is not specified. Maternity care is built on NICE and RCOG evidence-based guidelines, but protocols are developed locally by obstetric and maternity clinical governance teams, so there is no national consistency. Maternal experience indicates that care for older mothers is fragmented (O'Connor et al. 2014) with antenatal and birth options varying hugely, even between consultants within the same hospital. The aim of this chapter is to explore recent evidence relevant to first-time mothers over the age of 40. Of interest are women's experiences of pregnancy, birth and maternity care and how midwives fulfil the concept of 'with the older woman'.

Reasons for Advanced Maternal Age

There may be several reasons for delayed parenthood resulting in AMA and some studies have investigated cause and effect of this concept (Schytt et al. 2014; Aasheim et al. 2014; Nilsen et al. 2015; Waldenstrom 2016). Most studies on women having a first baby at an AMA were carried out in Sweden, which may provide data which needs to be considered in terms of the differences in cultures between Sweden and the UK. However, having a first baby at a later age is a universal trend, although reasons for this phenomenon may vary across countries.

The conclusions from the cited studies suggest that socio-economic reasons are usually associated with AMA. More focus on careers, finances and ensuring a stable standard of living usually has a bearing on having babies at a later age. Family background and negative and ambivalent attitudes to children in early adulthood is also a reason (Nilsen et al. 2015) together with a lack of partner, infertility problems and prioritising an independent life (Schytt et al. 2014). However, the consequences of AMA also include increased anxiety due to the added risks of stillbirth and preterm labour making pregnancy and labour difficult, resulting in a negative and more difficult childbirth experience (Aasheim et al. 2014; Waldenstrom 2016).

Perception of Risk

Midwives tend to consider an older nulliparous as 'high risk' and consequently perceive that care and outcomes for these women and their neonates may require increased vigilance and support. A study by Bayrampour et al. (2012) confirms that AMA is associated with adverse pregnancy and birth outcomes. The authors suggest, however, that there are several factors which influence how these women evaluate their pregnancy risk. This qualitative descriptive study, carried out in Canada, interviewed 15 women aged 35 and over in their third trimester who defined risk depending on their medical health but also on psychosocial elements to include a stable relationship and lifestyle, planning of the pregnancy, a supportive network and prioritising and controlling the situation. In addition, care providers' attitudes and opinions were also considered in defining their risk status.

Outcomes of Pregnancy and Birth

This section discusses current obstetric issues pertinent to older mothers in the UK and resulting complications of pregnancy and birth. Researchers based at the University of Manchester have generated several recent studies, using different methodologies, around AMA (Cooke et al. 2012; Lavender et al. 2015; Lean et al. 2017). Part of this group, Kenny et al. (2013), published a population-based cohort study examining AMA and adverse pregnancy outcomes: 215 344 singleton birth records from the North West England Perinatal Survey were analysed using log linear binomial regression. This quantitative research compared birth outcomes for women in three age groups (30–34, 35–39 and 40 plus years) with a reference sample of women aged 20–29 years. Outcomes examined were: stillbirth, preterm birth, small for gestational age (SGA), macrosomia and caesarean delivery. No statistically significant correlation between AMA and SGA was found; in fact, women over 40 years had an increased risk of larger babies and macrosomia. This was primarily due to raised body mass index (BMI) and social deprivation. The risk was not significant once adjusted for these confounders.

Preterm birth did, however, increase with maternal age with an increase of 24% in women over 40 compared to the reference sample. AMA also increased the risk of LSCS threefold for primiparae over 40 years. Stillbirth incidence for women in this group was also twice as likely, although no increase in neonatal deaths was noted. Strengths of the study were its large, relatively recent, sample (2004–2008). It was UK-based with data from 21 different hospitals in the north west, including areas at both ends of the socio-economic spectrum. This boosts the credibility and reliability of the data. Adjustments were made for parity, ethnicity, social deprivation and BMI across all the data to boost transferability. However, data for maternal smoking – now a key NHS care pathway (NHS 2019) – was only collected from 2007 so is not fully reliable. Additionally, smoking is a contributor to stillbirth rates so could skew the results (Marufu et al. 2015). The authors were also unable to adjust for co-morbidities such as hypertension or diabetes – particularly important due to their higher incidence as women age (Dietl et al. 2015). Additionally, no differentiation was made in the data between spontaneous or induced preterm labour. All these omissions reduce the rigour of the study and reliability of the results. However, the authors note that age-related risk is a continuum and acknowledge that increased surveillance of older mothers and real, or suspected, fetal compromise may provoke iatrogenic prematurity.

The increased risk of lower segment caesarean section (LSCS) with maternal age was a focus for Rydahl et al. (2019) who used Danish Medical Birth Registry data in their retrospective register-based study: 1 122 964 records between 1998 and 2015 were examined and the same reference and age ranges as Kenny et al. (2013) adopted. Adjustments were made via multivariate regression models for demographics, health and pregnancy-related issues, with results further divided by parity. The authors found that LSCS increases as women age, with nulliparity having a stronger association. Since adjusting for the confounders above had only a minor influence on the data, they suggest that obstetric culture may be partly responsible. Increased rates of elective surgery, induction and associated interventions which lead to higher rates of emergency caesarean are recommended as a potential area for further research. Qualitative or mixed method studies examining obstetric decision making would be extremely valuable, given the hugely varying rates of LSCS globally (Laopaiboon et al. 2014). The authors also urge further study into another potential variable – age-related physiological decline in uterine efficiency with the concomitant risk of labour dystocia.

The specifically increased risks for older nulliparous singleton pregnancies were a focus for Kahveci et al. (2018) who suggest that gestational diabetes mellitus, gestational hypertension, pre-eclampsia, SGA infants, spontaneous late preterm delivery and caesarean sections were factors in potential and significant maternal and neonatal outcomes for the effects of AMA in first-time mothers.

Women's Views

As previously discussed, there appears to be a growing trend for delayed childbearing beyond the age of 35 due to several factors. Some studies have explored women's views and experiences of having a first baby at an AMA. Cooke et al. (2012) indicated that AMA and delayed childbearing is rarely a conscious choice but dependant on life experiences and women perceiving childbearing as being beyond their control. Participants generally had a lack of understanding of associated risk factors with pregnancy over 35 years of age and that age alone had an association with poor outcomes. Lack of control over their circumstances such as finances, relationships and health may impact the timing of childbearing.

Women in Southby et al.'s (2019) study implied that they perceived conception of a first child at 35 years and beyond as a 'now or never' attempt to have a child. Both women and care providers understand this to be different to other, younger women and the perception of risk and associated care may limit choices for the woman with AMA. The authors suggest that women of AMA are seen to be more anxious during pregnancy and care providers lean towards conservative management of pregnancy and labour to minimise risk. These women expressed views of being judged for entering motherhood at an older age and may be reluctant to share news about their pregnancy due to anxieties over miscarriage and fetal abnormalities such as Down's syndrome. As a result, AMA may have an impact on psychological and mental wellbeing unless supported by healthcare professionals to improve outcomes. However, Aasheim et al. (2013) in a study of Norwegian women of AMA suggest that postponing childbirth to a later age only marginally effects the childbirth experience and older women coped with operative delivery better than their younger counterparts.

Finally, Mandel (2010) in a phenomenological study interviewing 11 single older women about their birth experiences as woman of AMA, implies that these participants related a sense of achievement when they became mothers and the challenges of becoming a single parent. However, support and being in control of decisions made for care was important in their journey and health professionals were key in providing that support.

Midwifery Care of the Older Mother

Limited literature exists about the views of healthcare professionals on women who experience childbirth at an advanced age. However, the literature from women's views is that they perceived midwives to be judgemental of their situation, as discussed previously, and are made to feel 'vulnerable, powerless and out of control' (Mandel 2010: 340). Bayrampour et al. (2012) suggests that although most healthcare providers do not usually disclose opinions, reaction and body language to women's age and perceived risks is observed by these women. Midwives should avoid stereotyping women of AMA and instead seek to normalise the psychosocial adjustments of transition to parenthood by these mothers (Guedes and Canavarro 2014) and the authors also recommend that healthcare professionals should promote realistic expectations through the interventions of antenatal psychoeducation.

Another study (Southby et al. 2019) suggests that the healthcare practitioners' attitude towards an increased risk of stillbirths (Kenny et al. 2013) may influence decision-making of the pregnant woman of advanced age, who may opt for early IOL and the use of pain relief, which may impact their birth experience. Midwives have a role to play when advising the pregnant woman in terms of physical activity, diet and nutrition and birth options and ensuring that they are psychosocially prepared through appropriate information. This enables these women to participate in their care planning and to maintain a sense of control (Mandel 2010).

Finally, it has been identified that antenatal depression levels are higher in the older woman, although postnatal depression and stress increases equally across all age ranges. However, Garcia-Blanco et al. (2017) found that higher stress-related cortisol was only present in the older woman in the postnatal period – although this effect was counterbalanced by increased social functioning such as maternal attitude towards the pregnancy and social support improved with age and delayed childbearing. O'Connor et al. (2014) suggest that the experience of older women varies according to the availability and delivery of maternity services. Some women experienced a lack of continuity of care due to understaffed and overworked health professionals. The authors suggest that further research is required to explore the needs of pregnant women of advanced age and how midwives can educate these women to enable them to achieve normality during their birth experiences balanced against the increased risks to both themselves and their neonates.

The literature has been examined through Rodgers' Concept Analysis framework and aspects of how attributes and consequences can impact the 'with woman' concept as identified within the studies (Table 10.1).

Table 10.1 Concept analysis of midwives 'with the older woman'.

'With the older woman' antecedents	Evidence	Attributes (A) and Consequences (C)
Reasons for advanced maternal age (AMA)	Schytt et al. (2014) over estimation of fecundity Waldenstrom (2016) exploring several aspects for delayed parenthood Nilsen et al. (2015) postponement of parenthood Aasheim et al. (2014) satisfaction with life in childbearing at an advanced age	Lack of partner and fertility problems (A) Childless (C) Lifestyle or socioeconomic factors (A) Anxiety (A) Satisfaction with life decreases with age (A) Childbirth experience more difficult (C) Increased risk of adverse pregnancy outcomes such as preterm birth or stillbirth (C) Negative overall birth experience (C)
Women's risk perception of being older	Bayrampour et al. (2012) women's knowledge of risk perception	Seen as low risk pregnancy by women (A) Limited physical activity (A) Anxiety (A) Unfavourable screening tests (A) Poor reproductive history (A) Improve the effectiveness of risk communication (C)
Outcomes for advanced maternal age	Kenny et al. (2013) adverse pregnancy outcomes Rydahl et al. (2019) CS increases for nulliparous more than multiparous women Kahveci et al. (2018) perinatal outcomes	Risks independent of parity and socio economic status (A) Increased SB, preterm births, macrosomia and CS births (C) GDM, Gestational hypertension, pre-eclampsia (A) Preterm births and CS significant adverse perinatal outcomes (C)
Women's views	Cooke et al. (2012) women's views of delayed childbearing	Stable relationship (A) Financial stability (A) Health and fertility (A) Risk status (A) No control over timing of childbearing (C) Pre-conceptual education (C) Sensitive information and support (C)

(*Continued*)

Table 10.1 (Continued)

'With the older woman' antecedents	Evidence	Attributes (A) and Consequences (C)
Women's experiences	Southby et al. (2019) women's experiences of pregnancy at advanced age	Worry throughout pregnancy (A) Better support for women in early pregnancy (C)
	Aasheim et al. (2013) marginally effects experience of childbirth	Manage better (A) With operative delivery (C)
	Mandel (2010) explores the lived experience of single older women	Importance of support (A) Stigma and changing priorities (A) Long-term concerns (A) Increased pregnancy risks (C) Physical and psychosocial support (C) Sense of control for women (C)
	Garcia-Blanco et al. (2017) impact of delayed parenthood	Depressive symptoms and increased stress (A) Maternal attitude and social support improved (C)
Midwifery care of the older mother	O'Connor et al. (2014) care provided by midwives for the older woman	Older women's midwifery needs not met (A) CPE and professional leadership required to develop skills (C)

Conclusion

On examining the studies relating to the childbearing older woman, evidence suggests that antecedents to the 'with the older woman' focus on reasons for AMA, women's perception of risk, birth outcomes for these women and their infants, their views and experiences and midwifery services for the older woman.

The attributes that relate to the childbearing older woman result from life-style and socio-economic factors such as fertility problems, lack of partner and focus on careers which consequently may result in increased anxiety and more difficult childbearing experiences resulting in increased risk of adverse pregnancy and birth outcomes. However, women perceived their pregnancies to be low risk and consequently it has been suggested that improving the effectiveness of risk communication by midwives and healthcare profession-als is required to support and educate the pregnant older woman. Studies on birth outcomes indicate that independent of parity and socio-economic status, there is an increase in stillbirths, preterm and macrosomic babies and births by caesarean section.

Generally, older pregnant women were found to be more anxious and worried throughout pregnancy. They highlighted the importance of eradicating stigmatisation of the older woman and changing care priorities by healthcare professionals. As a result, midwives suggest that the healthcare needs of these women, who require improved physical and psychological support, are not always fully met. The older childbearing woman is more likely to experience depressive symptoms and increased stress and therefore requires midwives to recognise these needs and manage care more effectively whilst providing women with a sense of control to fulfil the 'with woman' concept.

Midwife's Story

Clare's Story

I first met Kate* when she was 48 years of age and pregnant with her first baby, Adam. I was her community midwife and shared her care with an obstetric consultant. Kate's pregnancy was much wanted, but delayed, as she had not met the right partner until later in life. Having established that she was unlikely to achieve a viable pregnancy with her own eggs, she had been obliged to seek fertility treatment in Europe due to more stringent UK guidelines on maternal age. Kate looked fantastic throughout her pregnancy with no sign of pre-eclampsia, but scans showed poor placental perfusion and growth restriction from 24 weeks. Tragically, Adam was stillborn at 27 weeks and Kate gave birth to him vaginally following IOL. Visiting the couple at home after the birth, I was aware of such difficult and conflicting emotions: they were grieving for their little boy but acknowledging that they still wanted to try for another baby. In the background was the stressful tick of time plus worry about logistics and finances.

Kate is a strong and determined woman and within a year we met again for a booking appointment. In the intervening period, she had been diagnosed with antiphospholipid syndrome and advised to inject blood thinners and take aspirin. She had also been to hell and back but was always polite and positive. I was awed by her – and scared for her. Care was truly shared in this case: regular scans and obstetric reviews at the hospital were interspersed with as many antenatal reassurance examinations as Kate wished. The baby was growing normally. As a diagnosis of thrombocytopaenia was thrown into the mix at 37 weeks, Kate's consultant called time and recommended IOL. We didn't have a case loading team at that time (other than for home births) but I knew that true continuity would help in so

(Continued)

many ways – no explaining about her obstetric history to all and sundry and a friendly face in the environment where they had said goodbye to their son. I arranged to work on delivery suite for Kate's induction. An epidural was not an option given her low platelets, but Kate never needed one. She had some pethidine and some hours later pushed Oliver into the world at 37+5weeks weighing just over 3kg. I have never been so relieved to see a baby born. Some people are worth going that extra mile for and I will remember that day clearly forever.

Kate's story didn't end there: She describes below the emotional and physical journey she continued to have a sibling for Oliver. After a total of 18 implanted embryos and 6 vaginal deliveries, he now has a beautiful baby brother, and four lost, but never-forgotten, brothers and sister. Kate's pregnancies after Oliver were almost exclusively managed obstetrically, but being able to finally visit the family at home was magic.

Caring for older women is multi-dimensional. By their age alone, they are 'high risk' but don't necessarily feel it. Some have had fertility treatment; many have multiple pregnancies. Some do not want to see a consultant or have extra scans. Others compare notes and realise that their care pathways differ just because they have different consultants. Many will opt for elective caesarean; some will plan a candlelit water birth, only to abandon it at 40weeks when an induction is booked 'in case their placenta fails'. Continuity of care and carer is important for everyone, but none more so than for this fragmented group. I'm always struck by the number of women who anxiously ask to see me in addition to their consultant, because they need extra reassurance, or simply because it makes them 'feel more normal'.

Women's Stories

Kate*'s Story

My partner and I had always wanted children. We met relatively late by normal circumstance both into our 40s but neither of us had had children at this point. Almost from the start of our relationship our focus was on how we were going to achieve this. Might it by some miracle be natural, or would we need help? I was 45 when we embarked on our journey and my partner 42 and while I was fortunate to have everything gynaecological in good working order, we did in fact need a bit of medical help. Then ensued our long IVF journey to complete our family.

After several consultations and in particular the realisation that the only way to realistically achieve a successful pregnancy was for me to have a donor egg (fortunately we could use my partner's sperm), I became pregnant in 2014 with my first child, a little boy. We took a leap of faith and embarked on several trips to a clinic in Spain to achieve this. We were successful after the 4th transfer. During my pregnancy, which by all accounts was very positive and healthy, I regularly had appointments with my midwife which was helpful and reassuring especially as we were able to build a really positive rapport.

However, having achieved this longed for pregnancy, tragically we lost our son at 27weeks gestation due to a hitherto unknown blood condition which meant I should have been on anticoagulant for the duration of the pregnancy. I was told to stop taking this medication at 12weeks and without it the baby was starved of the necessary nutrients from the placenta and was very small. I found out there was no heartbeat at a routine check with the midwife who sent me straight to hospital where it was confirmed the baby had died. This was first thing on Wednesday morning. I finally delivered him on Saturday morning. The intervening three days were utterly devastating knowing then that at the end of my labour there was only going to be sadness then a long road to emotional recovery. Fortunately, the hospital offered a bereavement service which my partner and I took up to try and navigate the rawness of the loss. This did help us gradually come to terms with the tragedy.

When I gave birth in February 2015 I was 48. Despite the trauma of our loss, we did not wish to give up and this decision was fortified by our wonderful consultant who believed that I was physically capable, and we could achieve a successful birth if we wanted to try again.

In January 2016 I fell pregnant with my now 3 year-old. It was a wonderful pregnancy and the blood condition successfully managed. I was supported superbly by the same midwife with very regular checks and also regular scans at the hospital to make sure the growth in particular was fine and no other issues developed. Our second son arrived in September 2016 at just over 37weeks, completely healthy. Whilst you can never fully get over a stillbirth it made the loss easier to bear as we finally had a beautiful baby boy. I had just turned 50 when he arrived. My physical recovery was good and I returned to exercise after about three months.

We had always hoped for two children and on further consultation we continued to be supported by our consultant who believed it possible for me to have a further successful pregnancy should we wish. By now, because of my age, we had to switch clinics to one that would be legally able to do an embryo transfer because I was over 50. We took a further leap of faith using a fabulous European clinic which carried out the embryo transfers outside the European Union and was therefore not bound by the age restrictions. We just wanted to achieve one sibling for our son, knowing we are older parents. To our complete shock in April 2018 I fell pregnant

(Continued)

with triplets. A one in a million chance apparently. From the moment this happened we were faced with impossible challenges. Initially I had a major bleed at week five, just after I found out I was pregnant, so was simply hoping that my viability scan wouldn't reveal the pregnancy had failed. This added to the shock when all three embryos had survived. But then came the very tough decision as to whether to have a reduction, which has significant risks, or maintain the pregnancy, which also had major risks. After much deliberation we decided to let nature take its course. Having already suffered a traumatic stillbirth the thought of terminating one or more healthy embryos was a step too far even given very careful consideration of the potential challenges ahead.

This pregnancy, just as with my first and second, ran very smoothly (until we lost our first of course) and I was amazed at how similar the pregnancy symptoms were to my earlier two. I could not identify any particular worse symptoms due to the multiple status. I was again very supported by the same midwife who had looked after me during my two earlier pregnancies, so we were both very conscious of keeping note of anything untoward. However, it was not meant to be, as at just shy of 20 weeks my waters spontaneously broke around our little girl (the other two embryos were boys) and then ensued a significant run in hospital where for a good week we hoped the babies would be able to hold on. During this time, I remained as calm and positive as possible, but in the end it became apparent that all was going to be lost. I had developed sepsis and it was either the babies or me. Tragically I had to give birth to three beautiful tiny babies all of whom were alive (the two boys particularly thriving) just before their births. Nothing can prepare you for this kind of devastating loss.

After the birth, the placenta would not release, so I needed a general anaesthetic to complete the birth. This resulted in a large loss of blood and I became severely anaemic. I just managed to avoid a blood transfusion, opting for an iron transfusion instead. It took several weeks to recover from this scenario physically and even more to deal with the rawness of the emotions involved.

Despite the horrible trauma of losing four precious babies, after a few months we discussed trying one final time for our longed-for sibling for our son. As we still had support from the medical profession we made our decision to try after weighing up all the facts, risk factors, potential for success based on our second son and using gut instinct about whether we felt we could be successful. In April 2019, after this last attempt, and having just reached a point where I felt anywhere near capable of emotionally trying again, I became pregnant by the 18th embryo transferred. I was regularly monitored by the same midwife again. I had a precautionary stitch put in as with the triplets as my cervix was borderline too short. I then went on to have a good pregnancy without any major issues. The hardest part this time was that the stitch was rather bothersome and towards the end the bearing down pressure became very uncomfortable. None of the other potential risk factors for someone of my age – pre-eclampsia, gestational diabetes, anaemia, hyperemesis – affected me, thankfully, and we gradually edged towards full term always focusing on the likely success rather than possible further loss.

Towards the end of this pregnancy I started to have some bleeding episodes at week 32, which became increasingly significant over the next two-and-a-half-week period. I started contracting on the Friday before the birth on the following Wednesday, but on this first occasion I was stabilised. In the end our beautiful little boy decided it was time to make an appearance and he arrived at 34 + 3 weeks in November 2019, well and healthy – if a little small. Three weeks in special care baby unit (SCBU) gave him the growing time and we haven't looked back since. As I write he is now nearly 10 weeks old and doing extremely well. We are utterly relieved and grateful that he arrived safely and can now be our longed-for companion for his elder brother.

We are extremely grateful to those in the medical profession who supported us and believed that we could achieve both pregnancies on what was borrowed time. Whilst I know there have been women older than me having children, to be nearly 50 when you start the journey to have four pregnancies in quick succession is most likely still unusual and somewhat pioneering. That said, I envisage it will only become more common for women in their 50s to have children as medical advances make it easier and indeed societal attitudes consider it more 'normal'. Our journey to achieving our family was an extremely challenging one as no parent should have to bury one child, let alone four, but fortunately not without the delights of achieving our two beautiful boys. We simply believed it was possible to realise our dreams and so drew on every ounce of our resilience and determination to keep trying until we were told we had to stop.

Throughout this process it was vital for the medical profession to be supportive and non-judgemental and we were fortunate to experience this. Understanding that for some people the stars don't align to societal norms is critical for any professional coming across someone like me who fully understands the risks involved, has been thoughtful about the approach to be taken and believes success is possible based on clear medical guidance married with a strong gut feeling. A supportive, positive and thoughtful attitude from my midwife made all the difference on my journey – as did it with my consultants – to whom we will be eternally grateful for helping us achieve our dreams.

(Continued)

Lucy*'s Story

I was 43 when I became pregnant with our IVF baby. We had had a miscarriage prior to this pregnancy, which was discovered at a nine-week scan. Understandably we were both a bit jittery when it came to future scans with this pregnancy. One of the advantages of being an older mother is that you get monitored more frequently which, given our history, was great for peace of mind (I was so anxious each time we had a scan). It worked out that we were having a scan and follow up meeting with the doctor every 6 weeks or so after 12 weeks.

I was called a 'geriatric mother' the first time I walked into the NHS hospital for my 12 week scan; it was slightly shocking at first, and I never got over my dislike of the term, but at least I knew to expect it.

As the pregnancy progressed, I had the usual appointments with the community midwife, she told us what courses and workshops were available for us to attend (breastfeeding, hypnobirthing, active birthing workshop) and probably many more.

My birth plan stated that I wanted a natural birth, in the midwifery-led unit with very limited interference. At two separate post-scan meetings with the doctor and then later with the consultant I was strongly advised to have an induction. My age was brought up each time as one of the reasons for this recommendation. I was strongly against having an induction, as we had already been through IVF I wanted just one thing to happen naturally.

Our baby was due in October, in September I started to develop a very itchy rash on already swollen feet and ankles; as the month progressed, the rash did too. In October it was all up my legs and on my hands and wrists. At the end of October, I called the Maternity Helpline as I had a concern about reduced movement, we went into the hospital and a doctor recommended that I be induced that same day. That evening I went into labour and was transferred to the labour ward the following morning.

I was on gas and air for this bit so my partner has filled in some of the blanks for me. Unfortunately, despite drinking what felt like my own body weight in water I couldn't wee, so I had to be catheterised. I really liked my first midwife; she was friendly and down to earth and so easy to build a rapport with. This was a marked contrast to the second midwife we had when the shifts changed; whilst I have no doubt that she was competent at her job, I felt that she lacked empathy possibly due to the fact that it was an overnight shift. I didn't connect with her on any level and I feel that she made no attempt to connect with me. This lack of rapport is one of the overriding memories I have of that day.

I was in labour for a long time (approx. 36 hours) – stuck for eight hours at 8 cm dilation. At some point in this time I decided that enough was enough and that I would have an epidural. I remember being terrified of moving despite having contractions and it took a couple of attempts for the anaesthetist to find the right spot. Throughout this time my partner and I were continuously kept updated and he remembers more of what was said than I do.

Because the labour wasn't progressing it was decided that we would have to go to theatre for an assisted delivery (forceps). There were so many people around and I remember that I couldn't see my partner, after the low lights of the labour ward this was flood lit and packed and I hated every minute of it.

Everyone we spoke to at the hospital promoted the skin on skin post birth policy. I don't know why, but I didn't get to hold my baby skin on skin until I was in recovery and even then, I had to ask. I remember that he was given some formula as he was crying and wouldn't settle. I would have appreciated more time and assistance with breastfeeding, but again there were possibly reasons for this that I wasn't aware of at the time.

Post birth, I spent the next five days in hospital; the skin irritation got worse and spread to my stomach. We saw a dermatologist on day three, when the blisters had spread to the soles of my feet. I was fortunate to see her and am grateful that she took the trouble to see me. I also had issues with breastfeeding; everyone I spoke with had a different technique, so it was hard to work out what I was doing wrong. We later found out that our son was tongue tied which caused some of the issues – he had two operations to resolve this when he was just under a month old.

Our hypnobirthing leader (who also happened to be our NCT teacher) said one thing to us: 'keep your eye on the prize'. Whilst my birth plan turned out to be a work of fiction, at the end of the day we were blessed with a healthy baby boy and I am truly grateful to the entire team at hospital for looking after us.

Lessons Learnt

The needs of the older childbearing woman require some enhanced skills by healthcare professionals to enable the 'with woman' concept to be effectively achieved. Kate*'s birth account illustrates how these needs can be extremely complex and require compassionate and intuitive care by midwives to ensure that she achieved a safe and positive birth experience. Kate highlights how supportive and non-judgemental care was key through a positive and thoughtful attitude that made a difference to her birth outcomes.

Lucy*'s story is a little more complex and she did not experience the birth she anticipated due to additional complications. However, although she felt grateful for the care provided by hospital staff, she did remember the events and people who in some instances did not provide the support and reassurance that she needed. Whilst her physical needs during the pregnancy, birth and the postnatal period were fulfilled, her psychological needs of respect and empathy were overlooked.

References

Aasheim, V., Walderstrom, U., Rasmussen, S. et al. (2013). Experience of childbirth in first-time mothers of advanced age- a Norwegian population-based study. *BMC Pregnancy and Childbirth* 13: 53. http://www.biomedcentral.com/1471-2393/13/53.

Aasheim, V., Walderstrom, U., Rasmussen, S. et al. (2014). Satisfaction with life during pregnancy and early motherhood in the first-time mothers of advanced age: a population-based longitudinal study. *BMC Pregnancy and Childbirth* 14: 86. http://www.biomedcentral.com/1471-2393/14/86.

Bayrampour, H. and Heaman, M. (2010). Advanced maternal age and the risk of caesarean birth. *A Systematic Review Birth* 37 (3): 219–226.

Bayrampour, H., Heaman, M., Duncan, K.A., and Tough, S. (2012). Advanced maternal age and risk perception: a qualitative study. *BMC Pregnancy and Childbirth* 12: 100–113.

Campbell, P. (2011). Boundaries and risk: media framing of assisted reproductive technologies and older mothers. *Social Science & Medicine* 72 (2): 265–272.

Cooke, A., Mills, T.A., and Lavender, T. (2012). Advanced maternal age: delayed childbearing is rarely a conscious choice. A qualitative study of women's views and experiences. *International Journal of Nursing Studies* 49 (1): 30–39.

Decker, M. (2019). 30 celebrity moms who had kids after 40. https://harpersbazaar.com/celebrity/latest/g18196402/celebrities-children-after-40-infertility (accessed 6 May 2019).

Dietl, A., Cupisti, S., Backmann, M.W. et al. (2015). Pregnancy and obstetrical outcomes in women over 40 years of age. *Geburtshilfe und Frauenheilkunde* 75 (8): 827–832.

Fitzpatrick, K.E., Tuffnell, D., Kurinczuk, J.J., and Knight, M. (2016). Pregnancy at very advanced maternal age: a UK population-based cohort study. *BJOG : An International Journal of Obstetrics and Gynaecology* 123 (1): 100–109.

Fuchs, F., Monet, B., Ducruet, T. et al. (2018). Effect of maternal age on the risk of preterm birth: a large cohort study. *PLoS One* 13 (1): E0191002.

Garcia-Blanco, A., Monferrer, A., Grimaldos, J. et al. (2017). A preliminary study to assess the impact of maternal age on stress-related variables in healthy nulliparous women. *Psychoneuroendocrinology* 78: 97–104.

Guedes, M. and Canavarro, C.M. (2014). Psychosocial adjustment of couples to first-time parenthood at advanced maternal age: an exploratory longitudinal study. *Journal of Reproductive and Infant Psychology* 32 (5): 425–440.

Human Fertilisation and Embryology Authority (HFEA) (2018). *Fertility Treatment 2014-16: Trends and Figures*. London: HFEA.

Kahveci, B., Melekoglu, R., Evruke, I.C., and Cetin, C. (2018). The effect of advanced maternal age on perinatal outcomes in nulliparous singleton pregnancies. *BMC Pregnancy and Childbirth* [Online] Available at: https://doi.org/10.1186/s12884-018-1984-x (Accessed 19Sept 2019).

Kenny, L., Lavender, T., McNamee, R. et al. (2013). Advanced maternal age and adverse pregnancy outcome: evidence from a large contemporary cohort. *PLoS One* 8 (2): 1–9.

Laopaiboon, M., Lumbiganon, P., Intarut, N. et al. (2014). WHO multicountry survey on maternal newborn healthresearch network: advanced maternal age and pregnancy outcomes: a multicountry assessment. *BJOG* 121: 49–56.

Lavender, T., Logan, J., Cooke, A. et al. (2015). "Nature makes you blind to the risks". An exploration of womens' views surrounding decisions on the timing of childbearing in contemporary society. *Sexual & Reproductive Healthcare* 6: 157–163.

Lean, S.C., Derricott, H., Jones, R., and Heazell, A. (2017). Advanced maternal age and adverse pregnancy outcomes: a systematic review and meta-analysis. *PLoS One* 12 (10).

Loane, M., Morris, J.K., Addor, M.C. et al. (2013). Twenty-year trends in the prevalence of down syndrome and other trisomies in Europe: impact of maternal age and prenatal screening. *European Journal of Human Genetics* 21 (1): 27–33.

Mandel, D. (2010). The lived experience of pregnancy complications in single older women. *MCN: American Journal of Maternal Child Nursing* 35 (6): 336–340.

Marufu, T.C., Ahankri, A., Coleman, C. et al. (2015). Maternal smoking and the risk of stillbirth: a systematic review and mate-analysis. *BMC Public Health* 15: 293. https://doi.org/10.1186/s12889-015-1552-5.

Mills, T., Lavender, R., and Lavender, T. (2015). "Forty is the new twenty": an analysis of British media portrayals of older mothers. *Sexual & Reproductive Healthcare* 6 (2): 88–96.

National Health Service (NHS) (2019). *The NHS Long Term Plan*. London: NHS.

National Institute for Health and Care Excellence (NICE) (2008). *Antenatal Care for Uncomplicated Pregnancies*. London: NICE.

National Maternity Review (2016). Better Births: Improving outcomes of maternity services in England. [Online] https://england.nhs.uk/wp-content/uploads/2016/02/national-maternity-review-report.pdf (accessed 2 April 2019).

NHS Digital (2018). NHS Maternity Statistics, England 2017–18. https://digital.nhs.uk/data-and-information/publications/statistical/nhs-maternity-statistics/2017-18*key-facts (accessed 16 April 2019).

NHS England (2017). Implementing Better Births: Continuity of carer. https://www.england.nhs.uk/publication/implementing-better-births-continuity-of-carer (accessed 16 May 2019).

Nilsen, A.B.V., Waldenstrom, U., Espehaug, B., and Schytt, E. (2015). Still childless at the age of 32: an investigation of predictors in 22-year-old women and men. *Scandinavian Journal of Public Health* 43: 481–489.

O'Connor, A., Doris, F., and Skirton, H. (2014). Midwifery care in the UK for older mothers. *British Journal of Midwifery* 22 (8): 568–577.

Office for National Statistics (ONS) (2019). Births in England and Wales: 2017. www.ons.gov.uk and via NOMIS data generation on this site (accessed 16 April 2019).

Organisation for Economic Co-operation and Development (OECD) (2018). Age of mothers at childbirth and age-specific fertility. *OECD Family Database*. [Online] Available at: https://www.oecd.org/els/family/database.htm. (Accessed 5th May 2019).

O'Sullivan, J.F. (1960). The elderly Primigravida. *BJOG*. [Online] Available at: https://doi.org/10.1111/j.1471-0528.1960.tb06989.x (Accessed 27 May 2019).

Rahmanou, P., Caudwell-Hall, J., Atan, I., and Dietz, H. (2016). The association between maternal age and first delivery risk of obstetric trauma. *Australian Journal of Obstetrics and Gynecology (AJOG)* 215: 1–7.

Rydahl, E., Declercq, E., Juhl, M., and Maimburg, R.D. (2019). Cesarean section on a rise – does advanced maternal age explain the increase? A population register-based study. *PLoS One* 14 (1): e0210655. [Online] Available at: https://doi.org/10.1371/journal.pone.0210655.

Schytt, E., Nilsen, A.B., and Bernhardt, E. (2014). Still childless at the age of 28 to 40 years: a cross-sectional study of Swedish women's and men's reproductive intentions. *Sexual & Reproductive Healthcare* 5: 23–29.

Southby, C., Mills, T.A., and Lavender, T. (2019). "It's now or never" – nulliparous women's experiences of pregnancy at advanced maternal age: a grounded theory study. *Midwifery* 68: 1–8.

Sutcliffe, A.G., Barnes, J., Belsky, J. et al. (2012). The health and development of children born to older mothers in the United Kingdom: observational study using longitudinal cohort. *British Medical Journal* 345: e5116. https://doi.org/10.1136/bmj.e5116.

Waldenstrom, U. (2016). Postponing parenthood to advanced age. *Upsala Journal of Medical Sciences* 121 (4): 1–24.

Wood, M. (2008). Celebrity older mothers: does the media give women a false impression. *British Journal of Midwifery* 16 (5): 326.

11

'With the Bereaved Woman'

Anna M. Brown, Zara Chamberlain (Specialist Midwife);
Jennie (Student Midwife); and Kitty* (woman)

Introduction

A mother gives birth to her baby after many months of pregnancy, but her baby is dead. Few words are needed to convey the tragedy of stillbirth (Froon et al. 2011, p. 1353).

There is disparity in defining what constitutes a stillbirth. The World Health Organisation defines a stillbirth as the birth of a baby weighing 500 g or more, 22 or more completed weeks of gestation, or a body length of 25 cm or more, who died before or during labour and birth. In the UK this definition changes to a fetus who has died before or during labour and birth and is born at 24 or more completed weeks of gestation (WHO 2016).

The latest statistics from the Office of National Statistic (2019) state that in total there were 657 076 babies born in the UK in 2018. Of these, 4.0 per 1000 births were stillborn babies. This implies that one in nine babies were stillborn every day. However, the UK had the lowest rate of stillbirths, decreasing by a fifth, during this year as a result of new national guidelines on preventing stillbirth known as the Saving Babies' Lives Care Bundle (O'Connor 2016; Widdows et al. 2018). Educating pregnant women to practise mindfetalness, immediately reporting reduced fetal movement, which is perceived to indicate lack of oxygen to the fetus, could be preventative in reducing stillbirths (Radestad 2017). Conversely, according to a number of studies, about 60% of stillbirths are unexplained but underlying causes indicate an increased risk due to ascending infection, placental factors such as placental abruption and pre-eclampsia, congenital abnormalities and fetal growth restrictions. Other causes could be smoking during pregnancy, increased body mass index (BMI) of over 26 during pregnancy, gestational diabetes and advanced maternal age

Better Births: The Midwife 'with Woman', First Edition. Edited by Anna M. Brown.
© 2021 John Wiley & Sons Ltd. Published 2021 by John Wiley & Sons Ltd.

(Marufu et al. 2015; Ovesen et al. 2015; Schummers et al. 2015). In addition, women who are from a low socio-economic status are twice as at risk of having a stillborn child when compared to women from more advantaged backgrounds (Froon et al. 2011). Ultimately, it is the priority of health professionals to improve knowledge of possible causes and identify solutions for the prevention of stillbirths, as substandard care contributes to 20–30% of all stillbirths (Flenady et al. 2016).

The Consequences of a Stillbirth

Stillbirth impacts thousands of families' lives each year and the consequences of such a heartbreaking event remains with some women throughout the rest of their lives. Many women are twice as likely to suffer from increased anxiety and depression and are diagnosed with post-traumatic stress disorder (PTSD) after a stillbirth or neonatal death. In one study, women were found to have increasing anxiety up to 10 years after the death of their baby, severely affecting their mental health (Kokou-Kpolou et al. 2018). Women can begin to process the death of their baby if their loss is recognised and their baby is counted and acknowledged as equally important had it been born alive (Froon et al. 2011). In addition, the impact to the parents' psychosocial wellbeing, the parent's relationship (Avekin et al. 2013) and long-term consequences to future pregnancies (Hunter et al. 2017) and existing siblings have to be considered (Burden et al. 2016; Murphy and Cacciatore 2017).

In maternity units across the UK, psychological support is available although the evidence suggests that one in five women who has had a stillbirth will suffer from long-term depression, anxiety and PTSD (Pattinson et al. 2011). In general, healthcare providers support and respect women when a stillbirth has occurred, and many therapeutic services are available to ensure that the woman's emotional and psychological grief and pain is acknowledged, and she is not made to feel marginalised by the event. Essential empathetic encounters between the bereaved parents and caregivers will help to minimise the emotional and psychological effects of the death (Heazell et al. 2016). However, such support is not always available in other countries across the world and women's rights to register and acknowledge their stillborn baby are devalued and the baby not recognised as a unique and individual family member due to cultural and economic reasons. Many women remain disenfranchised, stigmatised and marginalised as they are seen by the communities to have failed at motherhood and in their role to produce children. Lovell (1983, p. 756) describes this as an *'unravelling of a woman's lived experience and rapid deconstruction of her motherhood'*. Men, on the other hand, as suggested by some studies, tend to hide their grief when they suffer a pregnancy loss or stillbirth. They perceive their role primarily as supporters of the woman and family before acknowledging their own loss, although they too feel overlooked and marginalised as a result of their less visible grief (Due et al. 2017).

Implications for Healthcare Providers

Overall, the impact of quality care provision may not always prevent a stillbirth. However, midwives can demonstrate the 'with woman' concept through respectful physical and emotional support for the parents in their time of grief and pain. Enabling the woman's rights and both parents' needs to make informed decisions about the final rituals for their child occurs through timely interventions based on education, evidence and training. In addition, quality bereavement care through trained professionals delivered sensitively through Birth Reflections services, may help to minimise the negative impact of a stillborn baby and offer a space in which parents can process their grief, share their story and set up supportive systems to cope with the long-term effects.

The impact of providing empathetic care and support for bereaved parents after a stillbirth needs to be considered. Emotional and professional involvement places a burden on midwives and other healthcare providers to the detriment of their mental wellbeing and has consequences for their personal and professional life. The psychological effect and impact on care providers, in the event of a stillbirth, is particularly prevalent when midwives and other carers seek to avoid emotional engagement with the experience through a sense of guilt, failure and powerlessness (Stadtlander 2012; Cacciatore 2013). Such negative effects can be ameliorated through education and training in dealing with death and bereavement and support, both formal and informal, from colleagues, managers and counselling/listening services can minimise this impact (Heazell et al. 2016).

One study which explored impact on carers after fetal loss found that healthcare providers may be at risk of compassion fatigue. The authors suggest that there is a need to identify interventions to help professionals to continue in their supportive role without detriment to their physical and mental health and wellbeing (Hutti et al. 2016). Mindfulness is one such recent intervention that is helpful for both maternity care providers and the grieving parents. There is a growing body of literature which explores the efficacy of mindfulness as an intervention in treating anxiety, depression and other mental health issues as well as to improve women's satisfaction with the psychosocial care provided. Mindfulness can be defined as a moment-to-moment awareness of one's thoughts, experiences and emotions without judgement and can be carried out through medication or exercise such as yoga (Huberty et al. 2018).

Cacciatore (2013) explored one such intervention model called ATTEND (attunement, trust, therapeutic tough, egalitarianism, nuance and death education) as a means to improve bereavement support through compassionate care afforded by this model. The model emphasises a move towards personalised care through which midwives are deeply self-aware of their physical and emotional presence, being attuned to the woman and her family. This is demonstrated through a willingness to witness the parents' grief whilst maintaining their own protective feelings towards the death of a baby. This enables parents to be empowered in having a greater sense of control over their grief, expressing their feelings and views in a mutually shared and honest relationship with the caregiver. More recent studies by Huberty et al. (2018) suggest that mindfulness practices through online streamed yoga may help to ameliorate the symptoms of PTSD after stillbirth for women and improve sleep quality, resilience and self-esteem. More research is needed in this area to understand how mindfulness application could improve wellbeing for these grieving women.

Parents' Perspective

The outcomes of a pregnancy, labour and childbirth are not only impacted by the physical, psychological and socio-economic situation of the parents expecting a baby but most crucially by the care that is provided throughout the childbearing continuum. The majority of literature from the UK and most other socio-economically stable countries indicates that quality of care for the prevention of stillbirths is progressively improving. One recent study suggests that women who receive antenatal care are more aware of the need to monitor fetal movements and the risk of stillbirth, although the information they received was inconsistent (Pollock et al. 2019). However, some literature suggests that women's views and perceptions of the care and support that is provided after the death of a neonate or that of a stillborn baby can be substandard (Cacciatore 2010). Women view suboptimum interpersonal care as crucial to the impact the death of their baby may have on their future wellbeing (Heazell et al. 2016). Parents judged that aspects of their care in the antenatal period with caregivers not spending enough time with parents to deliver care or provide information as pertinent to the outcome of their pregnancy. Some parents believed that they were not listened to and their concerns not taken seriously (Einaudi et al. 2010; Renfrew et al. 2014).

This appears to be a clear indication of when midwives and other healthcare professional were not 'with woman' in this life-changing event. In a study by Ellis et al. (2016) after the stillbirth, parents perceived that information and decision-making involvement was lacking as compared to their care before this tragic event. The behaviour and actions of staff had a memorable impact of long-lasting distress on the parents, who perceived staff to be taking avoidance strategies where midwives focused on physical tasks and distanced themselves emotionally as a coping strategy. Parents suggested that the way in which the diagnosis of a stillbirth was conveyed to them and not being given adequate time to come to terms with their loss – to make decisions about the birth options and dealing with a dead baby – had a negative impact on them. This was largely influenced by how sensitively they were treated by the staff, enabling parents to cope with the events. The authors conclude that supportive systems and structures need to be in place through improved training and clear care pathways to include continuity of care by the midwives and being emotionally and physically engaged with the unfolding events. Other studies concur with these findings and highlight the long-term importance grieving parents placed on their interaction with caregivers during this difficult time (O'Connell et al. 2016). Parents remember and value empathy and kindness, language that acknowledges the birth of their baby and staff who listen and keep them informed above all else (Henley and Schott 2008), evidence that is still relevant today.

Murphy and Cacciatore (2017) suggest that the decision by parent to see and hold their dead baby was associated with lower risks of depression and anxiety long term, although these feelings are temporarily reversed in subsequent pregnancies. However, Radestad et al. in an earlier study in 2009 found that the beneficial effects of holding and dressing their stillborn were only relevant to those babies born after 37 weeks gestation and that length of time spent with the baby could also impact on increasing depressive symptoms if the mother perceived this time period to be curtailed. However, overall a systematic review by Kingdon et al. (2015) reports that the role of the midwife and other carers was key in enabling the parents to see and hold their baby (Schott and Henley 2009; Erlandsson et al. 2013; Coffey 2016) and creating memories resulting in long-term positive outcomes.

Bereavement Care Services

Caring for families experiencing stillbirth can be physically and emotional challenging for staff, as previously identified. However, the actions and attitudes of staff, from conveying the diagnosis of a stillbirth to the parents, through to the management of labour and delivery of the baby and after care, can be critical to outcomes and coping needs of the family involved (Peters et al. 2015; Ellis et al. 2016). Awaiting the birth of a diagnosed stillborn is highly distressing and often painful. The systematic review by Peters et al. (2015) on caring for such families suggests that grieving parents want midwives and other caregivers to provide them with timely and ongoing information, support and guidance regarding culturally appropriate decisions concerning their baby, whilst validating their emotions and demonstrating respect, sensitivity and empathy. These findings have implications in setting care pathways that guide maternity care providers in their behaviour, actions and communication skills and are supported by more recent studies.

Shorey et al. (2017) suggest that perinatal death has a profound impact on healthcare professionals in terms of their psychological and physical wellbeing and perceive that their unmet needs need to be addressed through institutional support to acknowledge their stress after these events. Other studies reiterate these findings in terms of psychosocial factors that impact on midwives' confidence in providing bereavement support due to lack of knowledge and skills (Awgu Kalu et al. 2018). In addition, studies from a global perspective suggest that there is a continued need to improve standards and consistency of bereavement care and including bereavement education in pre-registration curricula for midwives and nurses may be the way forward (Steen 2015; Hollins Martin et al. 2016; Rivaldi et al. 2018).

The above literature was examined through Rodger's Concept Analysis framework to identify antecedents, attributes and consequences of the 'with woman' concept and the results are demonstrated in Table 11.1.

Table 11.1 Concept analysis of 'with the bereaved woman'.

Antecedents	Evidence	Attributes (A) and Consequences (C)
Psychosocial health	Burden et al. (2016) parents' psychosocial wellbeing after stillbirth Murphy and Cacciatore (2017) consequences to parental relation, siblings and future pregnancies after stillbirth	Acknowledging existence of birth event and baby improves outcomes (A) Reduces risk of marginalisation, depression, anxiety and PTSD (C)
Psychological health	Froon et al. (2011) long-term mental health issues after stillbirth Cacciatore (2013) engagement with bereaved parents after stillbirth Einaudi et al. (2010) parental experiences after stillbirth Renfrew et al. (2014) substandard care for bereaved women	Acknowledging stillbirth by professionals (A) Intervention models e.g. ATTEND (A) Midwives attuned to women's needs (A) Enabling women's rights to make decisions about the stillbirth (A) Women sharing their stories (A) Being listened to (C) Women begin the process of grieving the death of their baby (C) Decreases anxiety (C) Decreases risk of PTSD/depression (C)
Emotional wellbeing	Huberty et al. (2018) mindfulness and exercise for women grieving after stillbirth	Self-awareness (A) Mindfulness (A) Reduces symptoms of PTSD (C) Resilience (C) Improved self-esteem (C)

Table 11.1 (Continued)

Antecedents	Evidence	Attributes (A) and Consequences (C)
Knowledge	Cacciatore (2013) the psychological effect and impact on care providers in the event of a stillbirth due to lack of knowledge and training support	Avoid emotional engagement (A)
		Sense of guilt and failure (A)
		Education and training in dealing with death and bereavement (C)
		Avoidance strategy as coping mechanism by staff (A)
	Ellis et al. (2016) information giving and decision making after stillbirth	Memorable impact of long-lasting distress on parents (A)
		Training, care pathways, continuity of care resulting in sensitive treatment and enables coping (C)
	O'Connell et al. (2016) impact of care given	Formal and informal support from colleagues etc. (A)
	Heazell et al. (2016) impact on staff after stillbirth	Lack of knowledge and skills (A)
	Agwu Kalu et al. (2018) impact on midwives' confidence to provide bereavement support after perinatal loss	Respectful physical and emotional support for parents (C) Self-awareness and self-care (C)
Midwifery/ birth reflection services	Pattinson et al. (2011) supportive services for bereaved parents available but 1 in 5 women still suffer long-term consequences after stillbirth	Healthcare providers' support (A)
		Respect for women (A)
		Emotional and psychological pain and grief acknowledged (C)
	Heazell et al. (2016) empathetic relationships between caregivers and bereaved parents after stillbirth	Disenfranchised and stigmatised (A)
		Empathetic encounters between caregivers and staff (C)
		Minimises marginalisation and perceived failure at motherhood (C)
	Due et al. (2017) fathers after stillbirth	Supportive role (A)
		Grief not acknowledged (A)
	Kingdon et al. (2015) systematic review of seeing and holding baby after stillbirth	Staff acknowledging father's loss too (C)
		Midwives key in enabling parents to see and hold baby and make memories (A)
		Positive long-term outcomes (C)
		Better family outcomes (C)

Conclusion

Much of the literature explored examines the outcomes and consequences of a stillbirth from parents' and health professional's perspective. Studies identify bereavement services that are available now for women who have experienced loss and how midwives can support parents in this difficult time of grief. Other studies examined outcomes and impact on staff after involvement in stillbirth deliveries and midwifery care.

Much of the literature explores women's psychosocial and emotional wellbeing after a stillbirth as perceived by midwives and healthcare professionals. The importance of acknowledging existence of the birth event and the baby is an attribute displayed by midwives of the 'with woman' concept. Midwives become attuned to women's needs and grief at this difficult time and consequently empower women to make decisions about the stillbirth, reducing their stress and anxiety. They enable women to see, hold their stillborn baby and begin to process their loss and create memories, which enables resilience and decreases the risk of PTSD and depression.

The analysis of literature documenting women's perspective of this sad event indicates that not all women experience support from healthcare professionals, who due to a lack of knowledge and understanding of caring for women with a stillbirth resort to an avoidance strategy as a coping mechanism. The evidence suggests that midwives need further education, training and support to provide the necessary care and nurturing that bereaved women need. They need self-awareness and self-care to be able to truly fulfil the 'with woman' philosophy. Grieving women in general want to be listened to, to share their story of grief and loss, to feel less marginalised and experience emotional and psychological support from a caring midwife or healthcare professional. Midwives are key in being 'with woman' to ensure positive and better long-term family outcomes. The stories that follow are truly heartbreaking but illustrate some of this evidence and the lessons that can be learnt.

A Midwife's Stories

Zara-The Counsellor/Birth Reflection/Bereavement Midwife

Bereavement care and support has come a long way since I started in the NHS in 1980, much due to parents support groups and having a voice to improve the care given.

Allowing parents time to think about the choices they have is important so that they feel some control. Often parents feel totally overwhelmed by all the information they are trying hard to make sense of when they have just been given devastating news. It is important to ensure that this information is given in small stages; it is like planting seed by seed. Often parents have never seen a dead body before, they are frightened and may feel guilty about not wanting to see their baby. Explaining that this is quite normal is important and allows parents to move at their own pace. What is right for one may not be right for another and there is no right or wrong. Choices that are made are individual and must be respected.

Within a few days of parents discovering that their baby has died there is so much information to take in and decisions to be made. For example, how the pregnancy is going to be induced, where the mother will deliver, pain relief, the memories that parents may wish to have, whether they wish to see the hospital chaplain or a religious leader of their choice, what clothes they would like to choose for their baby, whether they wish to hold or see their baby, whether or not they wish to have photographs, whether older siblings may come and meet the baby they have been prepared to meet and hoped to take home, whether the parents choose to take baby home, should family and friends come to meet baby if they wish, funeral arrangements, the choice to have a post mortem, chromosome analysis, histology of the placenta . . . the list goes on.

So, it is not surprising that parents often need emotional support and help in their grief. Often the partner will return to work and the mother may be on maternity leave. At home, perhaps everything was prepared for their baby, all the clothes washed and hanging in a wardrobe, the nursery ready and a body that has all the signs of carrying life but no baby to hold. Just aching arms and broken hearts.

Support for these parents should be offered. A space for them to be able to grieve, to allow feelings of anger, envy, jealousy to be shared and to have reassurance that what they are feeling is normal. Support in future pregnancies is also often necessary and much appreciated by the parents. Understandably, any pregnancy after a pregnancy loss is one of anxiety and the unknown.

Staff also need care, kindness and help when caring for parents with a pregnancy loss or caring for a mother giving birth to death. It is emotionally draining and often the midwife may also have a labouring woman expecting a live baby and one of the happiest days of her life to care for at the same time. It is obviously best if this does not occur, but if the labour ward is busy, sometimes there is little or no choice. It is very important that staff, therefore, can offload and de-brief themselves. I have often seen staff holding it together for the sake of the parents and crying in a room away on their own. It is hard work and we need to be much kinder to ourselves and appreciate the difficult experiences that we as healthcare professionals face.

(Continued)

Grief can bring so many different emotions. Parents may be quiet in their demeanour, perhaps in a state of shock, not knowing what to ask or what to do. Some may be in denial, not able to believe the news that has just been given, perhaps asking for another scan to confirm the diagnosis – perhaps 'they had made a mistake, it can't be true'. Other parents may react very differently to the news that their baby has died. Often anger is a common emotion. Parents understandably look for reasons as to why their baby has died and there are often no answers at this early stage. A post mortem examination or placental histology may provide a cause of death, but these results can take several weeks.

It can be very helpful for parents to be offered a therapeutic birth reflection. This meeting should be held in a quiet room away from the maternity department if possible, or if the parents wish in their own home. Reflecting on their pregnancy from the beginning booking appointment and allowing the parents to ask any questions allows them to understand their experience. Often mothers feel guilty that they are at fault that their baby has died. Mothers can feel that it is their responsibility to carry the baby and bring the baby safely into the world. It can help tremendously to offer parents support at this most difficult and painful time. Counselling support is offered in some hospitals either separately or as a couple.

Many parents conceive again after a pregnancy loss and counselling and birth support is offered throughout the pregnancy working closely with members of the multi-disciplinary team.

Grief 50 years on

Whilst in my role as a midwife counsellor, birth reflection and bereavement midwife I received a phone call from an 85-year-old lady who wanted to know if she could buy a bench in her daughter's name 50 years after her death. It felt as if she were asking for permission to do so. I shall call this mother Lydia.*

It was evident from our conversation on the phone that she was talking about her daughter's death as if it had occurred recently and she shared that she had never really been able to talk about her daughter's birth and death to anyone. I offered her a space to meet and she gladly accepted.

Lydia was well dressed, slightly stooped, a mass of snow-white hair encasing her round kind face. She was accompanied by one of her four daughters who had brought Lydia to the hospital. I asked Lydia if she would like her daughter to accompany her into the counselling room, the reply was quick and to the point:

'No thank you. This is just for me. I have wanted to do this for so many years.'

I explained my role and tears welled in her eyes. 'There was no such thing as all this bereavement care when I had my daughter.'

Lydia and her husband had four babies, all girls. Lydia explained that she had no complications with any of her pregnancies. Her first daughter was delivered at term in a maternity ward; she stayed for several days where she was taught how to bathe, change and feed her daughter. All was well.

Her second daughter, who I shall name Mona, was also delivered at term. Lydia was accompanied to the hospital by her husband who waited outside the delivery room, as was the custom at that time. Mona's delivery was much quicker than the first, she explained, and there was no pain relief. She remembers a midwife and a doctor being present for the actual delivery. Mona was delivered and there was a silence in the room that haunts Lydia to this day.

'Why is it not crying' Lydia asked.

After what seemed like 'an awful long time', the midwife turned to Lydia and said, 'I'm sorry but your baby is not well'. She wrapped Mona in a towel and took her from the room.

Lydia said, 'all I could see was a mop of dark hair, just sticking out above the towel. That is all I could see.' The pain of grief was clear to see. Tears were streaming down her face as she recalled so clearly those moments and that one glance of her beloved daughter Mona, before she was briskly taken by the midwife from the room.

The doctor came to her left-hand side, knelt down beside Lydia on one knee and said very kindly 'I am sorry, but your baby was born dead'. In recalling these moments it struck me how Lydia was able to recall moment by moment in such detail. The blood on the doctor's gown, the glasses he wore that were sitting on the end of his nose, the stillness of the room, the absolute quietness. The feeling of shock, not understanding the words being spoken, the need for her to have her husband by her side.

Lydia rocked and wept for this child they named Mona that she never had the opportunity to hold and touch, to say goodbye to, to share the wonder of her beautiful baby, to create memories. The baby she had carried around inside her for the past nine months.

Instead, after 'I was made decent' her husband was allowed into the room and they embraced. The parents were told that they had a girl, but it was best for them if they put this behind them and tried for another baby 'as soon as possible'. It was felt that the best way forward was for Lydia's husband to take care of the funeral arrangements as that 'would cause extra stress for mother'. They never had the

(Continued)

opportunity to understand the reason why Mona was so cruelly taken from their family. There was no post mortem offered that Lydia can remember. Being told by one doctor 'It is just one of those things'.

Lydia did not attend Mona's funeral. Something she has regretted to this day, but at the time she just felt so overwhelmed with grief that she felt she couldn't go. So, her husband arranged the funeral and cared for Mona's grave. It was several years later that Lydia felt able to take herself to the grave and be near her daughter's resting place.

Two further pregnancies followed, both were quite physically straightforward as far as Lydia can remember. However, the emotional strain of 'hoping and praying that all will be well with the babies' certainly took its toll. Lydia explained how she was so afraid that something would happen in the pregnancies. The feeling of guilt that she has carried all these years that she had done something to cause the death of Mona has never left Lydia. 'It was my job to carry her safely into this world and protect her and I failed.'

Lydia and her husband received no bereavement counselling. Nobody talked about Mona. If her husband mentioned her name, Lydia would cry so he stopped, thinking that he was protecting his wife from further pain. Instead he tried his best to help with the household chores all he could, especially when Lydia was pregnant with their last two children. Not being able to take away his wife's pain, he helped in the way he felt he could. Lydia rested, left the house very seldom and grieved very much alone and in silence. Lydia had a desperate need to talk about Mona but there was no one to talk to. Her doctor prescribed sleeping tablets and something 'to calm me down'; there were no support groups or counselling available at that time for Lydia or her husband.

So, Lydia's desire to mark in some way Mona's existence for her 50th birthday was to buy a bench. Something that was visible to everyone who passed by. Something she wanted to leave behind her even after her own death.

Lydia asked me what we would do now if she had delivered Mona and how the care has changed.

I found this difficult as I was acutely aware that parents have so many more opportunities to create memories of their baby now. Parents in the hospital where I work are offered The Bereavement Suite away from the labour ward, so it is quieter. We help parents create memories, take photographs if they wish and hand and footprints. All are presented in a Memory Box donated by a charity. Parents are offered a post mortem examination for their baby to try and determine the cause of death, which may be helpful in planning the care for future pregnancies. They have an opportunity to speak with their consultant postnatally. As a bereavement midwife, I offer support to parents after they have left hospital and often they take the opportunity for counselling either as a couple or separately.

We understand that future pregnancies are going to be a very anxious time for parents. We work closely with the multi-disciplinary team and offer support throughout future pregnancies. Parents are invited to the annual Memory Day where grief is shared for the children who have died and are loved forever.

Parents do not forget their children who have died at whatever age. It is important to allow parents the space to talk about their feelings and express their grief. Often, family and friends are at a loss as to what to say or will say something inappropriate that parents find very hurtful. Offering parents a space to acknowledge their feelings of grief, their anger, jealously, envy and dislike at seeing pregnant mums and or babies is important. It helps them to make sense of their grief and to understand that their feelings are 'normal'.

How long does grief last? 'Somehow you'll get through it but you'll never get over it'

It was a Friday evening and I was ready to go home after a long and tiring week. The phone rang, and I answered it. It was a sister in the main hospital. Could I please come and see an elderly lady on the cardiac ward who was very ill but wanted to talk about her babies that had died.

My initial thought was 'I'm not a priest'; how could I help her? But what this woman really wanted was the opportunity to talk to someone who understood and who was willing to listen to her.

Lying in bed propped up with pillows, nasal oxygen being administered; I looked at this frail, fragile beautiful, 84-year-old woman. She told me that she was going to die soon, quite matter of fact, she didn't know when – 'the doctors won't tell me' – and that her dying wish was that her husband, whom she had always loved, would be with her when she died.

Then she began to tell me of her two babies she had given birth to. A girl, and three years later a boy, delivered when they were due, full term. Both babies were stillborn. Tears started to form in her eyes and the pain sketched on her face was as if she was experiencing the birth all over again as if it were happening at that moment. She explained that her first born, her daughter, was wrapped and taken from the room.

(Continued)

She never saw her baby again, it was never encouraged, 'the least you know the better'. She left hospital a few days later. 'Make another baby, it will make you forget this baby, it will be all right next time.'

Three years later she was pregnant and 'it was all just like before'. She delivered her son, there were no cries, just an icy silence and her baby was wrapped and taken from the room again. Her husband who was waiting outside the room was allowed to join her once 'she was all sorted'.

There were no 'hellos' or 'goodbyes', no cuddles, no photographs, no handprints or footprints, no blessing offered, no memories. Just told the sex of the beautiful babies she had given birth to. The babies were swiftly taken away as if nothing had happened. As if the nine months of pregnancy were an illusion.

She wept, and her husband did his crying on his own. He didn't want to cause his wife any further upset with his tears. They grieved inwardly, separately, afraid to upset the other for fear of causing the other more pain. They spoke about the children on their birthdays and always remembered the ages they would have been. The years went by, but the thought of living through another loss was unbearable so they never embarked on another pregnancy.

She took my hand in hers and asked me if I thought she would see her children again. It wasn't so much a question, more of a longing, a hope and a dream that she had carried within her all these years. She thanked me for helping her, for helping her feel at peace. For listening and for being there. She died three days later.

Another heartbreak...

Catherine* and Matt had experienced a very difficult obstetric history. Three years of unexplained infertility led them to explore in vitro fertilisation (IVF). It was during this process that Catherine conceived naturally. Feeling absolutely delighted, they shared their news with family and friends. Sadly, at seven weeks gestation Catherine started to bleed and she miscarried the baby. Understandably they were devastated.

They conceived a further three times following the first pregnancy and each time the pregnancy ended in a miscarriage between six and eight weeks, twice requiring surgical management of miscarriage. Tests and investigations took place and it was at this time that I met the couple.

The strain was beginning to affect Catherine and Matt. They couldn't think of a life without children and desperately wanted their own child. Their siblings were producing children; friends and work colleagues were sharing their pregnancies and scan pictures. There was no escape and it felt like torture.

Catherine and Matt had stopped telling their friends and family that they were pregnant as it had always been followed by 'we have lost the baby again'. They experienced the losses together and supported each other as best they could. At times, Catherine felt it was her fault for not being able to carry a baby to term and suggested to Matt that he found a woman 'with working parts that could carry his child and make him a daddy'. Every period that Catherine had signified a grief, a potential loss of a life that could have been.

Catherine conceived again and was seen frequently in the early pregnancy unit up to 12 weeks. Being able to have a scan every two weeks in the early stages was needed by the parents and offered some reassurance. A plan was in place, which included folic acid, aspirin and progesterone under consult-ant-led care. The couple were seen regularly, and Matt always came to every appointment, every scan. He didn't want to miss anything. We met frequently and had an agreement that they could contact me if they wanted to have a chat on the phone. The level of anxiety was palpable, and Catherine lived with this constant stress and worry which was exhausting. Mothers who have experienced early pregnancy losses like Catherine are very aware of any vagi-nal loss. Every time they go to the toilet they wipe and check for any blood. Any abdominal ache may signal uterine cramps. These mothers are super vigilant.

The pregnancy progressed well, and a plan was in place to wait for nature to take its course. If Catherine did not labour spontaneously, then an induction of labour was planned for 38–39 weeks gestation. The couple were at last beginning to prepare for their son, Alfred. They were very keen to have as normal a delivery as possible if all was well. Catherine was seen every week, and all seemed well. We wrote a birth plan together so that those caring for them were able to have an understanding of the very long and difficult journey that they had embarked on together.

At 37 + 3 weeks gestation Catherine and Matt contacted triage with reduced fetal movements that morning. They were told to come in straight away. The midwife was unable to find a fetal heartbeat. A scan confirmed that there was no heartbeat.

There are no words. Condolences seem so inadequate and the sadness is felt by everyone working on the labour ward, spreading to the antenatal clinic and the early pregnancy unit.

A post mortem found no cause of death.

A Student Midwife's Story- Jennie's Story

James*

On Thursday, James was born sleeping. I was at the end of my obstetric theatre week, which had been a challenge as I was once again learning new skills alongside the scrub nurse. I had missed working with the midwives and was looking forward to getting back to delivery suite shifts. My husband had been working away all week, and I had had very early mornings, dropping the kids off at a friend's and then arranging after school care for them all. I guess I was already exhausted. Our last c-section of the day was for an intrauterine death (IUD) at 36 weeks. The mother had come into the delivery suite after her community midwife was unable to hear a fetal heartbeat. A scan confirmed that baby James had already died.

The scrub nurse checked if I was ok to be there, and I felt I was. I knew this was something I would have to deal with as a midwife, and so I asked if I could shadow the midwife rather than the scrub nurse and help in any way that I could. The midwife explained that he would be beautiful but that he would just be asleep. As she said this, I felt tears prick my eyes, but my immediate reaction to this was to hold it all back. It didn't seem fair or valid. This was their grief, not mine. I continued to help prepare theatre and wait for the couple to come in.

Theatre was so quiet. It's usually quite noisy with the general hubbub of the procedure, with the operating department practitioner (ODP) and anaesthetist chatting away to the couple and to each other, and the radio on, usually playing music of the couple's choice. This time, it was totally quiet. Everything happened as it usually would but there was no joyful expectation. Just quiet. When James was born, he had no tone and was floppy. He was brought over to the resuscitaire just because we needed somewhere to dress him. He felt so warm and was indeed perfect but sleeping.

We wiped him down and then began to dress him. His clothes were cold, and I began to realise his temperature was dropping. In that moment, I wished the parents could have held him when he was warm. He seemed more alive when he was warm. I had had experience of babies being born flat, or needing help to breathe at birth, but all these babies began like James but then became more alive as the resuscitation worked. James just seemed more and more dead as the minutes went on. His pink colour began to fade. He really was sleeping, and it wasn't going to change.

The midwife passed him to his mother, all dressed in their outfit of choice and wrapped in the muslin they would have bought with such a different expectation.

Aren't muslins supposed to be comforters? My son still uses his at bedtime, but this one had become a shroud. James was handed to his father while his mother was moved on to her bed, and I felt heartbroken to see his face crumple momentarily, and then rally to say he was heavier than he thought he'd be. I pushed my grief down again. This was their moment not mine. He was snuggled back with his mother to leave theatre; they were wheeled out and he was gone.

My shift ended almost in the same moment. I knew I couldn't stay any longer. My kids needed picking up from their childcare and I had no one else to do it. The midwife had gone to care for the family and the scrub nurse was also gone. I stood there in theatre trying to assimilate in my mind what had just happened, and what I was supposed to do now. With no one else around, I went to the changing room, got my bags, went back to my car, and started the drive home, feeling like I was being strangled by my scarf.

And that was it. I picked up being a mummy. I stopped the children from arguing, made dinner, picked up my son from football and just carried on. There was no de-brief. No checking to see if I was ok. Of course, the midwife was where she should have been – supporting the family – but I felt I was in limbo. Who could I speak to in my normal run of life who could understand what I just saw? Was my grief valid? Should I have pushed away my tears? I couldn't find any answers to those questions. I just had to carry on.

A friend asked if we knew already that he would be stillborn, and when I said yes she commented that at least I had time to mentally prepare, but I don't think the preparation helped. Can anything help in those moments? I was required to be professional, which I did to the best of my ability for the mother and father, and for James, but that doesn't mean my heart didn't ache for them all. Surely, we are professionals in this arena because we care, and caring hurts. It certainly hurt on Thursday.

Postscript: The student alerted her personal tutor from the university about the incident and she was offered support and a de-briefing session a few days later.

A Woman's Story

Kitty*'s Story

The morning of the 24 December 1994 – Christmas Eve – 25 years ago today. My life was perfect but would soon become forever changed. My husband and I were happily married and our 4-year-old daughter was so excited for Santa's visit that night.

(Continued)

As I left for work all was well. Work was fun, dressed up in fancy dress and enjoyed Christmas lunch with the team. At the end of the day I went home as normal and played with my daughter before reading her a Christmas story and putting her to bed. We had some friends over for some drinks and nibbles to celebrate Christmas. Towards the end of the night I started to feel uncomfortable. It felt like indigestion, I thought nothing of it to begin with, but it gradually got worse. When everyone left, I wrapped the last of the presents and I went to bed hoping it would pass. It did not pass, it had in fact got worse and I hardly slept but, determined not to ruin Christmas, I did not say anything to my husband.

On Christmas morning my daughter was up early and despite being in pain I put my happy face on and watched her open her presents. Never once did I think anything was wrong with the baby, if I had I am sure I would have done things differently. Having had one happy healthy textbook baby I assumed that I would have another. We drove to my parents for Christmas lunch and as we sat for dinner the pain became unbearable. I excused myself from the table and I went to the toilet, I had some blood spotting but unlike what I had previously experienced in my first pregnancy as a 'show'. I was not due to have the baby quite yet and I became instantly concerned.

We called a locum GP who examined me and told me everything was OK. He advised me to take some paracetamol for the pain and prescribed me some antibiotics to prevent any infection. He told me to come back after Christmas if I was still concerned. I was young, I believed him that all was well and that I had nothing to worry about. On reflection he seemed annoyed that he had been called out possibly away from his own Christmas lunch. For many years I was angry towards him for what was about to come.

The pain did not really get worse or better. I slept intermittently. On Boxing Day, I had planned to be with my parents again, but I just wanted my own bed as I really did not feel OK. Not wanting to make a fuss, I laid on the sofa as my husband played with our daughter for the rest of the day at our house. On 27 December the minute I felt it was acceptable to go back to the surgery, I visited the GP. My blood pressure had dropped significantly, I felt dizzy and weak, the GP was concerned. He called an ambulance and I was blue lighted to hospital.

When we arrived at the General Hospital we were greeted by the obstetric team. I remember each of their faces to this day and the kindness and gentleness they showed me from the minute I arrived until I was discharged. The obstetrician was softly spoken, he sat on the edge of the bed, held my hand and broke the devastating news to us that our baby was dead. But I already knew I could not see him moving on the scan. Those words, however, brought the bitter sting of tears despite the comfort I was feeling from everyone around me.

This may have happened 25 years ago, but I have absolute recall of the devastation I felt in that moment. I could see the sadness and the compassion in his eyes and in his demeanour, he just seemed so caring, I'm not sure I've ever met another doctor like him in all my days. The sister in charge was the same. I remained in hospital for a few days because I had lost a high volume of blood whilst giving birth. During that time, I had many visitors and I would smile for all to see. But inside, I was dying. It was this sister herself that sat with me and listened to my grieving.

We had this tiny little boy who was ours and he died. In my everyday life I had to keep my grief hidden. I did not feel I could talk to anyone about my loss because no one knew how to act around me, I did not have the energy to deal with their reactions. Friends could not do right for doing wrong, but they would never have known because I never let it show. I had a friend who bought her new baby into visit me, I wanted to scream but I wore that same false smile; and another who didn't tell me she was pregnant because she was worried about upsetting me, again I wanted to scream when I found this out. At a time when everything just felt so hurtful, this lovely ward sister gave me all the time in the world. As a nurse myself, I now know that it was time she did not really have.

There was another plain clothed nurse who would visit daily and would listen to the outpouring of my broken heart. She would make me comfortable and make my bed with me still lying in it. I asked her why she wore plain clothes and she said she was a dual qualified nurse, meaning she was both a general nurse and a mental health nurse. I quizzed her further about her role. It was lying there in that hospital bed that I decided that when I had healed I would love to be a mental health nurse and give my unborn baby's life meaning. Perhaps one day, I thought to myself, I might be like that nurse and specialise in perinatal mental health – and that I did.

I believe this team gave me as much emotional care as they did physical care. They did this by giving me the space and permission to grieve, it was as simple as that. When I was discharged from hospital, I experienced panic attacks. They were emotionally excruciating, often with an overwhelming feeling that I was going to stop breathing and die myself. My grief was not only about the loss of my son it was about the loss of all the associated events and milestones that would have followed birth like a christening, graduating schools etc. I felt guilty that I had done something/failed to do something that had caused my

(Continued)

baby to die. The not knowing why it happened is the hardest despite being reassured that there is not always a medical reason. I also felt guilt that possibly my daughter would be an only child because I was too scared to go through another pregnancy.

My mental health was considered long after I left the hospital. I was discharged back to my GP who organised bereavement counselling. The hospital organised a remembrance service so I had an opportunity to say goodbye and lay my baby boy to rest. I am invited back to the chapel every year and each 27 December, the remembrance book is always open on his birthday. The love and care this team showed helped me to maintain my mental health throughout despite the utter distress and turmoil I felt.

The experience brought my husband and I even closer together. I did not think that was even possible. It also gave me a deeper appreciation of my beautiful daughter and life itself. My baby's name was Joshua and I thank Joshua every day for enriching my life in so many ways. His short life has had great meaning, he has been my drive and motivation for helping others who struggle with depression, anxiety and life in general. Joshua is a force that inspires me to get up every day and want to make a positive difference in the world.

Lessons Learnt

The above stories illustrate what is known from the literature about stillbirth, the role of midwives and healthcare practitioners and the consequences and outcomes for the grieving parents, their families and the midwives involved in these events. There are many lessons that have been learnt since some of the above events from years past have occurred, and currently most maternity services include a birth reflection or counselling service facilitated by specially trained and educated practitioners to provide the much-needed care and support for parents after stillbirth. Such care is generally provided in a sensitive and timely manner and the long-term impact of a stillbirth can be minimised to some extent.

Everyone copes differently with grief and parents and staff are no different. Sometimes parents can be stuck in their grief and it can be helpful to share these emotions with professional others outside of their family or friendship groups. It is now well recognised that allowing parents a safe place to cry and share their emotions without judgement can help them come to terms with their grief. Fathers and mothers often feel and cope very differently and this can sometimes cause stress in their relationship. Reassurance that this is 'normal' can be very helpful. It takes time adjusting to loss and grief, which can manifest itself in many ways. Some parents choose to attend support groups, for example SANDS, others withdraw and find it difficult to socialise with other people. Every parent has their unique story to tell.

Kitty's heartfelt story illustrates the pain and emotions that women experience when they have a stillbirth. It also highlights the importance of support and listening, giving time and space to women, by healthcare professionals. This is crucial in the healing process and women seem to remember vividly, even several years later, the kindness and compassion that is offered them at this extremely difficult time.

Staff are also very touched by these events and they too need support to be able to cope with emotions and stress as a result of stillbirths and other traumatic incidents during childbirth. Many trust providers offer staff a safe space to debrief with specialist counsellors and birth reflections midwives, as Zara relates in her story. However, as with the above case of the student midwife, immediate help and de-briefing is not always available and sometimes empathy from mentors and colleagues during the incident is the only support that can be offered.

References

Avekin, P., Radestad, I., Saflund, K. et al. (2013). Parental grief and relationships after the loss of a stillborn baby. *Midwifery* 29: 668–673.

Awgu Kalu, F., Coughlan, B., and Larkin, P. (2018). A mixed methods sequential explanatory study of the psychosocial factors that impact on midwives' confidence to provide bereavement support to parents who have experienced a perinatal loss. *Midwifery* 64: 69–76.

Burden, C., Bradley, S., Storey, C. et al. (2016). From grief, guilt, pain and stigma to hope and pride – a systematic review and meta-analysis of mixed-method research of the psychosocial impact of stillbirth. *BMC Pregnancy and Childbirth* 16: 9. https://doi.org/10.1186/s12884-016-0800-8.

Cacciatore, J. (2010). The unique experiences of women and their families after the death of a baby. *Social Work in Health Care* 49: 134–148.

Cacciatore, J. (2013). Psychological effects of stillbirth. *Seminars in Fetal & Neonatal Medicine* 18: 76–82.

Coffey, H. (2016). Parents' experience of the care they received following a stillbirth: a literature review. *Evidence Based Midwifery* 14 (1): 16–21.

Due, C., Chiarolli, S., and Riggs, D.W. (2017). The impact of pregnancy loss on men's health and wellbeing: a systematic review. *BMC Pregnancy and Childbirth* 17: 380. https://doi.org/10.1186/s12884-017-1560-9.

Einaudi, M.A., Coz, P.L., Malzac, P. et al. (2010). Parental experience following perinatal death: exploring the issues to make progress. *European Journal of Obstetrics & Gynaecology and Reproductive Biology* 151: 143–148.

Ellis, A., Chebsey, C., Storey, C. et al. (2016). Systematic review to understand and improve care after stillbirth: a review of parents' and healthcare professionals' experiences. *BMC Pregnancy and Childbirth* 16: 16. https://doi.org/10.1186/s12884-016-0806-2.

Erlandsson, K., Warland, J., Cacciatore, J., and Radestad, I. (2013). Seeing and holding a stillborn baby: Mothers' feelings in relation to how their babies were presented to them after birth- findings from an online questionnaire. *Midwifery* 29: 246–250.

Flenady, V., Wojciezek, A.M., Middleton, P. et al. (2016). Stillbirth: recall to action in high income countries. *Lancet* 387: 691–702.

Froon, J.F., Cacciatore, J., McClure, E.M. et al. (2011). Stillbirths: why they matter. *The Lancet: Stillbirth Series Steering Committee* 377: 1353–1366.

Heazell, A., Siassakos, D., Blencowe, H. et al. (2016). Stillbirths: economic and psychological consequences. *Lancet* 387: 604–616.

Henley, A. and Schott, J. (2008). The death of a baby before, during and shortly after birth: good practice from parents' perspective. *Seminars in Fetal & Neonatal Medicine* 13: 325–328.

Hollins Martin, C.J., Robb, Y., and Forrest, E. (2016). An exploratory qualitative analysis of student midwives' views of teaching methods that could build confidence to deliver perinatal bereavement care. *Nurse Education Today* 39: 99–103.

Huberty, J., Green, J., Cacciatore, J. et al. (2018). Relationship between mindfulness and posttraumatic stress in women who experienced stillbirth. *JOGNN* 47 (6): 760–770.

Hunter, A., Tussis, L., and MacBeth, A. (2017). The presence of anxiety, depression nd stress in women and their partners during pregnancies following perinatal loss: a meta-analysis. *Journal of Affective Disorders* 223: 153–164.

Hutti, M.H., Polivka, B., White, S. et al. (2016). Experiences of nurses who care for women after fetal loss. *JOGNN* 45: 17–27.

Kingdon, C., Givens, J.L., O'Donnell, E. et al. (2015). Seeing and holding baby: systematic review of clinical management and parental outcomes after stillbirth. *Birth Issues Perinat Care* 42: 206–218.

Kokou-Kpolou, K., Magalakaki, O., and Nieuviarts, N. (2018). Persistent depressive an grief symptoms for up to 10 years following perinatal loss: involvement of negative cognitions. *Journal of Affective Disorders* 241: 360–366.

Lovell, A. (1983). Some questions of identity: late miscarriage, stillbirth and perinatal loss. *Social Science and Medicine* 17: 755–761.

Marufu, T.C., Ahankari, A., Coleman, T., and Lewis, S. (2015). Maternal smoking and the risk of stillbirth: systematic review and meta-analysis. *BMC Public Health* 15: 239.

Murphy, S. and Cacciatore, J. (2017). The psychological, social and economic impact of stillbirth on families. *Seminars in Fetal & Neonatal Medicine* 22: 129–134.

O'Connell, O., Meaney, S., and O'Donoghue, K. (2016). Caring for parents at the time of stillbirth: how can we do better? *Women and Birth* 29: 345–349.

O'Connor, D. (2016). Saving babies' lives: A care bundle for reducing stillbirth. NHS England. http://www.england.nhs.uk/wp-content/uploads/2016/03/saving-babies-lives-car-bundl.pdf (accessed 23 July 2019).

Office of National Statistics (2019). Births in England and Wales. Office of National Statistics Publications. www.ons.gov.uk (accessed 23 July 2019).

Ovesen, P.G., Jensen, D.M., Damm, P. et al. (2015). Maternal and neonatal outcomes in pregnancies complicated by gestational diabetesA nation-wide study. *The Journal of Maternal-Fetal & Neonatal Medicine* 28: 1720–1724.

Pattinson, R., Kerber, K., Buchmann, E. et al. (2011). How can health systems deliver for mothers and babies. *The Lancet: Stillbirth Series Steering Committee.* https://doi.org/10.1016/S0140-6736(10)62306-9.

Peters, M., Karolina, L., Dagmara, R. et al. (2015). Caring for families experiencing stillbirth: Evidence based guidance for maternity care providers. *Women Birth* 28 (4): 272–278.

Pollock, D., Ziaian, T., Pearson, E. et al. (2019). Breaking through the silence: Fetal movement and stillbirth education. *Women and Birth.* https://doi.org/10.1016/j.wombi.2019.02.004.

Radestad, I. (2017). Mindfetalness: a method for structured observation on fetal movements. *Women and Birth* 30: 34–35.

Radestad, L., Surkan, P.J., Steineck, G. et al. (2009). Long-term outcomes for mothers who have or have not held their stillborn baby. *Midwifery* 25: 422–429.

Renfrew, M., Mcfadden, A., Bastos, M.H. et al. (2014). Midwifery and quality care: findings from a new evidence-informed framework for maternal and new born care. *Lancet* 384: 1129–1145.

Rivaldi, C., Levi, M., Angeli, E. et al. (2018). Stillbirth and perinatal care: are professionals trained to address parents' needs? *Midwifery* 64: 53–59.

Schott, J. and Henley, A. (2009). After a stillbirth- offering choices, creating memories. *British Journal of Midwifery* 17 (12): 798–801.

Schummers, L., Hutcheon, J.A., Bodnar, L.M. et al. (2015). Risk of adverse pregnancy outcomes by prepregnancy body mass index: a population-based study to inform prepregnancy weight loss counselling. *The Obstetrician and Gynaecologist* 125: 133–143.

Shorey, S., Andre, B., and Lopez, V. (2017). The experiences and needs of healthcare professionals facing perinatal death: a scoping review. *International Journal of Nursing Studies* 68: 25–39.

Stadtlander, L.M. (2012). The grief of caring: self-care in helping grieving parents of stillbirth. *International Journal of Childbirth Education* 27 (2): 10–13.

Steen, S.E. (2015). Perinatal death: bereavement interventions by US and Spanish nurses and midwives. *International Journal of Palliative Nursing* 21 (2): 79–86.

Widdows, K., Reid, H.E., Roberts, S.A. et al. (2018). Saving babies lives project impact and results evaluation (SPiRE) a mixed methodology study report. *BMC Pregnancy and Childbirth* 18 (1) https://doi.org/10.1186/s12884-018-1672-x.

World Health Organization (2016). International Statistical Classification of Diseases and Related Health Problems. 10th revision. Geneva: Switzerland

12

Global Midwifery Perspective of the 'with Woman' Concept

Julia Boon, Miriam Shibli and colleagues; Dina Ryan Davidson and colleagues; Elisabetta Colciago, Thorhild Borlaug, Natalie Papagiorcopulo, Alex Bell, Priscilla (midwives); and Annabel, Dina and Erin (women)

Introduction to Global Maternity Services

This chapter examines the importance of midwifery care to global health and illustrates how cultures and social factors have an impact on pregnancy and birth outcomes. Midwives play an essential role in the provision of high-quality care and improving health outcomes around the world (Renfrew et al. 2014).

Every year approximately 295000 women die as a result of pregnancy and childbirth (WHO 2019) and it is estimated that 80% of these women could be saved with high-quality midwifery care (Horton and Astudillo 2014). The threats to global maternal wellbeing are usually dependent on access to healthcare, poverty, lack of education, resources of staff and equipment, transport and infrastructure. Infection during childbearing in developing countries and over medicalisation of childbirth in developed countries are the extremes of the continuum. However, maternal death as a global concern is due to severe bleeding (mostly bleeding after childbirth), infections (usually after childbirth), high blood pressure during pregnancy (pre-eclampsia and eclampsia), complications from delivery and unsafe abortion (WHO 2019).

The 17 Global Goals were implemented in 2016 and one of the goals is to reduce maternal mortality and end preventable deaths of newborns (http://www.globalgoals.org). However, barriers to good midwifery care worldwide exist due to the low status of women in society, lack of understanding of the midwife's role, resources, global midwifery shortage, interprofessional rivalries, private maternity care sector and cultural expectations (Brodie 2013).

Better Births: The Midwife 'with Woman', First Edition. Edited by Anna M. Brown.
© 2021 John Wiley & Sons Ltd. Published 2021 by John Wiley & Sons Ltd.

The rest of this chapter gives a flavour of midwifery services across a few continents and midwives' and women's stories illustrate delivery of some of the midwifery services worldwide.

Midwifery Services in Israel

The Midwifery Division within Israel is regulated by the Israeli Nursing Division and is not a separate independent body. In cooperation with other midwife leaders, the President of the Israel Midwives Association acts as a consultant in advising the National Director of Nursing with regards to midwifery issues. In recent years, the consensus of this expert professional group has facilitated a significant achievement in updating evidence-based midwifery guidelines/policies to underpin the role of both nurses and midwives within the field of midwifery for contribution to safe and effective maternity services and mothers' satisfaction (Ministry of Health 2017, Nursing Division-Nursing Work plan).

The Israeli model of midwifery care is such that hospital-based midwives in Israel are usually only responsible for women during the intrapartum period. Antenatal and postnatal care is provided by nurses and obstetricians in different health sectors of the community such as *Kupat Huleem* or *Tipat Halav*. However, registered nurses in Israel are well prepared in the field of maternity nursing. Student nurses are required to attend 98 hours of theory and 144 hours of clinical practice during their obstetrics and gynaecology course (Nursing Division, Circular2012 - Core Nursing Program). Consequently, midwives are mainly based in labour and delivery rooms where they attend around 80% of all births (Cohain 2004; Nefesh B' Nefesh 2017). They generally work alongside physicians/obstetricians who have the final authority, make most of the important or serious decisions, provide additional medical intervention when necessary and are legally responsible for mother and baby (Ministry of Health Medical Administration, Circular 'Natural birth in Hospital' 2017). During the birth, the midwife is the professional who manages the birth. If an emergency arises during the birth, the midwife must inform the delivery room medical staff and the woman. As noted, responsibility for handling such emergencies rests with both the midwife and the doctor.

Unlike the United States, Canada and England, pregnant women in Israel who have a medical problem and are deemed 'high risk' during any stage of pregnancy are taken to the admission room of the delivery rooms rather than to the general emergency rooms of the hospital. There, they are seen by a midwife, who performs triage and initial care, before being seen by an obstetrician. This maybe the reason why caesarean section rates and other measures of quality obstetrical care — such as instrumental delivery, perineal trauma, obstetric anal sphincter injury (OASI), maternal mortality etc. – are among the best in the OECD despite the fact that the ratio of midwives to pregnant women in Israel is one to three whereas in other countries such as Finland, Sweden and England there is a ratio of one midwife to one or two women.

Since midwives do not usually care for women throughout the entirety of their childbirth (except for home births), being with the woman and supporting her is more difficult to achieve because the relationship has not been developed during pregnancy and cannot continue into the postnatal period. Midwives are therefore excluded from the opportunity of facilitating healthy pregnancies and childbirth or healthy parenting practices as recommended by WHO (2018). This is, however, likely to change soon, as the Nursing Division has recently acknowledged that the staff nurse on every shift in the high-risk pregnancy ward and gynaecology emergency room must be facilitated by a registered midwife.

In Israel, births are explicitly prohibited from taking place in locations which are not intended for admitting women for childbirth or, in other words, unlicensed medical institutions. However, Israeli law permits home births and obstetricians and midwives may attend them (Ministry of Health Circular No. 15/2017; 'Home Birth' Policy 2012) (Hebrew), because a woman's home is not in a place which operates with the intent of admitting women for childbirth. However, there is a very low rate of home births in Israel. According to the Ministry of Health, 181 000 births took place in Israel in 2016, (Central Bureau of Statistics 2016. Cited in The Knesset Research and Information Center, 2018) of which only 626 were home births. There are some midwives who have their own private practices providing assistance with births either at homes or at birthing centres. The position of the Ministry of Health is that births are safer for both the mother and the newborn in recognised and licensed delivery rooms. Only an authorised medical institution may operate a place intended for the admission of women for childbirth, i.e. hospital delivery rooms (Simon and Becker 2018).

To compensate for the discouragement of home birth and in response to women's increasing awareness of their rights in childbirth and their demand for autonomy, the vast majority of Israeli hospitals now provide designated birthing rooms that are more woman-friendly and provide a supportive environment for the purpose of encouraging natural birth within the hospital setting (Simon and Becker 2018; Ministry of Health, Medical Director Circular no. 17/2012, (2012); Ministry of Health Medical Administration, 'Natural birth in Hospital' 2017). The incentive to improve the reputation of childbirth within maternity units in Israel is encouraged by the large sum of money given to each hospital for every individual birth within the hospital setting (National Insurance Institute of Israel – Hospitalization and Maternity Grant 2019). This provision of secure finance motivates hospital managements to continually strive for improvement and to invest in services that attract women to give birth in their maternity units. As a result, Israeli women – both Arab and Jew – shop around, pursuing a service that appeals to them the most.

This has enhanced opportunities for choice and control in childbirth (The Knesset Research and Information Center, 2018). Eleven hospitals in Israel provide dedicated delivery rooms for natural birth. These rooms have a more home-like atmosphere and contain equipment to support the woman in natural birth, such as a birthing pool, physio ball, etc. Birth in one of these dedicated rooms is usually free of charge;

however, some hospitals may charge a fee. While an obstetrician is required to approve a woman's suitability for a natural birth, the midwife is the professional who manages the birth. Responsibility for handling emergencies rests with both the midwife and the obstetrician. If any intervention is required, the woman is transferred back to a normal birth track under the care of the obstetrician (Simon and Becker 2018).

Both Jewish and Arab Israeli women attend labour and delivery rooms. Both groups share Israeli residency, citizenship and the same rights to medical care (Rassin et al. 2009) but differ in language, religion, values, customs and lifestyle. Despite universal access to the Israeli healthcare system, Arab women are much less likely to attend childbirth preparation classes than Jewish women (5% versus 24%) (Halperin et al. 2014). Although Arab women report more birth trauma than Jewish women, another study by Halperin et al. (2015) reports more similarities than differences between Arab and Jewish women's birth experiences and no differences were found between them on the prevalence of post-traumatic stress disorder (PTSD) symptoms after birth.

Some independent birth centres enabling women to have natural births have operated without authorisation from the Ministry of Health. These centres have been contacted recently by the Ministry of Health and have been advised that they are operating in contravention of the law, and they must therefore discontinue their service. A petition was submitted to the High Court of Justice, and a hearing was expected in April 2018 (Simon and Becker 2018). Judgement on the proceedings has yet to be determined.

Midwives' Stories from Israel

Miriam's Story

Looking back over more than 35 years of experience in the field of midwifery, it becomes clear how important the learning process was for my growth both professionally and personally. Before working as a senior midwife, I worked as a midwife supervisor and clinical mentor and facilitated educational prenatal courses for parents for many years. I was consumed by my work assisting women during their times of labour and birth and found that supporting women's choices during childbirth proved to be positive, stimulating and, occasionally, challenging. I found that embracing rather than resisting my sense of vulnerability in the challenging moments was hard yet liberating. This developed in me a deeper sense of empathy and stronger connection to others as well as a stronger sense of belief in myself and a level-headed way of handling situations.

For many years, I have been giving prenatal classes and felt both a personal and professional interest in increasing women's awareness on the topic of childbirth. I also enjoyed listening to the birth stories of the women who had given birth; it was an opportunity for the women to verbalise and share their experiences. As Sam McCulloch states (2018): 'Telling the birth story is a way to make sense of it and to integrate the event into our lives.' The overall idea was to give women a supportive space in which to go over their experiences and piece together the event of childbirth.

Xenia*'s Birth Story

Xenia was 27 years old and had a normal delivery at 41 weeks. At 32 weeks, after her Oral Glucose Challenge Test (OGCT) came back positive and the ultrasound showed that she had a large baby, Xenia was diagnosed with gestational diabetes (GDM) and put on a controlled diabatic diet.

I had met Xenia in her antenatal classes and was coincidently involved in part of her labour and birth. As well as stabilising her blood sugar levels with a controlled diet, from 40 weeks onwards, Xenia was told that she needed to visit the delivery room every three days for an assessment of fetal wellbeing and an evaluation of her blood sugar levels. Her ultrasound showed a normal biophysical profile with the fetus having an estimated weight of 3800 g.

On each visit to the unit, Xenia was advised to have an induction due to her history of GDM and the large size of the baby, but she consistently refused on the grounds that her aim was to have a natural birth without medical interference. Her blood sugar levels were under control, she was 175 cm tall, the baby's weight was 3800 g and she was interested in having a spontaneous labour rather than being induced.

At 41 weeks, Xenia arrived at the delivery room at 02:00 in the morning after a spontaneous rupture of the membranes had been confirmed on her admission to the hospital. She didn't have any contractions but complained about having back pain. Her vital signs and blood sugar levels were normal, and her ultrasound showed a normal fetal presentation with a good amount of fluids and a healthy placenta. The monitor showed a reactive normal heartbeat.

Xenia's contractions began spontaneously 20 hours following the rupturing of the membranes; 46 hours after her admission, the labour had progressed nicely and she was fully dilated. Xenia had a spontaneous, normal birth without any medical intervention and delivered a healthy baby girl with a weight of 4.3 kg. Her coping methods for the pain during labour mostly included remaining mobile in an upright position, breathing and relaxation techniques, the physio ball and warm showers. Conversely, during the first 20 hours of ruptured membranes, Xenia was feeling quite anxious due to repeated doctors' advice to induce labour. Having already made acquaintance with Xenia throughout her antenatal classes, it was easy for me to connect with her during her labour and birth as we had already formed a relationship and she trusted me to be her midwife.

Miriam's Reflection

While supporting Xenia's choices and preferences throughout her last weeks of pregnancy, I was left feeling vulnerable and fearful of disagreements within the department. Even though births are often conducted by midwives without the presence of a doctor, it is the policy in Israel that the obstetricians have the authority over decisions regarding women who give birth in a hospital setting. As a result, I was left feeling uncertain about how to balance my support for Xenia's decisions and preferences with the protocols and opinions of others in the department.

In this particular case, Xenia was aware of what she had been advised to do and knew that she was fully in the right to do what she felt was best. She was aware of the implications of GDM and the consequences of having a large baby and had been advised to be observant of fetal movements and her blood sugar level. I believe that birth is a time where we can share our thoughts and feelings with each other which consequently makes us stronger and brings us closer together. Sometimes, as a midwife, I felt my strength turn to hopelessness when the feelings of the mother were disregarded and the decisions about how to progress were taken out of my hands.

While I do understand the doctors' obligation to the policies and their fear of receiving complaints which may lead to litigations or risk management issues, I believe that the focus on the risk of birth rather than on the joy of birth is a negative, disempowering shift which has the potential to make all of the doctors, midwives and women involved lose confidence in themselves.

Understanding and upholding the values and beliefs needed to create a humane birth practice in hospitals requires a theoretical knowledge of the social and cultural characteristics of childbirth. The application and explanation of this knowledge in a hospital setting would help to inform both the hospital staff's approach to birth as well as women's choices during childbirth.

Priscilla's Story

Dana,* a 33-year-old woman, came into the labour room in her third pregnancy at 40 weeks and for her third delivery. On admission, vaginal examination was 2 cm dilated and 70% effaced. The fetal station was minus two high and her amniotic fluid was intact. During this pregnancy, she had minimal antenatal care. She was a religious woman and the only tests she had completed in this pregnancy were ultrasound and the glucose challenge test. Both results were normal.

Dana did not come to the hospital with any written birth plan, but she verbally told me her expectations during the labour process. She desired an epidural, no perineal tears and wanted to breastfeed right after delivery. I told her that it was very good of her to let me know what she would like in her delivery, and I provided information on the different aspects of what she had planned for her delivery. I wanted her to feel in control of her birth plan and empowered in the birth process. Even though she was already given an epidural anaesthesia, I coached her through breathing with each contraction and how to relax her body after each contraction was over. I reminded her that she could go with what her body was feeling, but always remembering to breathe.

Concerning vaginal tears, I explained to her that there were different reasons for tearing. Skin type tissues played a role. Some skin types stretch well and are very elastic while others are not as elastic and are more prone to tearing. Fetal size also plays a role. I explained that there were several things I would do to help prevent perineal tearing. Her job was to focus on breathing, listening to her body, and pushing down her baby. I would apply warm water to soothe the perineum and perineal oil (almond oil) to reduce friction during the process of delivery. After saying these things, Dana said, 'What if we do all of these things and I still tear?' I encouraged her to think positively.

Dana progressed in labour with an epidural until her cervix was 6 cm, then stopped dilating for another three hours. I did change of position and told her the next steps, which were in two parts. The first step would be to perform an artificial rupture of membranes. After that, if her labour did not progress, we would give her Pitocin augmentation. She understood that if she did not progress in another hour after the rupture of membranes, then we would begin the Pitocin. In that moment, she was not comfortable with either option. The doctors came in, explained to the woman the options as well and gave the written order for Pitocin augmentation. We would not move forward until she gave her approval.

When the doctors left, Dana asked, 'When will I give birth'? I told her that hopefully it would be very soon. With my answer, she felt more empowered and gave a verbal consent to do the artificial rupture of membranes, hoping her baby would be in her arms soon. Therefore, I performed an artificial rupture of membranes and the amniotic fluid was clear. The fetal monitor showed that all was well with the baby, and soon Dana was having one contraction every 10 minutes. An hour later, on vaginal examination, she had not progressed in labour, but she was having two uterine contractions in ten minutes. She knew the next step was to augment with Pitocin. Her concern was that Pitocin would increase the pain. I reassured her that this next step would help to progress her labour and that she would not feel an increase in pain as she had already had an epidural. This gave her the peace she needed to move forward.

On that same shift, the labour ward was very busy. I had to leave her to attend to the other women periodically. The situation left her very uncomfortable and I felt it as well but had no choice because other women needed me. I handed her the nurses' bell to call me whenever she needed me and left her with her husband in the room, emphasising to him the need to call me whenever his wife needed me. I hoped that the trust she had gained from our relationship during the early interaction of the early shift would give her a sense of safety and empowerment,

(Continued)

knowing she could go through her labour without fears and distractions. An hour later, she accepted the Pitocin augmentation, which I immediately started after again explaining to her the process and its effect.

In a short while after starting intravenous Pitocin, the fetal heart rate started dropping. When this occurs, it is called variable decelerations. I stopped Pitocin and helped Dana into a different position. The doctor was called simultaneously, and the fetal heart rate became normal. I performed a vaginal examination and she was now 8 cm dilated, fetal head in zero station, and 90% cervical effacement. Dana was happy and relieved. She said, 'I am finally progressing in my labour!' I nodded my head and continued to give her words of encouragement to keep her relaxed. I left her room and attended to the other women equally. In the labour ward, we learn to juggle many women in different stages of labour.

Thirty minutes later, she rang the call bell and I immediately came into her room. She was feeling a strong sensation to bear down. I checked her and she was fully dilated. I was very happy for her. The reduction of anxiety and fear promoted courage, confidence and empowered her during the birth process. The delivery went well without vaginal tears and both she and the baby were in good health condition. She breastfed her baby just as she wanted immediately after delivery. She was elated and very thankful to the doctors and me.

Priscilla's Reflection

It was a great commitment to try to avoid perineal tears in a woman that had torn twice in previous deliveries, knowing fully that most vaginal tears are inevitable notwithstanding the midwife's years of experience. More so, the fact that I cannot be with the woman steadily throughout labour is very difficult for me, as my desire would be to stay at the woman's side throughout the entirety of the process. Nevertheless, it is a joy to help women like Dana overcome their doubts and fears in labour and assist them in achieving their desired plan birth, even when obstacles arise.

Gomer's Story

Rita* was 25 years old and 39+ weeks pregnant with her first child when she came to our ward for an external cephalic version (ECV); her baby was in breech position and she preferred to have a vaginal delivery. Following a successful ECV, she returned home for 2 weeks. By her 41st week, Rita's contractions had not yet started so she returned to the hospital for a check up. Fortunately, the baby's head was still in a downward position, so she began augmentation of labour.

Accompanied by her loving, young husband, Rita tried a number of methods to augment labour but, for the first few days, none of them helped in bringing on the contractions. On the third day, Rita had a vaginal examination and discovered that she was 3cm dilated; however, the baby's head was high in the pelvis which meant that it wouldn't be possible to rupture the membranes. The doctors suggested a caesarian section on the basis that they thought the baby was in malpresentation, but they were also willing to wait and see if Rita progressed on her own. Rita preferred to keep trying with the augmentation process and was hopeful and optimistic that the contractions would intensify in the following hours which might then push her baby downwards so that she could finally give birth. By the end of the day, however, Rita and her husband were disappointed once more by the lack of progress.

On the morning of the fourth day, Rita decided to try the Pitocin drip one more time but, by that point, she was already quite tired as the process was taking days. She was frustrated and wondered why her body wasn't responding. Throughout all of this time, doctors and midwives repeatedly explained to Rita what was happening, the processes that needed to occur in her body, the obstacles which might delay labour, how the baby encourages birth from within, and how all of those elements needed to work together in order for the labour to progress.

Slowly Rita started to understand and to accept that her ideal of having a spontaneous birth was no longer in her hands and so at noon, she gave up and asked to be operated on. Later in the afternoon, I went to visit Rita and her daughter: a sweet, lovely baby girl and a happy, proud mother.

Gomer's Reflection

I had met Rita prior to the birth which made me feel obliged to help her and I became very involved throughout the birthing process. I feel that meeting women prior to their arrival at the delivery room, getting to know who they are, what they see as meaningful and what kind of family they come from allows me to care for and treat women during birth in the best way I can.

Because I knew Rita's background, I accepted the fact the she needed to go through the birthing process all the way through to the end until she understood deep down from within herself that having a regular delivery wouldn't be possible with her baby. I also knew she needed to hear logical explanations about her situation so that she could understand what was going on.

All of this was fine, but what I found hard was trying to navigate between all of the caregivers who came and went as they weren't familiar with Rita like I was and therefore didn't offer good enough explanations or made biased remarks which I later had to present to Rita as being helpful and supporting. Due to the fact that the staff changes all of the time, the system isn't working as well as it could be, and women are experiencing a lack of continuity in their care.

Women's Stories

Annabel's Birth Story from Israel

For my first pregnancy, I didn't have a birth plan but had the idea that I would try and give birth as naturally as possible. I was both excited to meet our baby as well as nervous about how painful labour would be.

Two nights before our daughter was born, my mucous plug had come out and mild contractions had started. After coming across a small quantity of some unidentifiable liquid, I became nervous that my waters were leaking. Ringing the National Health Service helpline, the next day, I spoke to one nurse who suggested I go directly to the hospital as well as a second nurse who advised that all would be well if I waited until the contractions intensified. In hindsight, I probably should have taken the former advice but decided to wait instead.

The next day, my partner and I decided to go the hospital because the baby's movements felt uncharacteristically weaker. After a monitor and ultrasound check, the midwife suggested we take a more detailed ultrasound because it seemed the water in the amniotic sack was low. The second ultrasound confirmed this and the midwives at the hospital recommended that I stay the night and induce the labour with a balloon. While I didn't really like the idea of staying in a hospital when I wasn't yet dilated enough, I asked for a second opinion from midwives who we knew personally outside of the hospital. Both suggested that I remain in the hospital and drink plenty of water to see what the result showed in the morning. So, we went against the recommendation to get an induction and had to sign a form stating the fact.

It was recommended that I take antibiotics in case my waters were in fact leaking to avoid infection. The next morning a monitor check and ultrasound were taken, and it was found that the waters in the sack had returned to a normal level. This meant I was able to stop the antibiotics, go home and return to the hospital when the contractions were closer together or in the case that there was a bloody show.

And so, only around four to five hours later, I was back for a check up as I had had both the bloody show and stronger contractions. We were told that I was 4 cm dilated and I was relieved to learn that I could enter the birthing room. A midwife came in and gave me the option of an enema, which I declined, as well as a gymnastics ball, which greatly helped during the next four hours or so of contractions. I was surprised to learn that eating food (except for ice cream) was prohibited, as I felt the need to eat to receive energy for the upcoming labour. In any case, I was monitored every so often and found it very uncomfortable lying down with the monitor around my belly when the contractions came, but I understood the reason behind it.

I was advised to take warm showers to try and speed up the process but I'm not sure that it worked as around four hours after I had entered the birthing room I was only around 5 cm dilated. This came as a surprise as, considering the intensity of the contractions, I would have supposed the dilation to have progressed further. I was disappointed to learn that along with the pain of the contraction, I would have to strap the monitor on my belly from that moment until the birth of the baby. Something inside of me couldn't comprehend that I could manage both the intensity of the contractions and the tight monitor strap until I reached 10 cm dilation. My body was exhausted and so, when given the option of an epidural, I accepted.

I was disappointed in myself for not giving birth naturally at the start, but once the epidural took effect, I was very grateful for the break from the pain. Finally, my body could relax, I was put on a drip and told that lying down would be the only option as my legs began to tingle with numbness. Within the next hour or so of rest, I progressed quickly to 9 cm dilated. When the assistant came in to check, we stopped the epidural and tried to wake up my legs and lower muscles before it came time to push.

It was only when the morning shift of midwives came in that it felt like the time to push had begun. I was told to lie on my back and pull my knees up against my chest when the contractions came and to push. An incision was made to make the vaginal opening wider and assist the baby to come out more easily as it was noted that the baby's heartrate was getting weaker every time there was a contraction. A monitor was also attached to the scalp of the baby and finally the doctor decided that a vacuum would be necessary. While I pushed, two midwives helped hold my knees while another pushed down on my stomach and the doctor used the vacuum. Looking back on the scene now it seems very surreal and I almost can't believe that it was me in that room pushing. It seemed a case of mind over matter as the pain now seemed less important than getting the baby into this world. I am very grateful to this team for helping me birth my baby as well as my partner who stood by me through the whole process – massaging my back and offering support. I could not have planned or foreseen the decisions that were made in the final hour, but I respect that they were made with the health of mother and baby in mind.

Following the birth, our daughter was taken to have a scan because the midwives and doctor noticed she had difficulty breathing. This was another shock but thanks to the doctors in the intensive care unit, spontaneous pneumothorax was diagnosed and treated immediately and in the following days she became stable and we were able to return home.

(*Continued*)

Dina's Birth Story from Israel

I was pregnant with my first son. I was clear that I wanted a natural birth and I did not want any medication. I hired a doula to be with me and I knew that I wanted her along with my husband to be with me during the birth. I chose the hospital which I wanted to give birth in. I visited the hospital when I was in my sixth month and I was given a form to fill in saying what I wanted and what I did not want to have in my birth.

When I was in week 39.5 all of a sudden my water broke at 3 a.m. I called the doula, she asked me to relax and sleep since I did not have any contractions and wait till the morning. I knew then that even when the water breaks, not all of it goes out and there will be still water around the baby – so I knew this (not going to the hospital immediately) was safe for the next 18 hours. At 3.30 p.m., I began to have contractions by the time we arrived at the hospital (with a lot of traffic on the way), we arrived at 7.00 p.m. to the department at the hospital.

The midwife was shocked when she knew that my water had broken at 3:30 a.m. They wanted to give me antibiotics for the baby and I refused. I said I know the baby was safe. Then while being on all fours on the bed trying to breath and focus on myself and contractions, the gynaecologist was standing next to me asking me questions to fill a form and repeating my answers. I was really angry because I felt my privacy and space had been invaded. Luckily my husband took her out of the room and answered her questions.

Then the pain started to be more intense, I decided that I needed the hot water to help me with the pain. I went to the bath tub, by then there was a new midwife on the shift. She was afraid that I was going to the toilet – they wanted to tie me to the monitor and I refused, I could not stay in the bed and be in pain, I needed to help myself deal with the pain so I knew water would help me. Then the midwife kept coming to the shower from time to time; first she asked me not to fill the bath tub with the water because my water already broke and this might not be healthy for the baby, then she came back again and again asking me to be put on the monitor. From 11 p.m. till the next day 6 a.m. I was in the bath tub using hot water to help me with the pain – and the midwife never stopped coming and interrupting me to come and ask me to be put on the monitor.

My husband said we had to go back to the room. And we did eventually, but by then I was really tired. I started to cry and say I am tired, and I was trying to explain what I was feeling but I was lost for words. The midwife started suggesting taking medication to take. My husband started to be angry with me, and I was lost. Then the doula looked at me. She was sitting with me on the floor and asked me what I felt – she tried to help me express myself. Then I said: 'I feel I need to empty my bowels but I can't, so the doula said maybe what you feel is the head. So I relaxed, I calmed down. I was able to go up to the labour bed and then a new midwife came and started to get ready. I looked at her and asked her what she was doing, and she said you are going to push this baby out. And this gave me a lot of power to push and in one hour the baby was out at 8:00 a.m. in the morning.

I did not want them to wash him nor to give him milk in bottles. I wanted him to sleep with me in the same room and breastfeed him. All the time the nurses tried to convince me to put him in the nursery room so I could sleep and they would give him the bottle and I refused. I felt all the time under pressure and all the time I felt I needed to explain and every new nurse on the shift would try to convince me to put my baby in the nursery.

Then there was a situation in which my son was crying and not sleeping and we realised that he had a dirty nappy and I did not know that I needed to change his nappy. The nurse was scolding me and saying I was a careless mother. It was very painful for me to hear this. I was a new mum and I knew nothing about taking care of a baby and this was the first remark I received after giving birth. It was very painful. I needed a lot of support and tenderness and what I got from that nurse was judgement.

Midwifery Services in Italy

Elisabetta's Reflection

The Italian National Healthcare System (NHS) provides universal services, largely free of charge at the point of service, regardless of origin or income. The Italian birth context has a classification system for levels of maternal care for Obstetric Units, comprising Level I Maternity Units providing care for low-risk pregnancies or with minor complications and Level II Maternity Units dedicated to women with high-risk pregnancies. Women with low-risk pregnancies may choose to give birth in either a Level I or II Maternity Unit.

Italian maternal care is quite medicalised throughout the childbearing continuum (Euro-Peristat Project 2018; Istituto Superiore di Sanità, Sistema Nazionale Linee Guida 2011) and there is a notable difference between the north and the south of the country – where the caesarean section rate can reach 50%. Although the national guideline on normal pregnancy recommends midwife-led care (Istituto Superiore di Sanità, Sistema Nazionale Linee Guida 2011), obstetricians are the primary providers of all antenatal care with the majority of women having a private doctor. Very few women are cared for by a midwife within the NHS service or choose an independent midwife during their pregnancy. There are mainly obstetric-led antenatal clinics and only a few that are led by midwives, based either in hospital or in the community. Almost all births in Italy, 99.7%, take place in hospital (Lauria et al. 2012; Ministero della Salute - Direzione Generale della Programmazione Sanitaria - Comitato Percorso Nascita Nazionale 2017).

Different birth settings, such as midwife-led units, are not available and home birth is not guaranteed by the NHS and discouraged by doctors. Continuity of caregiver through antenatal, intrapartum and postnatal care is rare in Italy (Lauria et al. 2012). The NHS midwives work in the community or in hospital and they rotate between labour areas (where they are quite autonomous if a woman has a normal labour and birth), antenatal and postnatal wards. Independent private midwives usually provide midwifery continuity of care.

The absence of national intrapartum guidelines leads maternity units across the country to write their own protocols, resulting in a very heterogeneous panorama with regard to midwifery practice among institutions with no mapping available at present. However, an interesting document has been realised by the Ministry of Health in 2017 (Ministero della Salute - Direzione Generale della Programmazione Sanitaria - Comitato Percorso Nascita Nazionale 2017), recommending offering low-risk women midwife-led care throughout the childbearing continuum. This should include also the intrapartum care period, with a room or a dedicated area both within the labour ward, where low-risk women are looked after during normal labour and birth.

Due to the high-risk culture surrounding birth, midwives are far from being the primary caregiver for women and families and their key role for women's health and their babies is not well recognised. However, in this historic moment, the midwives' professional body is strongly committed to building up a robust common identity, in order to be the ones to promote, support and look after women, babies and families.

Betty's Birth Story from Italy

Being 'with woman' is a central tenet of midwifery philosophy and practice. As a midwife I have always cared for women and their family, focusing on their needs and providing evidence-based information with the aim to allow them to make a well-informed choice during the childbearing continuum.

My birth story is quite different to the majority of Italian women's childbirth experiences. I feel very lucky to be a midwife and to be surrounded by very special colleagues. When I found out that I was pregnant, I was in the position to choose my midwife and I already knew who I wanted to be with me, my baby and my partner. I wanted as little interventions as possible and a home birth, so I wanted a midwife who believed that pregnancy is a normal event, that women can give birth naturally, a professional with experience with home births, but also someone who could stay with us in case we needed hospital care. (Most of the time women who want a home birth, have to choose a private midwife. In case they need to be transferred to the hospital, sometimes their midwife is not allowed to stay.) These are the reasons why I chose a midwife who works as a ward manager in hospital; however, she works also in community once a week looking after pregnant women and she attends home births too.

My pregnancy was straightforward. We didn't know the sex and we were so excited to meet our baby. My labour started on my due date and as soon as I felt I needed my midwife, I called her. She stayed with us during the night and during the day. A second midwife also arrived, who was known by me and my partner. The labour was quite long and after 12 hours with little progression (from 4 to 6 cm) and with very irregular contractions, we decided to go to the hospital. At that point I was really frustrated. I wanted my home birth with all my strength and, although my midwife spoke with us about the 'unexpected' aspects and tried to modulate my expectations while I was pregnant, I did not expect this. However, the midwife remained with us in the hospital and gave me even more support. She trusted my body more than I did and helped me to give birth in a calm, peaceful and dimly lit environment. My partner was the first to see our baby and to tell me that he was a boy.

Although I still had in my mind and in my heart the desire to have my home birth as I planned, I could not thank my midwife enough, who had helped me to feel safe and supported at all times, made my birth emotional and allowed us to have a positive experience.

When I become the mum-to-be, everything changed. I discovered how being a mother could make me different; all my knowledge, my confidence to know the physical changes of the pregnancy, the development of the baby and what is normal and what is not, were not enough. I realised how much the women–midwife relationship is important to ensure this period of calm and serenity. From my perspective, being 'with woman' means shared knowledge and competencies in a professional, sensitive and supporting relationship, and being a trusting guide. During pregnancy I could always count on my midwife's professional advice and most of all I felt reassured during the entire process.

Midwifery in Norway

Thorhild's Reflection

Midwifery education in Norway is now a master's degree. In order to start midwifery education, one needs to be a registered nurse and have practised a minimum of one year as a nurse. Two years of a course that combine theory and practical training gives new midwives authorisation to practise midwifery.

There are approximately 2500 midwives practising in Norway, they practise as community midwives responsible for pregnancy follow ups in cooperation with general practitioners, in women's clinics, midwifery-led units, or they can be private practitioners. The majority of midwives are organised in an independent midwifery union, some within the nursing organisation.

Home birth midwives are private, and they cater for less than 1% of around 58 000 births per year in Norway.

Midwives try to keep birth normal and find that the increased medicalisation and sometimes inaccurate use of technology, strict procedures and regulation can be a threat to women's choices and midwives' autonomy.

At the universities we try to educate caring, conscious, independent midwives who are team workers with integrity and who will protect normal birth.

Midwifery Services in Canada

Dina's Reflection

Long before the first registered midwife began practice in the northern part of Turtle Island now known as Canada, there were traditional indigenous midwives caring for their communities. During the colonisation process, many aspects of traditional culture were lost, yet indigenous midwifery has been an unbroken line throughout history.

Canadian midwifery is currently a community of approximately 1700 direct-entry midwives practising across 10 provinces and 3 territories. Regulations, scope of practice and registration processes differ from jurisdiction to jurisdiction. Midwives are integrated into local health systems as autonomous primary caregivers, and their services are covered by the Canadian National Health Service. They work in diverse models from caseload 'solo' practice, to team-based care, in collaboration with the rest of the maternity care team that may include perinatal nurses, family physicians, and obstetric and paediatric consultants. Care is provided in clinics, birth centres, hospitals and community settings. Prenatal, intrapartum and postpartum care is provided to dyads from early pregnancy through to between 6 weeks and 12 months after birth.

Across Canada, Midwives facilitate approximately 11% of births. Indigenous midwives make up an important part of communities, where they often act as leaders, passing on knowledge about ceremony and health to the next generations. Canadian midwifery is rooted in not only evidence-based and person-centred care, but also continues to uphold and strive for increased social justice, anti-racism and inclusivity for all people.

Maternity Services in Australia

Natalie's Reflection

Australia has a universal healthcare system where medical care is provided free of charge under a system called Medicare, together with a very popular private healthcare sector. Midwifery in Australia had traditionally had a medical model, where obstetricians provide all antenatal care, attend deliveries and have daily contact with patient input in the postnatal ward: this is still currently the model of care for women who elect to give birth in the private health system.

Midwifery care started to change in Australia after the 1986 nurses and midwives strike, which resulted in the profession receiving pay and conditions that aligned with being a medical profession. Around this time, midwifery training moved to university and the degree was recognised as a profession rather than a vocation.

In the 1990s, midwife-run family birth centres began opening, mainly in major hospitals with the support of sympathetic obstetricians, focusing on natural birthing practices. Over the years, many of these family birth centres closed down to be replaced by what today is called the Maternity Group Practice (MGP), a model of care where a midwife is allocated a number of patients per month for whom she is totally responsible, being on call for the delivery, which in some areas can be a home birth. If delivered normally in a hospital setting, early discharge of four hours is the norm and the midwife will continue the care in the patients' home. Midwives who work in MGP are employed by hospitals, but they are not part of the staffing within that hospital.

Another popular model of care is team midwifery. A group of midwives work together as a team and care for women who elect to be part of this model of care in the hospital setting. The concept is that the patients are more likely to meet the same midwives and have continuity of care. These midwives work normal shifts in hospital, rotating through the antenatal clinic, delivery suite, postnatal wards and domiciliary home visits.

The remaining patients are cared for in the standard model of care: they elect to be seen by a combination of midwives and doctors in the antenatal period and are delivered by midwives unless delivery is instrumental or surgical. Many high-risk patients seek this model of care to avail themselves of specialist obstetricians as required.

Australia also has a small number of independent, private midwives not associated with any hospital who care for women who elect to have home births; these independent midwives take complete responsibility for these families.

Australia is a vast country and the above models of care are common primarily in main cities, such as Melbourne. Other models of care may be available for families living in rural or bush settings, especially ones that have a large Aborigine and Torres Straight Islanders.

Maternity Services in North Adelaide

Aboriginal Family Birthing Programmes (AFBP) in South Australia (SA) aim to offer Aboriginal and Torres Strait Islander (ATSI) women and non-ATSI women carrying an ATSI baby the option of accessing culturally-specific and safe maternity care. Supported by Aboriginal Maternal Infant Care practitioners (AMIC) and midwives working in partnership, these programmes improve access and engagement with maternity care, therefore promoting and enhancing best practice in partnership with the AFBP team.

The AFBPs in SA are available to ATSI women and non-ATSI women carrying an ATSI baby, birthing within their relevant local health network, of which there are four in South Australia. Broadly, these programmes aim to address prevalent risk factors, improve experiences and close the gap in mortality and morbidity between ATSI and non-ATSI people, within the context of acknowledging the historical intergenerational trauma and continued barriers that exist for many ATSI people and communities.

Recently, the Australian Federal and State Governments' initiative 'Closing the Gap – the First 1000 days' (CtG), has provided funding to health networks, including the Northern Adelaide Local Health Network, which aims to make significant improvements in engagement and reductions in the health inequalities for ATSI people, compared to non-ATSI people, by improving access to health services from pre-conception up to the first two years of life, thus reducing the risk of poor outcomes and improving morbidity and mortality, e.g. babies born less than 37 week gestation or below 2.5 kg. Improvements in this pivotal time frame of the first 1000 days have been demonstrated to positively affect life expectancy and health quality for these communities.

Alex's Reflection

My role as the midwifery unit manager for the North Adelaide Birth Programme (NABP) within North Adelaide Local Health Network (NALHN), under the Closing the Gap First 1000 Days funding, is to increase recruitment of and develop an Aboriginal workforce of AMIC trainees/practitioners and to embed the role in the wider maternity and paediatric service. Government targets to increase the

Aboriginal workforce in Australia are an ongoing initiative and NALHN has a target of 4%. It is well documented that Aboriginal communities are more likely to engage and attend health services if there are Aboriginal practitioners available. The long-term aim of the improved programme is also to develop future community and postnatal services. The programme existed historically as a smaller service managed by an AMIC practitioner and a midwife. The service provides maternity care and support for approximately 230 women a year.

Essentially, the programme has been and is currently an antenatal programme, given the high level of psychosocial considerations and complex obstetric needs many ATSI people face; e.g. ATSI women are seven times more likely to have their babies removed from their care. The role of the NABP is intended to foster partnerships with consumers and communities to understand their specific needs and to design a service that will engage and offer flexible care and support to optimise positive outcomes. Since starting this role, we have introduced a multi-disciplinary clinic with a dedicated obstetrician, the AMIC practitioner/trainee and NABP midwife. Mother carers, with the woman's permission, discuss the most appropriate pathway of care. Historically, many ATSI women have been on a high-risk obstetrics pathway; this clinic looks at the whole picture and in partnership with the woman and her family make the decision based on her individual medical and psychosocial needs – thus reducing the risk of non-engagement with the service.

As a service, the NABP works closely with the Aboriginal Health Services within NALHN, non-government organisations (NGOs) and other relevant services and organisations that sit outside NALHN but are a part of SA Health. In addition to this, NABP have fostered excellent working relationships with the Child Protection Service – CPS (Health), and the Department for Child Protection – DCP (Government Statutory Implement). Women accessing the NABP therefore have a comprehensive wrap-around service that is individually tailored to the specific needs and challenges they live with.

The NABP midwife provides midwifery care to ATSI and non-ATSI women carrying an Aboriginal baby birthing within NALHN. They work primarily in the provision of antenatal care through the outpatient clinics and are registered to practise within the guidelines of the 'Midwifery National Competency Standards' 4 and 'National Midwifery Guidelines for Consultation and Referral' 5, Australian College of Midwives. The NABP midwife provides direct and/or indirect supervision for the AMIC practitioners and trainees.

Evidence also demonstrates that midwifery-led and coordinated antenatal care positively impacts pregnancy outcomes. Although the NABP is a multi-disciplinary, all-risk programme, most of the care will be given by midwives and AMIC team. Community-based antenatal care is deemed an effective mechanism to meet the diverse emotional, cultural, social and physical needs of women and their families. It includes the assessment and management of women who are impacted by high-risk psychosocial considerations, such as mental health concerns, domestic violence, substance use, cigarette smoking and inadequate nutrition. However, all women identifying as ATSI or non-ATSI women carrying an Aboriginal baby, who are high and low risk both medically and psychosocially, will be automatically included in the NABP. Following discussion with women at their first antenatal appointment, the option to opt out of the programme will be given, thus gaining informed consent. Improving access and engagement to early antenatal care, particularly for Aboriginal women and people of low socioeconomic status, is pivotal to increasing birthweights and improving maternal and infant mortality and morbidity as per CtG First 1000 Days evidence.

Alex's Story from AFBP

Sonia*'s Birth Story

Sonia was a 19-year-old Aboriginal primigravid woman with a monochorionic diamniotic twin (MCDA) pregnancy. She was far from her home, which is in remote country, and where most of her family reside. As Sonia's pregnancy was high risk, she had been advised to travel to a metro area to access the care of the obstetric high-risk team. Sonia lived with a family member but was waiting to be temporarily rehoused as a priority as her living situation was untenable. Sonia's partner offered limited support as he was a minor and lived at home with his parents who were not supportive of the relationship and the pregnancy. Sonia had been assigned a case worker from social work who supported her with day to day activities such as shopping and paying bills etc.

Sonia was sent a first booking appointment to see a midwife at 13/40 which she cancelled as she had no means of transport. At the first booking appointment with the midwife, Sonia alerted the midwife that she has no way of getting to the hospital and public transport would take too long, so through the Closing the Gap programme the organisation was able to support her to attend her appointments and offered this to Sonia.

The maternity service offers Midwifery Group Practice (MGP) as an option for women for their pregnancy, which is an all risk model and prioritises Aboriginal and Torres Strait Islander women and babies. This option was offered to Sonia and following a discussion she opted for this pathway as it meant that some of her appointments could be done in the community. Sonia was also reviewed in the dedicated Northern Aboriginal Birthing Programme obstetric clinic at 15/40 to ensure all obstetric needs were met and a recorded plan made moving forward. This multi-disciplinary clinic provided Sonia with further support from the AMIC team and midwife.

Following her booking in appointment, arrangements were made for Sonia to attend an ultrasound scan (USS) for fetal wellbeing and dating as Sonia's last menstrual period (LMP) was unclear. Sonia then came to meet with the AMIC manager at the hospital NABP clinic to establish a relationship and rapport, particularly in context to cultural and psychosocial support. The AMIC manager offered local supports and groups for Sonia to contact and also referred her to NGOs who offer support specifically to Aboriginal women and babies, including transport, housing, social activities and mental health support. This in addition to Sonia's social worker and MGP midwives.

At 21/40 Sonia's MGP midwife had made three attempts to contact Sonia at her home, unsuccessfully, after which a meeting was held with the Consultant lead for NABP and a further USS was arranged. The MGP midwife made contact with Sonia by phone and arranged a visit and offered her the USS appointment.

Sonia was not at home when the MGP midwife arrived for the appointment. The MGP midwife met with the lead midwife and arranged to visit Sonia together at home to offer further support and to make a plan with Sonia to support her needs more appropriately.

The vignette above illustrates the diverse aspects of maternity services across Australia; as a very different story demonstrates below.

A Woman's Story

Erin's Birth Stories

I went through the private hospital system with an obstetrician in Melbourne, so I only had contact with midwives during labour and delivery and my hospital stays. Max was born via emergency c-section so there were about 10 people in theatre and I had no idea who was who. The midwives afterwards were great though, Max went into the special care nursery as he was very small and had some issues maintaining oxygen levels and regulating his heartbeat. He remained in the nursery for 11 days and I was discharged after 5; it was so hard leaving but I knew the nurses would take care of him. We went back every day a few times a day to feed and cuddle. Pierre, my husband, might remember the head nursery midwife was amazing, who gave us lots of support and reassurance.

Luca, my second son, was a VBAC birth, so I spent more time in labour with the midwives, but they changed shifts in early stages of labour, so I got to know one lady then another started. By that stage my contractions were pretty bad, so I

(Continued)

> *didn't really pay attention to names. I went from 2 to 9 cm in two hours and Luca was born 15 minutes later. During that time, I remember the midwife rubbing my back, getting me a heat pack, helping me on and off the bed and finally coaching me through the pain (at times I forgot Pierre was there as I was so focused on her voice!). It was such a different experience with Luca, he was in my room and I could see/touch him whenever I wanted, they helped me breastfeed and we took him home the day I was discharged. I actually had to go back into hospital about a week after having Luca as I had a uterine infection, so I ended up in the same hospital but on a normal ward with Luca. The midwives still came up each day to check on me and were very apologetic about me not being able to return to the maternity ward due to lack of space.*

Lessons Learnt

Some of the above stories illustrate the different approaches and influences of midwifery alongside cultural practices in countries other than the UK. Most midwives perceive that the birth experience is a special event in women's life and their need for support and nurture echoes ethical principles and expectations in every other country during the childbirth event. Insensitive behaviour by health professionals is deeply felt and may have lasting impressions on the women giving birth. Equally, those that feel that midwives have been in tune with their needs and expectations will forever recall the highlights of a joyous birth and how in some cases across the globe the 'with woman' concept was truly accomplished.

References

Brodie, P. (2013). 'Midwifing the midwives': addressing the empowerment, safety of, and respect for, the world's midwives. *Midwifery* 29: 1075–1076.

Cohain, J.S. (2004). Midwifery in Israel. *Midwifery Today International Midwife*, [online] 71: 50–51. Available from https://www.ncbi.nlm.nih.gov/pubmed/15536943 [Accessed 28 August 2019].

Euro-Peristat Project (2018). European Perinatal Health Report. Core indicators of the health and care of pregnant women and babies in Europe in 2015. https://www.europeristat.com/images/EPHR2015_Euro-Peristat.pdf (accessed 3 July 2000).

Halperin, O., Sarid, O., and Cwikel, J. (2014). A comparison of Israeli Jewish and Arab women's birth perceptions. *Midwifery* 30 (7): 853–861.

Halperin, O., Sarid, O., and Cwikel, J. (2015). The influence of childbirth experiences on women's postpartum traumatic stress symptoms: a comparison between Israeli Jewish and Arab women. *Midwifery* 31 (6): 625–632.

Horton, R. and Astudillo, O. (2014). The power of midwifery. *The Lancet* 384 (9948): 1075–1076.

Hospitalization and Maternity Grant (2019). Maternity benefits [Hebrew]. www.cbs. gov.il/he/pages/default.aspx (accessed 28 August 2019).

Istituto Superiore di Sanità, Sistema Nazionale Linee Guida (2011). Linee Guida. Gravidanza fisiologica. Aggiornamento 2011. www.salute.gov.it/imgs/C_17_ pubblicazioni_1436_allegato.pdf (accessed 20 May 2000).

Lauria, L., Lamberti, A., Buoncristiano, M., et al. (2012). Percorso nascita: promozione e valutazione della qualità di modelli operativi. Le indagini del 2008–2009 e del 2010–2011. Roma: Istituto Superiore di Sanità; 2012. (Rapporti ISTISAN 12/39). http://old.iss.it/binary/publ/cont/12_39_web.pdf (accessed 20 May 2000).

Midwifery in Israel - Nefesh B' Nefesh (2017). Midwifery. www.nbn.org.il/ aliyahpedia/employment-israel/professions-index-employment-israel/medicine-health/midwifery (accessed 15 August 2019).

Ministero della Salute - Direzione Generale della Programmazione Sanitaria - Comitato Percorso Nascita Nazionale (2017). Linee di indirizzo per la definizione e l'organizzazione dell'assistenza in autonomia da parte delle ostetriche alle gravidanze a basso rischio ostetrico (BRO). www.salute.gov.it/imgs/C_17_ pubblicazioni_2836_allegato.pdf (accessed 20 May 2000).

Ministry of Health, Medical Administration Notice No. 15/2017 (2017). Natural birth in a hospital, 22 Iyar 5777—18 May 2017 [Hebrew]. www.health.gov.il/hozer/ mr15_2017.pdf (accessed 28 August 2019).

Ministry of Health, Medical Director Circular no. 17/2012 (2012). Home births, 3 Sivan 5772—24 May 2012. [Hebrew]. www.midwivesil.co.il/_Uploads/ dbsAttachedFiles/Homebirth_Nohal_2012.pdf (accessed 28 August 2019).

Ministry of Health, Nursing DivisionCircular no. 20/2012 (2012). Core nursing program. [Hebrew]. www.health.gov.il/hozer/ND91_11.pdf. (nursing division circular no. 2012 – core nursing program). [Hebrew] (accessed 15 August 2019).

Ministry of Health, Nursing Division (2017). Nursing work plan. [online] https:// www.health.gov.il/English/MinistryUnits/Nursing/Pages/default.aspx (accessed 28 August 2019).

Rassin, M., King, E., Nathanzon, H. et al. (2009). Cultural differences in child delivery: comparisons between Jewish and Arab women in Israel. *International Nursing Review* [online] 56 (1): 123–130. Available from https://onlinelibrary.wiley. com/doi/full/10.1111/j.1466-7657.2008.00681.x> (accessed 15 August 2019).

Renfrew, M.,.M.F.,.A.,.B.,.M.H. et al. (2014). Midwifery and quality care: findings from a new evidence-informed framework for maternal and newborn care. *The Lancet* 384 ((9948): 1129–1145.

Simon, S. and Becker, E. (2018) 'Birth Centers: A Comparative Review'. [online] Jerusalem: Knesset Research and Information Center. Available from https://m. knesset.gov.il/EN/activity/mmm/eng120318.pdf >[28 August 2019]

WHO (2018). WHO recommendation on continuity of care for a positive childbirth experience. https://extranet.who.int/rhl/topics/preconception-pregnancy-childbirth-and-postpartum-care/care-during-childbirth/who-recommendation-continuity-care-positive-childbirth-experience (accessed 14 November 2019).

WHO (2019). WHO recommendation on continuity of care (February 2018). https://www.who.int/news-room/fact-sheets/detail/maternal-mortality (accessed 15 August 2019).

Some Useful Websites

https://www.globalgoals.org/3-good-health-and-well-being
www.internationalmidwives.org
www.rcm.org.uk/midwives/news/global-midwifery-shortage
www.rcm.org.uk/gmtp/global-blog
http://www.unfpa.org/sites/default/files/resource-pdf/SOWMY-Factsheet-Key%20 messages-English-web.pdf
www.un.org
www.who.int

Conclusion: Reflections on Midwifery Practice: Does Professional Regulation Promote a 'With Woman' Philosophy?

Melvyn John Dunstall

Before reading this chapter, the reader must ensure that they are familiar with the requirements of midwifery professional regulation applicable to the country in which they practice.

Introduction

After 40 years of working in the National Health Service (NHS) within the United Kingdom (UK); 35 years as a practising midwife with a varied and wide experience of practice, management, education, research and professional regulation (as a supervisor of midwives and a Nursing and Midwifery Council [NMC] visitor); this chapter is my own personal reflection upon my own midwifery practice and what a being 'with woman' philosophy means to me with regard to professional regulation. Rather than just present an explanation of the documentation produced by NMC (regulatory body for midwives practising in the UK), I have focused on the content and themes of the documents that can be utilised in promoting and enacting a being 'with woman' philosophy.

At the time of writing this chapter, the NMC had published an updated 'Standards for proficiency for midwives' (NMC 2019a) and although being 'with woman' is not explicitly mentioned in the text, the document is rich in statements and language that can be interpreted as promoting and advocating a being 'with woman' philosophy. There are too many to reference and quote them all directly; this chapter is my own interpretation and understanding, through my own personal reflection. All practising midwives in the UK need to scrutinise this document carefully and utilise it to develop and promote being 'with woman' in their own practice and the practice of other professionals.

Better Births: The Midwife 'with Woman', First Edition. Edited by Anna M. Brown.
© 2021 John Wiley & Sons Ltd. Published 2021 by John Wiley & Sons Ltd.

Globally, maternity services have undergone many changes and transitions as societies develop and will continue to evolve with technological advances and the assimilation of empirical evidence. The nature and essence of maternity care is difficult to capture, let alone align, alongside a philosophy of being 'with woman' especially within such constantly changing environments. I make no apologies for assuming the reader has an understanding of what a philosophy of being 'with woman' encapsulates. Is it just midwives who should embrace a 'with women' philosophy? Should it not be a multi-professional approach within the maternity services setting? We need a greater focus on this whole concept of being 'with woman' which has foundations in the much wider concepts of being 'with person', 'with human' and ultimately being 'with nature'; being with the world in which we exist. Is it applicable just to birthing or should we look at this concept not just occurring at birth but throughout life and only ending in death? Just as midwives are privileged to be present at the birthing of a baby soul, healthcare professionals are 'with person' at the time of their dying, and this is a concept that requires further exploration within the nursing paradigm.

From a physiological perspective, a woman can give birth in isolation and without assistance. However, childbirth is not just a straightforward physiological and biological function, it is a rich mixture of human interactions, emotions, reactions and behaviours. The concept of being 'with woman' is a fundamental element of childbirth with roots deep in the history of human evolution, culture, society and religion, entwined with stands of femininity, masculinity and humanity. By its very nature it cannot be defined by science because it is an art; an expression, not of form, but of spontaneous, innate, cultural and social behaviours, emotions and reactions in individuals responding to triggers within the birthing environment.

Many publications have explored aspects of the concept of being 'with woman' in detail and there is no universal model that can define what being 'with woman' means, but it does mean so much more than just being physically present at the birthing of a baby. Being 'with woman' is a spontaneous and unique experience for everyone present at the birthing of every baby; it cannot be predicted or planned: to do so implies elements of planning, control and intervention. For all of us who have experienced being 'with woman', it is a truly 'magical', emotional and spiritual experience.

When exploring professional regulation globally, internationally, nationally, regionally and locally, it is difficult to identify an explicit, applicable and meaningful definition of being 'with woman' and how it could be applied in practice. There are many forms of professional regulation that are applied in many ways, forming a complex multi-layered 'web'. Being 'with woman' cannot be universally defined; each individual midwife and birthing mother will form their own distinctive definition, and this will continuously be reformed by each birthing experience. So, the concept of being 'with woman' can only be constructed through experiential learning and by exploring the expression of feelings, manifestation of behaviours, both positive and negative, and physical reactions and responses experienced. Being 'with woman' cannot be taught directly but individuals can be taught systems, processes and frameworks in how they can explore, examine, integrate and shape their own thoughts, feelings, reactions, emotion and behaviour to be 'with woman'.

Midwives should not label being 'with women' as an issue of femininity or take the view that it means 'woman' being 'with woman'. Midwives should culture their perceptions of femininity as a human quality rather than a female only quality. Please forgive me for using this cliché, but for me personally it is not just a case of me connecting with my feminine side. It is about allowing my subconscious self to recognise, and react, to the needs of women as they birth, through the emotional and behavioural cues that the women exhibit; it is more than just verbal communication. I believe that there may be some 'truth' in John Gray's *Men are from Mars, Women are from Venus* (1991) account which theorises on the differences between the sexes. I have observed reactionary fear and distress in many men at the birthing of their baby and yet most women react differently, not just being 'motherly' but naturally and spontaneously 'with woman'. This phenomenon needs further investigation; for example, through observational analysis. How much of this behaviour is socially constructed rather than biologically determined? Does society perpetuate social norms; for instance, men should not attend births, birthing is a painful, physical ordeal (labour)? Such a big question to be explored further outside of this chapter.

Professional regulation sits within a scientific paradigm, whereas a 'with woman' philosophy sits in a paradigm grounded in the humanities. The challenge here is to establish evidence that demonstrates improved outcomes for mothers and their families by adopting a 'with woman' philosophy. The key to untangling this web is to focus on the nature of some of the elements of professional regulation rather than just on the demands of them. It is not a case of complying with mandatory rules and regulations in order to practise as a midwife; what midwives must also do is learn to utilise and apply the 'tools' within professional regulation to develop, deliver and embrace the concept of being 'with woman' as a fundamental element of their own individual practice. Only then can the concept be transformed into a philosophy and become the heart and soul of midwifery practice and within the wider context of maternity service provision. Midwives must not only learn how to utilise professional regulation to enhance their own practice in being 'with women', but also how they can influence the practice of others and ultimately influence professional regulation at the highest levels. Being 'with women' must not be confined to spontaneous, natural childbirth; however complicated and difficult the birthing situation becomes, midwives must always 'be with woman' because they are all humans interacting with humans.

Self-Professional Regulation

Self- or personal professional regulation sits at the centre of the 'web' model mentioned above. Practising midwives must retain their registration by demonstrating and evidencing ongoing learning and experience. Within the UK, the NMC sets out these requirements for midwives within the NMC Revalidation requirements (NMC 2019b). Although individuals are regulated externally, in order to keep up with these external requirements, there is a need for personal commitment to comply with the mandatory requirements. Each individual midwife must ensure self-regulation to remain on the NMC register; nobody can act on their behalf to do this. The challenge to every midwife is to seek out and develop knowledge (through empirical research) and evidence to promote a 'with woman' philosophy within practice.

With the integration of both pre- and post-registration midwifery education and training within the higher education framework within the UK, midwives can now actively research at all levels not only to inform their own practice but also the practice of others as well. It is not enough that midwives should be actively informing their practice through research, they need to develop robust skills to identify, evaluate, apply, review and measure outcomes continuously as more research by other practitioners is undertaken and published. Such skills enable self-regulation to occur and the use of such skills is required by the NMC UK regulatory body (NMC 2019a) resulting in the accumulation and application of evidence-based practice.

Another key requirement of the NMC Revalidation guidance is 'reflection' (see also section 1.7 Standards of Proficiency for Midwives, NMC 2019c). Reflection is primarily a learning tool though which individuals identify how practice can be enhanced through structured analysis of past real events. Midwives could reflect on their understanding, application and outcomes arising from adopting a 'with woman' philosophy in practice as part of this process. Personally, I use a Cognitive Behavioural approach to reflect on a 'with woman' philosophy as it enables examination, exploration and integration of the thoughts, emotions and behavioural and physical responses to triggers experienced within a specific situation. For midwives who struggle to reflect systematically, this is a simple but structured approach and enables analysis, but it is down to personal choice and the NMC does not dictate how reflection should be analysed, only that it must be done. The overall aim of reflection is to use past experiences to help you develop your professional practice in preparation for future challenges. Midwives can reflect upon a 'with woman' philosophy and as a result use it to modify and improve their own understanding of this concept. Whilst the research process sits within a scientific paradigm, reflection is not so easy to place as it is unique to not only each individual but also every situation that is reflected on.

Another important aspect of learning in practice is the gathering and application of tacit knowledge, which is basically acting on impulse and intuition or spontaneously doing what needs to be – without consciously knowing why you did or made such decisions. Instinct and intuition are powerful 'tools', but they must be used wisely and with caution and reflected upon. As experience grows, tacit knowledge also grows, but in ways that are not implicit to the requirements of professional regulation, which are formal and structured. I often reflect on those 'tacit' moments: those moments when I acted on impulse, asking the question: what triggered those spontaneous responses and why and, in hindsight, how, did it affect the situation – either positively or negatively? With regards to a being 'with woman' philosophy, it is possible that this is primarily built on the accumulation of tacit knowledge rather than the 'learning' of it. It may not be possible to teach, but it is necessary to reflect on it to inform and develop your practice as a midwife.

Within the UK, the NMC require that, as part of the Revalidation guidance, registrants evidence that they have undertaken a discussion around their reflections of practice with a fellow registrant of the same profession. Reflection has a variety of models that facilitate the process and it is widely used within higher education as a tool of 'learning'. There is no requirement to provide details of such a discussion, only confirmation that it has taken place.

One final point I would like to make on reflection is: don't limit your reflections to situations that were negative; when things went wrong with sub-optimal outcomes. These situations should be reflected on, but individuals also need to be kind to themselves; they need to reflect on the 'good times' and congratulate themselves; being 'with woman' needs to be celebrated as it is a fantastic prize that can easily be won even in the most difficult times.

How can we square a being 'with woman' philosophy with that of the statutory requirement of being professional at all times? The word professional has connotations of being an expert; undertaking a specific and defined role in a defined situation: that is exactly what professional regulation requires – and for good reasons. Midwives are professionals and must always remain professional, but we must not allow this to hinder and suppress our own humanity. Ask yourself: is it wrong for a midwife to cry tears of joy or sorrow alongside a mother and her family? The true art of being professional is to recognise and be human, be true to yourself and others; being human should not restrict your practice: it should enhance it.

How many times in practice have you felt afraid, worried or anxious, and hopeless? These feelings are all emotionally driven – even professionals have emotions; what is important is that you recognise and understand why you feel like this and what you need to do; remember feelings are 'telling you something', so do something about it! This is so common in practice; for example, how do you react to the high-parity mother with a history of previous lower segment caesarean section

(LSCS) with a twin pregnancy expressing a need to birth at home? The point here is not to let your fears justify a refusal of home birth, but use them to inform and be 'with woman' in explaining the risks and problems that could potentially arise and what can be done to mitigate against such risks. A frequent phase that is used in professional regulation is 'in partnership' – and that is exactly what is required; being 'with woman' is a partnership, but it is not just about working with the woman. This partnership can only be made by the 'self', it cannot be imposed on by factors external to the 'self' – such as professional regulation – as individuals cannot be told how to be 'with woman' but external factors can influence and promote the 'self' to achieve the being 'with woman' philosophy.

An element of practice that must be used to negotiate this 'conflict' is care planning and documentation, not just because of the legal requirements of record keeping, but also as a contract, declaration of expectations and a method of communication inter-professionally and with women. Care plans are not set in stone; they often need re-discussing and refining, but they should never be confused with treatment plans or protocols which, by their nature, are rigidly applied to the condition and not necessarily the person with the condition. The NMC stress the importance of continuity of care and carer. Care plans are pivotal in providing continuity of care because they can be accessed and actioned by all professionals involved in the individual's care in a systematic and uniform approach. Simply, all are informed by the care plan through inter-professional contribution and working. But can being 'with woman' be incorporated into a care plan? A care plan tends to focus on defined problems and interventions but being 'with woman' is a human relationship and not a defined problem.

A birth plan is only a small part of this process: why focus on just the birthing of a baby? Being 'with woman' does not just happen at birthing but throughout the whole pregnancy continuum and postnatal period. Midwives need to facilitate a more holistic approach to care planning; as well as recognising problems and identifying interventions, they must plan how best to meet the wants, needs, wishes, family, social, cultural and religious factors of women and their families. This has to be a two-way process; for a woman to 'know her midwife' the midwife must 'know the woman' – without this a midwife cannot formulate care plans that facilitate a being 'with woman' philosophy. So, whilst care plans are formulated by the team, each individual of that team must be guided by their own professional regulatory requirements balanced with the individual wants, needs and wishes of all the individuals in their care.

Continuity of carer is a different concept to continuity of care. Carer implies that only one person always provides care to each individual at all times. To achieve a named midwife providing total care for each woman under her care, would be the pinnacle, gold standard in achieving holistic care and so facilitating a being 'with woman' philosophy; but is achieving this realistic? Within the new proficiency standards (NMC 2019a), section 2.5 states that midwives at the point of registration must:

> *demonstrate the ability to provide continuity of midwifery care across the whole continuum of care and in diverse settings for women and newborn infants with and without complications and additional care needs.*

The key point here is that the NMC does not say you must provide continuity of carer, what it is saying is that all midwives must be able to demonstrate they are proficient throughout the pregnancy continuum and be able to provide care, at any point and time. It is having the ability, not the need or requirement, to provide continuity of carer. So, a midwife is accountable to ensure she can always demonstrate all the proficiencies required by the NMC at all times. There can be no such thing as a prenatal midwife, antenatal midwife, intrapartum midwife and postnatal midwife; to be labelled as such goes against the NMC (2019a) requirements. I am not saying that midwives cannot specialise in practice – for example, diabetic, epileptic, vulnerable individuals, high-risk conditions, etc. – they can and they do practice across the whole pregnancy continuum for women with identified needs and problems. The introduction to Domain 1 states:

> *Midwives are fully accountable as the lead professional for the care and support of childbearing women and newborn infants, and partners, and families . . .*

This is a powerful statement that empowers midwives. All midwives are experts in maternity care provision, but they can only be experts by being proficient in every area of their practice domains at all times.

There is another important point to be made that has not yet been covered and that is the role of the individual in overall professional regulation. The NMC not only represents registrants; it is a professional body made up of all the practising registrants on the NMC register. Members of council are elected by registrants and not appointed. When elections occur, members use their votes for their preferred council members in a democratic way. The NMC also consults widely – including with all registrants – in a variety of ways, when proposals and changes are made are made to key standards, codes and rules relating to professional regulation.

The NMC have to coordinate a top-down approach of statutory professional regulation with a bottom-up approach of self-professional regulation and have the difficult job of balancing 'the how we wish to practice' with 'the law in which we have to practice'. A being 'with woman' philosophy is not explicitly required by law, but if we are serious in developing the concept then the NMC will 'hear' our views – but we have to tell them and not assume they know what is required outside the statutory framework underpinned by law.

Peer Professional Regulation

In 2017, statutory supervision of midwifery ceased; before that, it had been a key component of midwifery professional regulation since the original midwives' act of 1902. Supervision is no longer a part of midwifery regulation; however, I would like to briefly revisit this concept. Supervision as we knew it is now gone but the essence of supervision survives and, in my opinion, requires revival and careful consideration but in a different form. The framework that defined midwifery supervision was removed from statute in 2017 but the NMC remains accountable to set rules and standards to regulate midwifery practice. Midwifery supervision was historically in place to uphold the NMC rules, codes and standards. The NMC standards, codes and rules, although they may change, still exist as required under statute. Every NMC registrant must uphold these rules, codes and standards, not only for themselves, but for all midwives and other health professionals that they work with. Professional regulation refers to this as 'accountability'.

One of the many problems of midwifery supervision was the label of supervisor, implying that seniority and expertise came with the title. However, the role of midwifery supervision evolved significantly during its lifetime and in the simplest terms required supervisors to apply the NMC professional requirements in everyday practice situations, to enable individuals to be accountable. This has always been and still is a statutory requirement of every individual NMC registrant, and so statutory supervision may be dissolved but the requirements that supervision focused upon remain the same. It is clearly the responsibility of every registrant to meet these statutory requirements, not just individually but with regard to their colleagues as well. This needs to be embedded within professional preparations programmes: every registrant must be able to act as a 'supervisor' to ensure professional regulatory requirements are met; by the nature of being a professional, you are always accountable.

Role modelling is also an important element of professional regulation expressed in the NMC code of conduct (2015, amended 2018) and the new standards of proficiency for midwives (NMC 2019a), see section 5B. It is not enough to be the perfect role model, but individuals at all levels need to learn from how others behave and conduct themselves in practice, including how one self-manages difficult situations and errors made in practice. Such conduct is defined within the NMC codes, standards and rules; for example, in the standards for student supervision and assessment (NMC 2018), section 3 states that practice supervisors *serve as role models for safe and effective practice in line with their code of conduct.*

Can role modelling be utilised in developing and promoting a being 'with woman' philosophy?

In the current NMC code of practice, it states that registrants must

> *act as a role model of professional behaviour for students and newly qualified nurses, midwives and nursing associates to aspire to. . .*

The NMC have disassociated themselves from using the term 'mentor', which is often associated with a more formal transfer of knowledge and experience from senior to junior personnel. Acting as a role model is passive compared to the active role of the mentor, so why the change and how does this impact on learning in the practice environment? Answering this question is beyond the scope of this chapter but passive learning from observation is well documented (De Waal 2001). Social learning and social constructs are passively 'taught' in this way; they are not innate but are often learnt subconsciously through repetitive observation. Psychologists refer to this as the formation of 'memes' passed on from generation to generation by observation of behaviour, rather than innate behaviour which is inherited genetically. This is linked to the earlier reference to the social construction of norms: being 'with woman' may be innate, but rather than be suppressed by social norms we can construct social norms that encourage it.

The only way student midwives can develop their own being 'with woman' philosophy is to observe the practice of other midwives. The 'art' of midwifery is passed on by observation and not taught. The most important caveat to this is: how can we ensure that students do not observe and therefore learn bad practice habits? The key point here is that if midwives incorporate a 'with woman' philosophy into their practice, then they must be accountable for being 'with woman'. In observing this, students can incorporate a 'with woman' philosophy into their own practice for which they are accountable. To be accountable requires professional regulation, and professional regulation is in place to protect against suboptimal and unsafe practice.

Non-statutory Professional Regulation

Most midwives working in the UK practice within the environment of the NHS under a contract of employment. Although employers do not have a statutory requirement to ensure professional regulation, it is in their best interests to promote and facilitate it. Many aspects of job descriptions will reflect the requirements of professional regulation. The NMC do require employers to validate that registrants have fulfilled the Revalidation requirements and have provided employers guidance to undertake this (NMC 2019c). What employed midwives need to do is use the organisational processes, such as appraisals, to 'communicate' a 'with woman' philosophy in practice and their place of employment as an essential element in maternity service provision. Midwives can take this further by ensuring that the 'with woman' philosophy is embraced in organisational mission, vision and values statements.

Appraisals are not just a way that individuals are told how they must do their job, but an opportunity for individuals to say how they think the job should be done; and if appraisal is undertaken effectively, these messages will be conveyed throughout all levels of the organisation.

Individual midwives can promote a being 'with woman' philosophy but midwives need to work together to build and strengthen this philosophy at team, organisational, national and international levels. The Royal College of Midwives (RCM) is pivotal in driving national standards for midwives and provide a wealth of material from which a being 'with woman' philosophy can be developed; for example, on the RCM website there is a whole section dedicated to continuity of carer

(www.rcm.org.uk/promoting/professional-practice/continuity-of-carer).

The advantage of the RCM is that it is not just a professional body but also a trade union and so is uniquely placed to influence the NHS as an employer in how midwifery practice can and should be shaped. It is also proactive in providing guidance, information and research findings for individuals to utilise in their own practice development.

Government Policy

Reflecting on my own career, Changing Childbirth (DH 1993) was the first major governmental report that directly influenced my own personal development. To explore how government policy has influenced practice over the years is not possible in one chapter; however, I would like to focus on the recent report: Better Births: Improving outcomes of maternity services in England. A Five Year Forward View for Maternity Care (NHS England 2016)

(https://www.england.nhs.uk/2016/02/maternity-review-2)

Baroness Cumberlege (Chair of National Maternity Review Committee) – 20 years after producing Changing Childbirth (DH 1993) – has produced another thought-provoking and detailed vision for future maternity service provision within the UK. Every midwife should read this document and use it to help develop and frame their own being 'with woman' philosophy. The advantage here is that this document aligns itself with my own personal reflections and, hopefully, of every midwife's aspiration to develop a being 'with woman' philosophy. When the 'top' matches the 'bottom' with similar drives, ambitions and philosophies, change is easier to enact. Better Births is an opportunity for the midwifery profession to do this in relation to being 'with women'.

I have had the privilege to meet Baroness Cumberlege on several occasions through my previous work as supervisor of midwives. Her vision and passion for maternity care is not only inspirational but genuine and sincere. Baroness Cumberlege is not only 'with woman', she is 'with midwife' as well. Better Births clearly gives a realistic view of the challenges the maternity services currently face. By developing a being 'with woman' philosophy, many aspects of these challenges could be addressed, but it can only be achieved by individual midwives working together and with other professionals to achieve the vision of Better Births. On reflection, I think the biggest mistake midwives, as a professional group, made with Changing Childbirth was the expectation that it would be imposed top down. Midwives missed the empowering opportunity that Changing Childbirth offered them; Better Births is another empowering opportunity for midwives. My message to midwives is not to make the same mistake as my 'generation' of midwives. Embrace Better Births and drive it forward – and a big part of this is has to be 'with women'.

International Influences and Regulation

Superficially, professional regulation is often observed as a set of rules, standards, competencies and knowledge to be obtained through a defined educational programme and maintained throughout professional life.

> *Midwifery regulation is the set of criteria and processes arising from the legislation that identifies who is a midwife and who is not and describes the scope of midwifery practice. The scope of practice is those activities which midwives are educated, competent and authorised to perform. Registration, sometimes called licensure, is the legal right to practise and to use the title of midwife. It also acts as a means of entry to the profession. The primary reason for legislation and regulation is to protect the public from those who attempt to provide midwifery services inappropriately. In some countries midwifery practice is regulated through midwifery legislation whilst in others regulation is through nursing legislation. It has become increasingly apparent that nursing legislation is inadequate to regulate midwifery practice.*
> *Framework for midwifery legislation and regulation (2011) ICM*

Within the United Kingdom, this role is the statutory responsibility of the NMC (2019a). This statutory responsibility is required currently under European Law (WHO 2009) but, with the UK set to leave the European Union, the statutory requirements may be subject to 'local' statutory requirements as defined by Parliament. It is outside the scope of this chapter to explore in detail how leaving the EU will impact on midwifery regulation. In the short term, it is likely that the government will adopt all the EU requirements and in the long term local statute will mirror European statute.

The NMC (2018a) clearly references the EU directives that define statutory professional regulation within the UK. The NMC also acknowledge that the proficiency document is based on the ICM Essential Competencies for midwifery practice (2018). This is another document that all midwives should be familiar with as it sets a global standard for midwifery. The NMC and ICM do pose an interesting question: what is the difference between competency and proficiency and which term is suited for the formulation of a being 'with woman' philosophy?

Competencies comprise the knowledge and attitudes that are required to undertake a task or skill. Proficiencies build on competencies by defining and measuring outcomes through observable behaviours and a flexible and adaptive approach. Simply, proficiency is an advanced form of competency. Competency training tends to be externally led; for example, 'this is how things will be done', whereas proficiency comes from questioning 'within'; for example, 'why do I need to do this, how should I do this, what factors are present that may influence or affect what needs to be done and was what I did effective and do I need to do anything different next time?'

The NMC (2019a) requires midwives to be autonomous practitioners, so they must be proficient in their ability to practice; therefore, to use the word proficiency is appropriate. If midwives were not proficient, they would not be able to self-regulate, identify problems and establish interventions and recognise, facilitate and understand the uniqueness of being 'with woman'.

Conclusion

Regardless of where you practise as a professional midwife, professional regulation is an important and necessary framework to ensure you practise safely, effectively and continually develop as a registered midwife. Do not feel constrained by professional regulation; it is a powerful tool for change management, and it begins with every individual registrant. If individual midwives cannot grasp and utilise the concept of self-regulation then, at a professional level, the midwifery profession will never truly be 'with woman'.

References

Department of health (1993). *Changing Childbirth. Part I. Report of the Expert Maternity Group*. London: HMSO.

Gray, J. (1991). *Men are from Mars, Women are from Venus*. Thornsons Publications.

International Confederation of Midwives (2011). Global standards for midwifery regulation: framework for midwifery legislation and regulation. www.internationalmidwivs.org (accessed 23 January 2020).

International Confederation of Midwives (2018). Strengthening midwifery globally: essential competencies for midwifery practice. www.internationalmidwivs.org (accessed 23 January 2020).

NHS England (2016). Better Births: Improving outcomes of maternity services in England. A five year forward view for maternity care. https://www.england.nhs.uk/wp-content/uploads/2016/02/national-maternity-review-report.pdf (accessed 23 January 2019).

Nursing and Midwifery Council (NMC) (2018). *The Code: Professional Standards of Practice and Behaviour for Nurses, Midwives and Nursing Associates*. NMC Publications.

Nursing and Midwifery Council (NMC) (2019a). Standards for proficiency for midwives. www.nmc.org.uk/globalassets/sitedocuments/standards/standards-of-proficiency-for-midwives.pdf (accessed 10 January 2020)

Nursing and Midwifery Council (NMC) (2019b). *Revalidation: How to Revalidate with the NMC: Requirements for Renewing your Validation*. NMC Publications.

Nursing and Midwifery Council (NMC) (2019c). *Revalidation: Employers' Guide to Revalidation*. NMC Publications.

Waal, F.D. (2001). *The Ape and the Sushi Master: Cultural Reflections by a Primatologist*. Allen Lane: The Penguin Press.

WHO (2009). European Union Standards for Nurses & Midwives: Information fro Accession Counties, 2nd Ed. (ed T. Knighley), Demark: WHO publications.

Further Reading

Bennett-Levy, J., Thwaites, R., Chaddock, A. et al. (2009). Reflective practice in cognitive behaviour therapy. In: *Reflective Practice in Psychotherapy & Counselling* (eds. R. Dallos and J. Stedmon). Maidenhead: McGraw-Hill Education Publications.

Berg, M. (2005). A midwifery model of care for childbearing women at high risk: genuine caring in caring for the genuine. *Midwifery* 14 (1): 9–22.

Department of Health (2016). *Safer Maternity Care: Next steps towards the national maternity ambition.* http://www.gov.uk/dh.

Hoope-Bender, P., Tavares Castro Lopez, S., Nove, A. et al. (2016). Midwifery 2030: a woman's pathway to health. What does it mean? *Midwifery* 32: 1–6.

International Confederation of Midwives (2016). *Revalidation Toolkit* https://www.researchgate.net/publications/303519543.

NHS England (2017). *Advocating for Education & Quality Improvement: A-Equip: A model of clinical midwifery supervision.* Publications Gateway Ref No: 06612.

Nursing and Midwifery Council (2015). *Practice Standards for Midwives.* Dublin: Nursing & Midwifery Board of Ireland.

Nursing and Midwifery Council (2018). *Realising Professionalism: Standards for Education & Training Part2: Standards for student supervision and assessment* www.nmc.org.

Parliamentary & Health Service Ombudsman (2013). *Midwifery Supervision & Regulation: Recommendations for Change.* The London Stationary Office.

Royal College of Midwives (2018). *Midwifery Care in labour Guidance for all Women in all Settings RCM Midwifery Blue Top Guidance.* RCM Publications.

WHO (2009). *European Union Standards for Nurses & Midwives: Information for Accession Countries,* 2e (ed. T. Keighley). Denmark: WHO Publications.

Better Births: The Midwife 'with Woman', First Edition. Edited by Anna M. Brown.
© 2021 John Wiley & Sons Ltd. Published 2021 by John Wiley & Sons Ltd.

Index

Better Births: The Midwife 'with Woman', First Edition. Edited by Anna Brown.
© 2021 John Wiley & Sons Ltd. Published 2021 by John Wiley & Sons Ltd.